Climate Change and Urban Health

This book describes a theoretical framework and related technical skills for investigating climate change and its public health consequences and responses with a focus on urban settings, and in particular Hong Kong, a subtropical metropolis in Asia.

Specifically, the book examines the impact of climate change on health in terms of mortality, hospital admissions and help-seeking, as well as key response strategies of adaptation and mitigation. Many existing books tend to consider the relationship of climate change and public health as two independent issues that are divided into various discrete topics. Conversely, this book explicitly applies public health concepts to study the human impact of climate change, for example, by conceptualising climate change impact and its alleviation, mitigation, and adaptation in a public health framework. Overall, this volume summarises what is known about climate change and health in Hong Kong and intends to ignite further debates in the area, especially for urban subtropical communities from a wider global perspective.

This book will be of great interest to students and scholars of environmental health, public health, climate change, urban studies, and Asian studies.

Emily Ying Yang Chan serves as Professor, Head of Division of Global Health and Humanitarian Medicine and is Assistant Dean of Faculty of Medicine at The Chinese University of Hong Kong. She concurrently holds academic appointments as Visiting Professor (Public Health Medicine) of Nuffield Department of Medicine, University of Oxford, UK, and is Co-Chair of the WHO Thematic Platform for Health Emergency and Disaster Risk Management Research Network. She is the author/editor of numerous titles and articles, including *Public Health Humanitarian Responses to Natural Disasters* (Routledge, 2017).

Routledge Studies in Environment and Health

The study of the impact of environmental change on human health has rapidly gained momentum in recent years, and an increasing number of scholars are now turning their attention to this issue. Reflecting the development of this emerging body of work, the *Routledge Studies in Environment and Health* series is dedicated to supporting this growing area with cutting edge interdisciplinary research targeted at a global audience. The books in this series cover key issues such as climate change, urbanisation, waste management, water quality, environmental degradation and pollution, and examine the ways in which these factors impact human health from a social, economic and political perspective.

Comprising edited collections, co-authored volumes and single author monographs, this innovative series provides an invaluable resource for advanced undergraduate and postgraduate students, scholars, policy makers and practitioners with an interest in this new and important field of study.

Ethics of Environmental Health
Edited by Friedo Zölzer and Gaston Meskens

Healthy Urban Environments
More-than-Human Theories
Cecily Maller

Climate Information for Public Health Action
Edited by Madeleine C. Thomson and Simon J. Mason

Environmental Health Risks
Ethical Aspects
Edited by Friedo Zölzer and Gaston Meskens

Climate Change and Urban Health
The Case of Hong Kong as a Subtropical City
Emily Ying Yang Chan

For more information about this series, please visit: www.routledge.com/Routledge-Studies-in-Environment-and-Health/book-series/RSEH

Climate Change and Urban Health

The Case of Hong Kong as a Subtropical City

Emily Ying Yang Chan

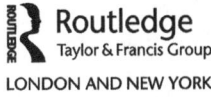

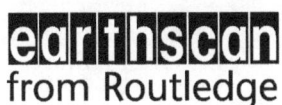

Routledge
Taylor & Francis Group

LONDON AND NEW YORK

earthscan
from Routledge

First published 2019
by Routledge
2 Park Square, Milton Park, Abingdon, Oxon OX14 4RN

and by Routledge
605 Third Avenue, New York, NY 10017

First issued in paperback 2020

Routledge is an imprint of the Taylor & Francis Group, an informa business

British Library Cataloguing-in-Publication Data
A catalogue record for this book is available from the British Library

Library of Congress Cataloging-in-Publication Data
Names: Chan, Emily Ying Yang, author.
Title: Climate change and urban health : the case of Hong Kong as a
subtropical city / Emily Ying Yang Chan.
Description: Abingdon, Oxon ; New York, NY : Routledge, 2019. |
Series: Routledge studies in environment and health | Includes
bibliographical references and index.
Identifiers: LCCN 2018061141 (print) | LCCN 2019011814 (ebook) |
ISBN 9780429427312 (Master) | ISBN 9781138385139 (hbk) | ISBN
9780429427312 (ebk)
Subjects: LCSH: Medical climatology–China–Hong Kong. | Climatic
changes–Health aspects–China–Hong Kong. | Human beings–Effect of
climate on–China–Hong Kong. | Hong Kong (China)–Climate.
Classification: LCC RA793 (ebook) | LCC RA793 .C4375 2019 (print)
| DDC 616.9/880095125–dc23
LC record available at https://lccn.loc.gov/2018061141

ISBN 13: 978-0-367-72936-3 (pbk)
ISBN 13: 978-1-138-38513-9 (hbk)

Typeset in Goudy
by Wearset Ltd, Boldon, Tyne and Wear

To my father Professor Chok-wan Chan who believes in human goodness and resilience

Contents

Figures

Tables

Boxes

Case Boxes

Knowledge Boxes

Contributors

Author

Emily Ying Yang Chan, MBBS (HKU), BS (Johns Hopkins), SM PIH (Harvard), MD (CUHK), DFM (HKCFP), FFPH, FHKAM (Community Medicine), FHKCCM, serves as Professor and Assistant Dean, Faculty of Medicine, and Associate Director, JC School of Public Health and Primary Care, The Chinese University of Hong Kong (CUHK); Director, Collaborating Centre for Oxford University and CUHK for Disaster and Medical Humanitarian Response (CCOUC), Centre for Global Health (CGH) and Centre of Excellence (ICoE-CCOUC), Integrated Research on Disaster Risk (IRDR); Co-Chairperson, WHO Thematic Platform for Health Emergency and Disaster Risk Management Research Network; Member, Asia Science Technology and Academia Advisory Group (ASTAAG); Visiting Professor, Oxford University Nuffield Department of Medicine; and Fellow, FXB Center, Harvard University. Her research interests include disaster and humanitarian medicine, climate change and health, global and planetary health, human health security and health emergency and disaster risk management (Health-EDRM), remote rural health, implementation and translational science, ethnic minority health, injury and violence epidemiology, and primary care. Awarded the 2007 Nobuo Maeda International Research Award of the American Public Health Association, Professor Chan has published more than 200 international peer-reviewed academic, technical, and conference articles and eight academic books. She also has extensive experience as a frontline emergency relief practitioner in the mid-1990s spanning 20 countries.

First author of Chapter 5

William B. Goggins III, BA (Brandeis), SM, ScD (Harv), joined The Chinese University of Hong Kong as an Instructor in Biostatistics for the Centre for Epidemiology and Biostatistics of the JC School of Public Health and Primary Care in October 2003. He was promoted to Assistant Professor in September 2004 and is now Associate Professor. Professor Goggins obtained his doctorate in Biostatistics from Harvard University in 1997. His current research focuses on the health impact of meteorological conditions in subtropical climates and the impact of urban design on health. In addition, Professor Goggins serves as a collaborator and statistical consultant for numerous projects within the JC School of Public Health and Primary Care and other departments of the CUHK Faculty of Medicine. Professor Goggins is a statistical advisor for the *Hong Kong Medical Journal* (from 2005 onwards), Associate Editor of the *International Journal of Biometeorology* (from 2014 onwards) and a member of the Grant Review Board of the Hong Kong SAR Government Food and Health Bureau's Health and Medical Research Fund (from 2013 onwards).

Case contributors

Donald K. T. Li, SBS, CStJ, JP, MBBS, FHKCFP, FRACGP, FHKAM, FHKDS, FFPH, FAFPM, FACP, FRCPT, FAMS, is a specialist in Family Medicine and President of the World Organization of Family Doctors (WONCA). Dr Li is also Past President of Hong Kong Academy of Medicine and Chairman of the HKJCDPRI Governing Board. Dr Li is Censor of the Hong Kong College of Family Physicians. Dr Li graduated with his first degree (BA) in 1975 from Cornell University, USA, and second degree (MBBS) in 1980 from the University of Hong Kong. He is an Honorary Fellow of the Hong Kong College of Family Physicians, the Hong Kong Academy of Medicine, the Hong Kong College of Dental Surgeons, The Chinese University of Hong Kong, the University of Hong Kong, the Royal Australian College of General Practitioners, the Academy of Family Physicians of Malaysia, the Royal College of Physicians of Thailand, and Fellow of the Faculty of Public Health, the Academy of American College of Physicians, and the Academy of Medicine, Singapore. He is a registered medical practitioner in Mainland China.

Christine Loh, LLB (Hull, UK), LLM (City University, Hong Kong), obtained her Master of Law in Chinese and Comparative Law. She has spent over three decades in public policy and politics, last serving as the undersecretary for the environment in the Hong Kong SAR Government. Her current work includes being the Chief Development Strategist, Institute for the Environment at Hong Kong University of Science and Technology (HKUST), as well as teaching at the Anderson Graduate School of Management at the University of California at Los Angeles.

Chao Luo, MBBS (Shandong University), MPH (CUHK), PhD candidate (CUHK), is a year-4 PhD student in the JC School of Public Health and Primary Care of The Chinese University of Hong Kong. Her MPH concentration was epidemiology and biostatistics and her research project was about the impacts of gaseous air pollutants on the occurrence of myocardial infarction. After graduation, she worked on a children's physical activity study as a research assistant. In 2015, Miss Luo started her doctoral study focusing on the association between weather and injuries in Hong Kong.

Chao Ren, BArch (XJTU), PhD (CUHK), BEAM Pro, is an associate professor in the Faculty of Architecture at the University of Hong Kong. Her research interest is Sustainable Urban and Environmental Design and Urban Climatic Application in Urban Planning. She serves as the editorial advisor for *Cities & Health* and is an associate editor for *Urban Climate* (2018–2020). She is a board member of the International Association for Urban Climate (2017–2021). She is a registered BEAM Professional and joined the Working Group of BEAM Society in 2011.

Namgay Rinchen, MBBS (University of Kelaniya), MPH (CUHK), works as a Medical Officer at Tsimalakha General Hospital, Ministry of Health in the Kingdom of Bhutan. Dr Rinchen received his Master of Public Health from The Chinese University of Hong Kong, majoring in population and global health. He obtained a Bachelor of Medicine and Bachelor of Surgery degree from University of Kelaniya, Sri Lanka. He has participated in field-based assessments and interventions in Nepal organised by CCOUC and also presented his research project at the Research Summit on Health-Related Emergency Disaster Risk Management in 2018.

Amos P. K. Tai, BSc (MIT), PhD (Harvard), is an assistant professor in the Earth System Science Programme at The Chinese University of Hong Kong, specialising in atmospheric chemistry and physics, eco-climatology, and biosphere–atmosphere interactions. He obtained his BSc from MIT, and PhD in Environmental Science and Engineering from Harvard University.

Associate editors

Holly Ching Yu Lam, BEng (CUHK), MSc (CUHK), PhD (CUHK), is a postdoctoral fellow at the Collaborating Centre for Oxford University and CUHK for Disaster and Medical Humanitarian Response (CCOUC). With a background in engineering, she went on to obtain her Masters in Data Science and Business Statistics, and then her PhD in Public Health from CUHK. Having joined the JC School of Public Health and Primary Care in 2010, Dr Lam's research experience encompasses cancer epidemiological projects and environmental health-related studies. Her current research focuses on the impact of meteorological factors on health and the health co-benefits that can result from the carbon-reducing behaviours of Hong Kong people.

Chi Shing Wong, MSc (LSE), has a background in Journalism and Communication. He received his Master in Comparative Politics at the London School of Economics and Political Science, focusing on democratisation, ethnic politics, and nationalism with regional foci in China and Southeast Asia, and researched on political identity at the University of Oxford afterwards. Having worked in various teaching, research, and administrative positions in universities, he is now the Publications Manager of the Collaborating Centre for Oxford University and CUHK for Disaster and Medical Humanitarian Response (CCOUC).

Forewords

In recognition of the importance of research and evidence-based scientific and technical information for disaster risk reduction policy and practice, United Nations Office for Disaster Risk Reduction (UNISDR) established a Scientific and Technical Advisory Group (STAG) to provide technical advice and support in the formulation and implementation of activities carried out by the disaster risk reduction community. As Chairman of this group and her long-time academic collaborator, I congratulate Professor Emily Chan for coming up with this research monograph on climate change and urban health, particularly when climate change-related disaster risk is on the rise globally and the health impacts of these disasters have been direly experienced all over the world.

The environmental consequences of climate change, such as extreme temperatures, changes in precipitation patterns and rise of sea level, are impacting on health and the public health system directly and indirectly. Health has also been recognised as an expected outcome and goal of various disaster-related international policy initiatives including the Sendai Framework—four out of its seven global targets directly relate to health, including reducing disaster mortality and numbers of people affected. As the frequency and severity of climate-related disasters are both surging, there is an eminent need to understand, prepare for, mitigate, and adapt to the subsequent health risk in order to protect human health and well-being. Moreover, rapid urbanisation (two out of three people are expected to live in cities by 2030) complicates and exacerbates the public health impact of climate change on the one hand (e.g. urban heat island effect), while providing opportunities for mitigating this impact on the other (e.g. the smart city initiative). The work of Professor Chan and her team in the past decade provides a timely scholarly response to the current knowledge gaps in the health impacts of climate change in urban settings in Asia, which is the continent with the largest and fastest growing urban population. It is exemplary in using science for disaster risk reduction, which will inform relevant policy- and decision-making in alleviating and mitigating the health impacts of climate change.

Climate Change and Urban Health: The Case of Hong Kong as a Subtropical City presents not only findings on a wide range of health-related consequences of and response strategies to climate change, but also methodological details of health-related climate change research and in-depth discussions of the health implications of climate change on individual and policy levels and the challenges and limitations of the current research frontier in this subject area, which makes it a must-read for both seasoned and young researchers, as well as students and policymakers of climate change and health.

Rajib Shaw

Professor, Keio University, Japan

Since the publication of the *First Assessment Report* by the Intergovernmental Panel on Climate Change (IPCC) in 1990, climate change and its health consequences have gradually emerged as huge global health challenges. The UK Climate Change Act, the first of its kind worldwide, is now 10 years old.

A landmark report *Health Effects of Climate Change* was published in 2012 by the then Health Protection Agency, the predecessor of Public Health England (PHE). As highlighted by the former UK Special Representative for Climate Change Sir David King in the inaugural distinguished lecture on climate change and planetary health at the 2016 PHE Annual Conference, "climate change is the biggest challenge that our civilization has ever had to face up to". From the UK, PHE in partnership with the Met Office issued many warmer weather forecasts in 2018 for parts of England prompting warnings to take care. Such actions are summarised in the Heatwave Plan for England, which is intended to protect the population from heat-related harm to health. By continuously assessing knowledge and conducting research, where necessary, on public health impacts associated with climate change-related extreme weather events such as flooding and cold weather, it ensures lessons are learned and where relevant can be incorporated into policies and planning.

So it is very encouraging to see that parallel scientific efforts have been made by Professor Emily Chan and her team at the Collaborating Centre for Oxford University and CUHK for Disaster and Medical Humanitarian Response (CCOUC) in another part of the world for more than a decade to look into the health impact of extreme weather events in a subtropical urban setting. The fruits of this decade-long effort are nicely presented in Professor Chan's new book *Climate Change and Urban Health: The Case of Hong Kong as a Subtropical City*, a locally focused yet globally oriented resource for students, researchers, practitioners, and policymakers in climate change and health.

As her long-time collaborator in both academic and international policy levels, I am impressed by Professor Chan's academic rigour amidst her responsibilities in classroom and field teaching, research, knowledge transfer, and policy consultancy activities all the way from school and university to regional and global levels. Her new book will prove to be a timely and valuable academic contribution to this rapidly developing subfield of global health, where Professor Chan introduces the basic concepts, principles, and methodology in this multidisciplinary arena where climate change meets health and demonstrates how they can be applied in actual research projects to generate evidence to inform policies and practices.

Among the first to record and discuss the health impact of extreme weather events in a subtropical urban setting, I believe that this book will help readers from various parts of the world to foster a coherent view toward the commonalities and differences in the human health impact of extreme weather events as a result of climate change, thereby develop insights in understanding, mitigating, and reducing related health risk tailored to needs and issues unique to their own countries and regions.

Therefore, I recommend this book as a very useful resource for students, practitioners, and policymakers of health and non-health background alike who shared the common interest in this global issue, and a must-read for anyone seeking to develop a deeper understanding of the human consequences of climate change in the decades to come.

Virginia Murray
Professor, Head of Global Disaster Risk Reduction, Public Health England

The Intergovernmental Panel on Climate Change released the Special Report on Global Warming of 1.5°C on 8 October 2018, calling for policymakers to take rapid, far-reaching, and unprecedented changes in all aspects of society to limit global warming to 1.5°C above the pre-industrial levels. The Special Report clearly presents the multiple benefits of limiting global warming to 1.5°C, including lower climate-related risks to health. Warming of 1.5°C or higher will increase health and other risks associated with long-lasting or irreversible changes, such as the loss of some ecosystems. Given the current global trend, this is likely even taking into consideration the Paris Agreement. Against the backdrop of global warming, the warming trend in Hong Kong has been exacerbated by local urbanisation. Over the last 100 years, temperature in the city has increased by 1.2°C, with extremely hot days and hot nights and extreme rainfall becoming more frequent. Our mean sea level is rising 3 mm per year, and this rate will further increase. Professor Emily Ying Yang Chan's new book *Climate Change and Urban Health: The Case of Hong Kong as a Subtropical City* thus serves as a very timely reminder for practitioners and policymakers alike regarding the health impact of climate change in cities similar to ours, and the need for urgent and concrete actions in mitigation and adaptation.

Professor Chan has been a member of Hong Kong Observatory Strategic Advisory Committee since 2016 and we have had collaborations in temperature warnings and public education of the health impact of extreme temperatures, including the development of the Hong Kong Heat Index for enhancing the heat stress information service of the Hong Kong Observatory. The pioneer study of Professor Chan and her team at The Chinese University of Hong Kong on help-seeking behaviour during periods of elevated temperatures in the city found that routine emergency help calls to the "Personal Emergency Link" Service of the Hong Kong Senior Citizen Home Safety Association started to increase around 30–32°C. This study is a fine example of the real social impact of academic studies, as potential programmes could be developed to protect vulnerable people from the adverse health impact of elevated temperatures.

By compiling her team's studies on climate change and health in the last decade, Professor Chan has provided not only scholarly contribution to the academia in a crucial aspect of climate change, but also an invaluable reference to practitioners and policymakers in health, meteorology, and environmental protection. It vividly depicts the impact of climate change at a level closer to people's first-hand personal experience and will definitely provide a strong argument for curbing human-caused carbon emissions and global warming to ensure a safe and sustainable world for us and for our future generations. I congratulate Professor Chan for this achievement and highly recommend this title to those who are concerned with the imminent impact of climate change on human beings.

Chi-ming Shun
Director of the Hong Kong Observatory

While the world is waiting anxiously for the upcoming *Sixth Assessment Report* of the Intergovernmental Panel on Climate Change (IPCC) scheduled to be released in 2021, the IPCC released a Special Report on the impacts of global warming of 1.5°C above pre-industrial levels in October 2018, urging policymakers to realise rapid, far-reaching, and unprecedented changes in all aspects of society to lower climate-related risks to health, among other adverse environmental impacts of climate change. The report warns that more extreme weather events have been witnessed as a result of the current 1°C of global warming above pre-industrial levels and a global warming of 3°C is very likely by the end of this century, with dire consequences for humanity. More evidence regarding these adverse impacts of climate change is urgently needed to convince the public and the policymakers that drastic actions are required, the sooner the better. Among these adverse impacts, negative health outcomes are no doubt most directly experienced by individuals as well as the community and can potentially generate public opinion strong enough to help realise the required policy changes.

The Chinese University of Hong Kong (CUHK) has long encouraged academic staff to engage in various global initiatives, which will not only inform their academic research, but also benefit students' education and contribute to the well-being of local, regional, and global community. We have scholars from a broad range of disciplines studying different aspects of climate change and its impacts. In particular, I am glad that we have an excellent expert team in CUHK, which is at the forefront of climate change and health research. Professor Chan and her team at the JC School of Public Health and Primary Care, with strong support from the Faculty of Medicine, took up this challenge in 2007 to explore the theoretical and methodological issues of the human health consequence of climate change to inform the scientific study of this crucial public health crisis for the 21st century. Working with multi-national partners, they are among the leading teams in the region and the world in terms of studying the climate change health impact in subtropical urban settings and producing relevant evidence to inform policy. They strengthen their capacity to explore the academic frontier via building up global academic network. With academic strength in health study, Professor Chan and her multi-national academic partners do not limit themselves to the academic study of climate change and health, but also support various global engagements related to climate change practice and policy. The study of the impact of climate change on health in subtropical urban setting is still in its infancy and multidisciplinary academic leadership is urgently needed to ensure a rapid development of this subject area in a complementary and synergetic way. Professor Chan's new book *Climate Change and Urban Health: The Case of Hong Kong as a Subtropical City* serves as an interim report of this endeavour and will no doubt advance our knowledge in climate change and its negative impact, thereby contributing to the global effort in containing them.

I congratulate Professor Chan and her team on their academic achievement in building up this field of study and we at CUHK are happy to see the publication of more of this kind of evidence-based research monograph, which will also inform practitioners, policymakers, and the community and serve as a basis for global engagement and dialogue.

Tai-fai Fok
Pro-Vice-Chancellor/Vice-President, The Chinese University of Hong Kong

Acknowledgements

This work originates from the author's climate change and health teaching and research at the JC School of Public Health and Primary Care (JCSPHPC), Faculty of Medicine, The Chinese University of Hong Kong, and the Collaborating Centre for Oxford University and CUHK for Disaster and Medical Humanitarian Response (CCOUC) in the past decade, with the generous support and encouragement from the two universities and their former and incumbent Vice-Chancellors, Professor Andrew Hamilton, Professor Louise Richardson, Professor Joseph Sung, and Professor Rocky Tuan, the former and incumbent Deans of CUHK Faculty of Medicine, Professor Tai-fai Fok and Professor Francis Chan, the former and incumbent Deans of JCSPHPC, Professor Sian Griffiths and Professor Eng-kiong Yeoh, and Associate Head of Oxford University Nuffield Department of Medicine (NDM), Mr Darren Nash.

The author acknowledges with gratefulness the assistance of Dr Holly Ching Yu Lam and Mr Chi Shing Wong for preparing the manuscript for submission and the patient facilitation from Ms Annabelle Harris, Mr Matthew Shobbrook, and their colleagues at Routledge. I also wish to thank the climate change and health research team at the JCSPHPC who have been working so hard and contributed to the various studies cited in this title, including Professor William B. Goggins III—who is also a co-author of Chapter 5, Dr Gemma Yang Gao, Dr Holly Ching Yu Lam, Dr Alpin Pin Wang, Ms Janice Ying-en Ho, Mr Zhe Huang, Ms Po-yi Lee, Mr Kevin Sida Liu, Mr Eugene Siu Kai Lo, Ms Chao Luo, Ms Janice So-kuen Yue, as well as all contributors and friends who have assisted in the publication of this research manuscript for their valuable assistance and friendship at various points in this book project. Special thanks go to Professor Rajib Shaw of Keio University, Professor Virginia Murray of Public Health England, and Mr Chi-ming Shun, Director of the Hong Kong Observatory for their support. Last but not least, special thanks must go to Eric Yau and our children Ellie and Ernest.

Emily Ying Yang Chan

1   Introduction

Climate change affects all geographic regions around the world. Its implication on health and well-being of human beings is an essential topic for public health and environmental health practice in the 21st century. Extreme temperatures, changes in precipitation patterns, and the rise of sea level, are some main environmental consequences of climate change that affect global health and the public health systems. Rapid urbanisation (two out of three people are expected to live in cities by 2030), population movement, ageing, and globalisation further complicate and exacerbate the public health impact of climate change on the one hand (e.g. urban heat island effect), while providing opportunities for mitigating this impact on the other (e.g. the smart city initiative). In addition, with surging of both frequency and severity of climate-related disasters, the understanding and preparation for related events will matter to the survival of individuals and communities in urban context.

This book presents a public health conceptual framework and the latest research findings of the climate change impact on human health in Hong Kong, a subtropical metropolis in Asia. It also aims to introduce essential concepts and methodologies in the field to non-specialists, as well as discuss local and global policy implications of climate change-related health impact. It will help readers understand, study, and discuss climate change impact on urban health in the context of public health; explore what could be done to minimise health impact of climate change from public heath perspectives; and appreciate recent research findings and local and global policies in relation to climate change and health.

The book starts with describing the basic concepts and principles of climate change, disaster, and public health. It goes on to discuss the association between climate change and natural disasters, trends of the occurrence of the climate change-related natural disasters, as well as the public health and vulnerability of the populations exposed to the risks, with a specific focus on urban subtropical Asian context. Issues regarding the challenges of health impact assessment and future extreme weather event trend prediction are also discussed. Research methodologies that are commonly used to study climate change and health impact will be examined. A substantial part of the book is devoted to discussing the latest research evidence in climate change health impact in terms of mortality, hospital admissions, help-seeking behaviours, adaptation, and mitigation in Asian urban settings. This book explicitly explains and applies public health concepts to examine the human impact of climate change, i.e. conceptualising climate change impact and its alleviation, mitigation, and adaptation in a public health framework.

Chapters 2 to 4 of the book provide an overview of the concepts of public health, climate, and its impact on health and well-being. Chapter 2 discusses the common theoretical principles that are useful for understanding the relationship among health, public health, and climate change. Chapter 3 examines the general health-related impact of climate change on human population. Chapter 4 describes how climate change might affect natural disasters. The following three chapters describe the study context and research methodology for the evaluation of health impact of climate change in urban context. Chapters 5 and 6 provide a general description of the research methodologies for impact-health outcomes modelling and climate in urban context. Chapter 7 describes Hong Kong as the main study context of research outcomes reported in this book. The subsequent three chapters present a range of studies related to analysing how health of population in Hong Kong, as a subtropical highly urbanised city, is being affected by climate change. Specifically, impacts of temperature on various health outcomes are examined. Chapter 8 describes the findings of how mortality is being affected by temperature, its extreme and urban heat island effect in Hong Kong. Chapters 9 and 10 further present findings of how temperature might affect various communicable disease-related hospitalisation outcomes and non-communicable disease-related hospitalisation outcomes in the city. Chapters 11 to 13 discuss how strategies and programmes in adaptation, mitigation, and policymaking might facilitate future planning and programme implementation to mitigate the adverse health outcomes for urban communities. Chapter 11 delineates help-seeking, health, and information-obtaining behaviours of at-risk communities in Hong Kong. Chapter 12 shares studies that inspect adaptation strategies that might be adopted from top-down (e.g. temperature warning from the authority) as well as bottom-up (e.g. self-help behaviours) approaches. Chapter 13 examines mitigation strategies with specific discussion of findings of health-environmental co-benefit (HEC) patterns in the local study context. Crucial global climate and health agreements such as the Sendai Framework for Disaster Risk Reduction 2015–2030, Paris Agreement under the United Nations Framework Convention on Climate Change, and New Urban Agenda (Habitat III) are explored. Chapter 14 is the epilogue of this book, which summarises and concludes the current knowledge of climate change and health in Hong Kong.

2 Principles of health, public health, and climate change

This chapter provides an overview of the common theoretical concepts in health, public health, and climate change. It highlights how the health implication of climate change might be conceptualised and potentially examined systematically.

Health and public health principles

Health and public health

World Health Organization (WHO) defined **health** as: *"a state of complete physical, mental and social well-being and not merely the absence of disease or infirmity"* (WHO, 1946, p. 1). The definition includes both *negative* (e.g. illness and disease) and the *positive* dimensions of human well-being. It implies that there are always actions that may *minimise* diseases and *maximise* attainment of potential health (WHO, 1946). Whilst clinical medicine aims to protect health from diseases of *individuals*, public health focuses on approaches to protect and improve the health of *communities* and *populations*. **Public health** is defined as *"[t]he science and art of preventing disease, prolonging life and promoting health through the organised effort of society"* (Acheson, 1988, p. 1). Fundamentally, public health concerns about preventing and tackling health risks and challenges resulted from biophysical characteristics, human behaviour, and living environment.

The three domains of public health

Academic subjects related to public health might be conceptualised in three key domains and their methodological approaches. Public health as a science-based academic/subject discipline is grounded with methodological branches such as epidemiology, biostatistics, law, and ethics, and research approaches such as clinical trials. **Health protection** describes the prevention and control of health risks and hazards. Examples of core topics in health protection include infectious diseases, the regulation and monitoring of environmental hazards, such as quality of air, water, and food, and response to chemical emergencies.

Health improvement involves approaches and strategies that might improve health and well-being, as well as how health inequality may be reduced. Activities and interventions in health improvement often work best when multi-sectoral collaborative efforts with health are involved (e.g. education, housing, and social services). **Health services** identify the best ways to organise, deliver, and mobilise resources to address needs in policy and service arrangement (e.g. service planning, improving evidence-based practices, clinical effectiveness, governance, and resource allocation) (Frumkin, Hess, Luber, Malilay, & McGeehin, 2008; Griffiths, Jewell, & Donnelly, 2005). Figure 2.1 shows a conceptual diagram of how public health might be conceptualised.

Health determinants

Health outcomes and well-being of individuals and communities are affected by multiple health determinants. Figure 2.2 illustrates the determinants of health. It hypothesises that individuals have only partial control over many of these determinants and whether people are healthy or not is determined by both modifiable and non-modifiable risk factors across one's lifetime (WHO, n.d.). **Non-modifiable health risk factors** include age, sex (with physiological

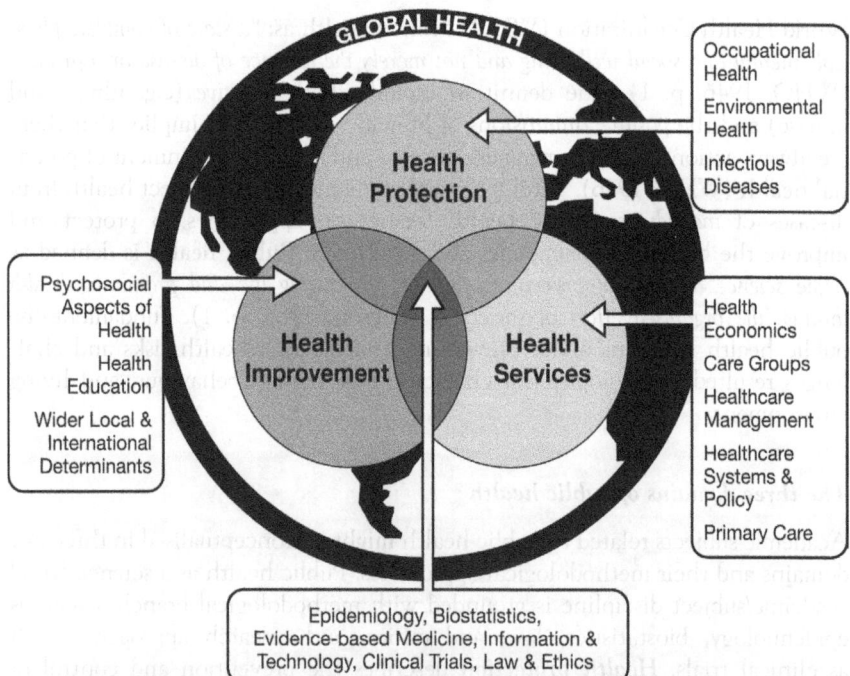

Figure 2.1 The three domains of public health.
Source: Chan (2017).

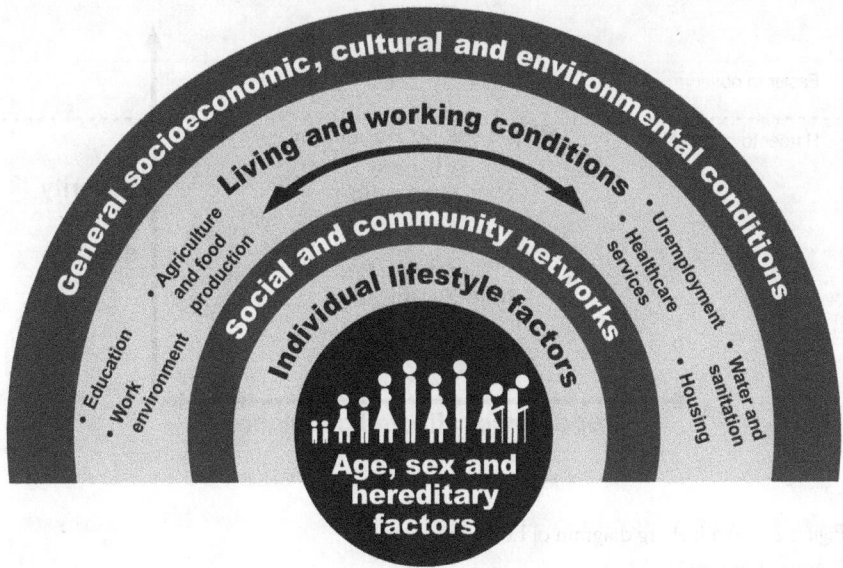

Figure 2.2 Determinants of health.

Source: Adapted from Dahlgren and Whitehead (1991).

difference), and genetics (the likelihood of developing certain illnesses), while **modifiable health risk factors** involve personal belief, behaviour, and coping skills; dietary habit, exercise, smoking, and stress coping methods; income level and social status; education level; social support networks (e.g. availability of community support); context and location of residence; access to health service; and macro-determinants (e.g. cultural, religion, and political systems).

Measuring health effects

Measuring health effects of a condition/context on a person or in a community requires the quantification of relationship between health outcome severity and the proportion of the population experiencing the effect/impact. Figure 2.3 shows how health outcomes might be affected by the same condition. Health outcomes may be measured in a diverse way. They can be assessed by physiological outcome measures (e.g. mortality rate and clinical symptoms), psychological aspects (e.g. depression patterns), or service utilisation outcomes as a result of impact severity (e.g. hospital admission rates and health-seeking behaviour). Measuring health effects are often based on the best estimate and the choice of health outcomes affects how policymakers decide what types of intervention might be prioritised or invested. For most conditions/diseases/situations, whilst most people might experience no or mild symptoms, a few individuals might experience the more severe health effects, which may result in resource

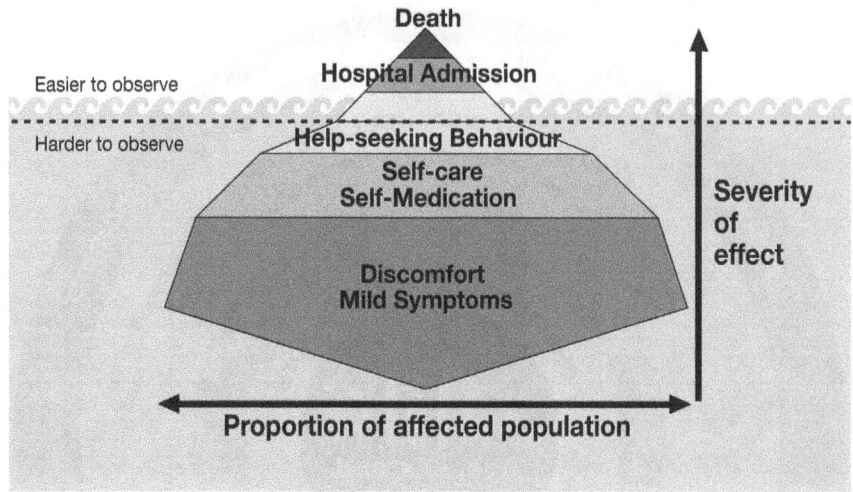

Figure 2.3 An iceberg diagram of health outcomes.
Source: Chan (2017).

utilisation (e.g. hospitalisation). Nevertheless, the most common reported outcomes are associated with mortality. For example, WHO assessment estimated that among the additional 250,000 climate change-related deaths per year between 2030 and 2050, about 38,000 will be attributable to heat exposure among older people, 48,000 to diarrhoea, 60,000 to malaria, and 95,000 to childhood undernutrition (WHO, 2018).

Weather, climate, and climate change

Weather and climate

Weather is the atmospheric conditions, such as wind, rain, snow, and temperature, at a particular time and place while **climate** is the average state of the atmosphere in a specific region over a long period of time (World Meteorological Organization [WMO], 1992). Interactions of climate elements (**atmosphere, hydrosphere, cryosphere, surface lithosphere, and biosphere**) determine the earth's climate system. Atmosphere is the envelope of gas surrounding the earth. Hydrosphere comprises all surface and underground water in liquid form (including fresh and saline water). The cryosphere contains frozen water (e.g. glacier and snow). The surface lithosphere is the upper layer of solid earth on land and oceans. The biosphere contains all living organisms and ecosystems over land and oceans.

What is climate change?

The world's climate has always been changing since the beginning of earth time. However, the current and ongoing issue is based on accelerated global warming and climate change due to increased human-induced greenhouse gas emission since the 1950s (Intergovernmental Panel on Climate Change [IPCC], 2013). **Climate change** is "*a change in the state of the climate that can be identified by changes in the mean of its properties, such as temperature, precipitation, or wind patterns, that persists for an extended period, typically decades or longer*" (IPCC, 2007b, p. 30). Factors that influence climate are often categorised into "**natural internal processes**" or "**external forces**". Changes in the sun's intensity (e.g. El Niño) and changes within the climate system (e.g. ocean circulation) are classified as natural internal processes or known as "internal climate variability". External forces refer to human activities, also known as **anthropogenic** drivers, which influence key elements in climate systems, e.g. composition of the atmosphere changed by burning fossil fuels and the land surface by deforestation and urbanisation.

What is global warming?

Global warming is an average increase in the temperature of the atmosphere near the earth's surface. Although global warming causes change in climate system, temperature change is only one of the main aspects of climate change. Extensive scientific evidence has pointed out that increased emissions of **greenhouse gases (GHGs)** from human activities have contributed to poor air quality and temperature increase.

Greenhouse gases and greenhouse effect

The atmosphere is the envelope of gas surrounding the earth and contains various gases, such as water vapour, nitrogen, carbon dioxide, and methane (see Table 2.1), which are collectively known as **greenhouse gases** (GHGs). **The greenhouse effect** is a natural process to maintain energy balance in the climate system. When the sun's energy reaches the atmosphere, some energy is reflected back to space and the rest is absorbed and re-radiated by GHGs in the atmosphere to keep the earth's surface warm around 14°C. Without any GHGs, the earth's surface would be cold at around –19°C and become inhabitable (Le Treut et al., 2007, pp. 96–97).

The **natural greenhouse effect** is caused by the natural amounts of GHGs in the atmosphere, while **the enhanced greenhouse effect** refers to the additional radiative forcing due to increased concentrations of atmospheric GHGs. The increased GHG concentration intensifies the natural greenhouse effect and results in increasing of the global average surface temperatures, i.e. **global warming** (see Figure 2.4).

Table 2.1 Major greenhouse gases of concerns to living systems

GHGs	
Water vapour	Most abundant GHG Short lived in the atmosphere and little impact on humans
CO_2 (carbon dioxide)	Mostly released by human activities, such as burning fossil oil Long-lived in the atmosphere
CH_4 (methane)	Produced from agriculture
N_2O (nitrous oxide)	Produced from agriculture
Fluorinated gases (hydro fluorocarbons)	The man-made compounds produced for industrial use, in refrigerants and air conditioners. Regulated under Montreal Protocol to stop its effect on ozone layer.

Source: IPCC (2013).

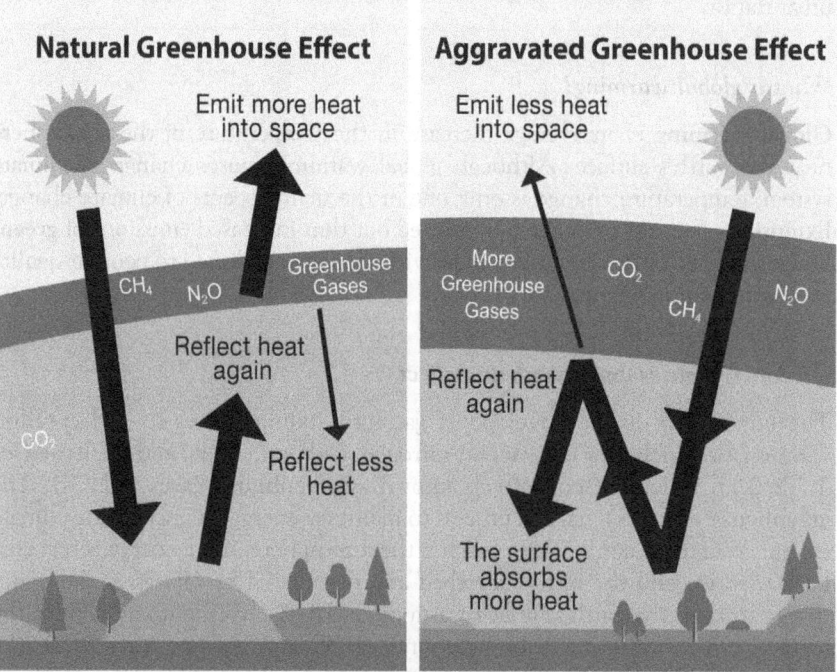

Figure 2.4 The natural and enhanced greenhouse effects.
Source: Adapted from Walter (n.d.).

Observed changes in climate

Climate observations in temperature and other variables at the global level have been reported since the 1950s. Direct measurements and remote satellite sensing have provided scientific evidence of the ongoing changes in weather variables worldwide. The world's climate is becoming warmer with stronger tropical cyclones, longer and more intense heatwaves, more frequent and severe droughts, heavier and more frequent precipitation events, flooding, and changes in sea level at coastal regions. Table 2.2 shows some of the evidence reported in the latest report by the Intergovernmental Panel on Climate Change (IPCC).

Uneven impacts of global climate change

Although all regions of the world are affected by climate change, its human impacts vary according to topology, meteorology, geography, and socio-economic

Table 2.2 Summary of observed major evidence for climate change

Climatic variables	Descriptions
Atmospheric carbon dioxide	Atmospheric carbon dioxide (CO_2) concentration has increased by over 40% since pre-industrial times. The increase is primarily due to burning of fossil fuels and secondarily due to deforestation. Present-day concentration of CO_2 is the highest in the last 800,000 years.
Temperature	The global mean surface temperature has risen by 0.85°C during the period of 1880–2012. Most parts of the world have experienced a warming trend throughout the 20th century.
Melting of ice and snow	Warming temperature has contributed to widespread melting of snow cover, ice caps, mountain glaciers, and ice sheets over Greenland and West Antarctica. Reduction in ice and snow surfaces may increase heat absorption as the earth's ability to radiate sunlight back to space is reduced. This is expected to accelerate the melting of ice and snow.
Sea-level rise	Thermal expansion of sea water and melting of land-based ice and snow contribute to global sea-level rise. The rate of sea-level rise since the mid-19th century has been larger than the mean rate during the previous two millennia. Global average sea level rose at 1.7 mm per year during the period 1901–2010. The rate accelerated to 3.2 mm per year for the period 1993–2010.
Extreme heat	The number of cold days and nights has decreased, and the number of warm days and nights has increased on the global scale. The frequency of heatwaves has increased in many parts of Europe, Asia, and Australia.
Precipitation	Ocean warming leads to more evaporation of sea water. A warmer atmosphere has the capacity to hold more water vapour, thereby increasing the chance of heavy rain. More land areas have experienced an increase in heavy precipitation since the mid-20th century.

Sources: Hong Kong Observatory (n.d.); IPCC (2013).

contexts. Hence, although the same public health protection principle might apply to generate solutions for addressing human vulnerability in climate change, *population vulnerability specific analysis* should always be attempted as coping capacity might vary in different at-risk communities.

Main impacts of climate change

Average temperature rise and extreme temperatures

Most regions around the world have been affected by the rise of average temperatures. From 1880 to 2012, the average surface temperature rose 0.85°C (IPCC, 2013). Although the world is experiencing fewer cold days and nights and more hot days and nights, some regions are also experiencing extreme cold spells and erratic temperature patterns.

Temperature patterns vary with other climate variables. If the average temperature rises more than 2°C, the level of climate disruption will be increased throughout this century. Based on observation of climate and economic activities, it has been predicted that temperature may rise by 4°C by 2060 (Anderson & Bows, 2011). Thus, if the global community fails to act urgently, climate change may pose an unacceptably high and potentially catastrophic risk to health (Watts et al., 2015).

According to the Paris Agreement reached in December 2015, countries expressed their commitment to reduce GHG emissions so as to limit the average global temperature rise for this century below 2°C over the pre-industrial average. Figure 2.5 illustrates the potential impacts of rising temperature without aggressive GHG mitigation efforts.

Extreme precipitation

Global warming has direct impact on precipitation. When the temperature increases by 1°C, air may contain approximately 7% more water vapour. When the total content of water vapour in the atmosphere increases, the global average precipitation changes. The change in annual average precipitation from 1951 to 2010 is more serious than the change from 1901 to 2010 and the frequency and intensity of heavy rain increases (see IPCC, 2013, Figure SPM.2). Heavy rain is intense precipitation in a particular region, which is far higher than the annual average for that region at that time. Since heavy rainfall can be a single event, an episode of intense rainstorm might not increase the total annual precipitation in a certain region (IPCC, 2014).

Sea-level rise

Climate change might cause sea-level rise through two important factors. **Ocean warming (thermal expansion)** describes how sea water might be heated and expand its volume when the globe gets warmer, and about 50% of the sea-level

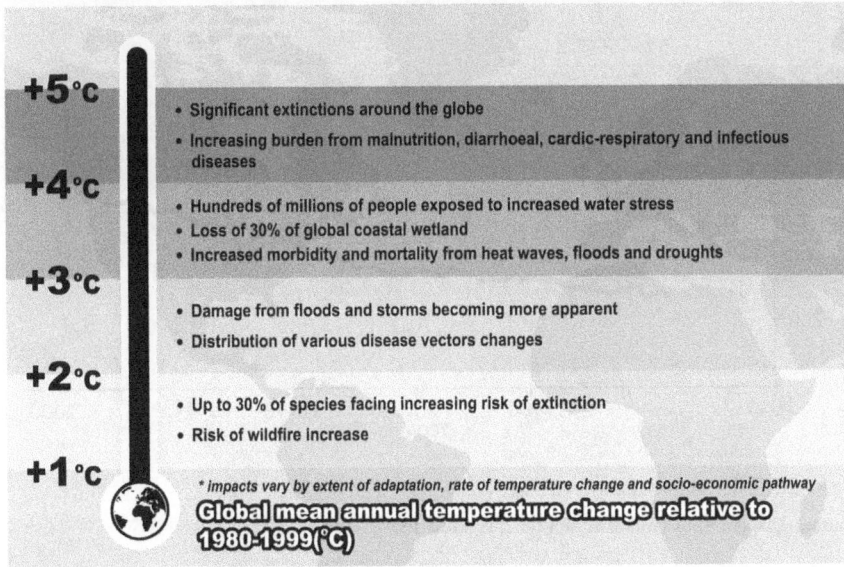

Figure 2.5 Rising impacts of global warming.
Source: Adapted from IPCC (2007c, Figure SPM.2).

rise phenomenon happens because of this effect. **Glacier and ice sheet melting** is another result of global warming, which speeds up the melting rate, diminishes snowing, and thereby upsets the balance of glacier accumulation and melting. More melted fresh water thus flows into the ocean. Although ocean warming and melting glaciers and ice sheets are the main factors that lead to a rise in sea levels, the **increasing amount of underground water usage** by humans also has an effect. The demand for underground water for agricultural, industrial, and domestic water usage increases every day, and more and more underground water is extracted. This water ultimately finds its way into rivers and ends up flowing into the sea, leading to a rise in sea levels.

Lowland and coastal areas will be swallowed by a rise in sea levels, which also leads to general flooding, seawater intrusion, and soil salinisation. This poses a huge threat to the economic, social, and environmental situation in coastal areas. Sea levels have been rising faster over the past 160 years than the average increase in levels over the previous 2,000 years (IPCC, 2013). Since the 20th century, the global average sea level has been rising 1.7 mm each year (Bindoff et al., 2007). Figure 2.6 illustrates the global mean sea-level rise from 1870 to 2000.

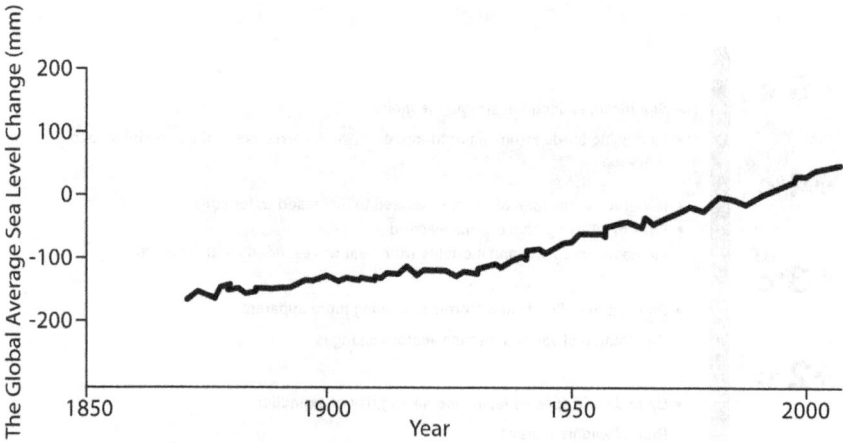

Figure 2.6 Global mean sea-level rise.
Source: Adapted from Bindoff et al. (2007, Figure 5.13).

Disasters and extreme weather events

Climate change phenomena, such as temperature increase, sea-level rise, and extreme precipitation, may bring more natural hazards (such as flooding and drought) that affect extensive areas. Figure 2.7 shows the time trend comparison of geophysical and climate-related disasters.

Drought

Drought might be caused by prolonged absence or marked deficiency of precipitation or a period of abnormally dry weather sufficiently prolonged for the lack of precipitation to cause a serious hydrological imbalance (World Meteorological Organization, 1992). In general, drought may happen when: (i) there is no rainfall for a long period of time; (ii) during the period without rainfall, the demand of water exceeds its supply; and (iii) usable water resources are polluted.

Flooding

Flooding describes the impact of floodwaters on humans. It may be defined as: (i) the overflowing by water of the normal confines of a watercourse or other body of water; or (ii) the accumulation of drainage water over areas that are not normally submerged (World Meteorological Organization, 2011). Apart from consistent heavy rain, anthropogenic, topographic, and other climatic factors also cause flooding. Table 2.3 describes the common types of flooding.

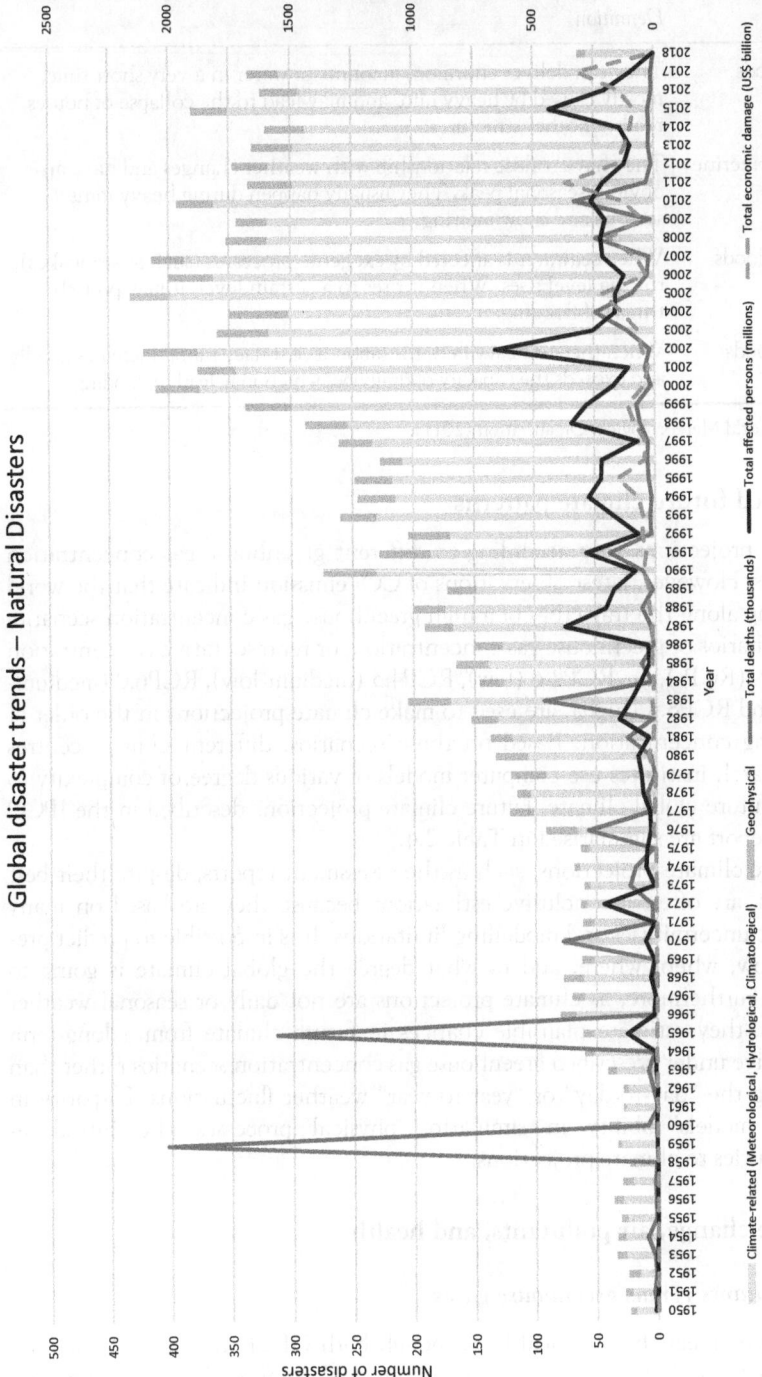

Figure 2.7 Time trend comparison of geophysical and climate-related disaster 1950–2018.

Source: Guha-Sapir, Hoyois, Wallemacq, and Below (2016).

Table 2.3 Common types of flooding

Type	Definition
Flash floods	They can deliver enormous amounts of water in a very short time, mostly caused by heavy rain, and may lead to the collapse of houses, roads, or other structures.
Fluvial (riverine) floods	They have a close relationship with weather changes and have an obvious seasonal peak. They usually happen during heavy rains seasons and snow melting.
Coastal floods	When seawater is affected by exogenic processes (such as seaquakes), the sea level rises. When it rises to a certain level, it may pose the threat of flooding.
Urban floods	When there is heavy rain, the amount of surface runoff increases rapidly and exceeds the capacity of drainage, which may lead to flooding.

Source: World Meteorological Organization (2011).

Projected future climate patterns

Climate projections vary according to different greenhouse gas concentration scenarios. However, latest observations of CO_2 emission indicate that the world is moving along the trajectory of a high greenhouse gas concentration scenario. Four scenarios of greenhouse gas concentration, or representative concentration pathways (RCPs), i.e. RCP2.6 (low), RCP4.5 (medium-low), RCP6.0 (medium-high), and RCP8.5 (high), are used to make climate projections in the order of increasing concentration. Based on these scenarios, different climate centres and research institutes use computer models of various degree of complexity to project future global climate. Future climate projections described in the IPCC (2013) report are summarised in Table 2.4.

Future climate projections, such as the assessment reports, despite their best attempts, are often inconclusive estimations because they are based on many scientific uncertainties and modelling limitations. It is impossible to predict precisely how, when, where, and to what degree the global climate is going to change. Furthermore, as climate projections are not daily or seasonal weather forecasts, they estimate plausible changes in future climate from a long-term perspective under prescribed greenhouse gas concentration scenarios rather than depicting the "day-to-day" or "year-to-year" weather fluctuations. Disparity in climate models' ability in simulating physical processes also introduces uncertainties to climate projections.

Climate change, air pollutants, and health

Air pollutants versus greenhouse gases

Air quality affects human health. Although both GHG and air pollutants are by-products of human activities, poor air quality and climate change are

Table 2.4 Summary of climate variable projections

Climatic variables	Projections
Temperature	Under this scenario, global mean temperature is expected to increase by 4°C by 2100.
Sea level	Under the high greenhouse gas concentration scenario, global mean sea level toward the end of the 21st century (2081–2100) is likely to rise by 0.45–0.82 m relative to the average of 1986–2005.
Extreme weather events	It is virtually certain that there will be more hot and fewer cold temperature extremes. It is also very likely that heatwaves will occur with a higher frequency and longer duration despite the occasional episodes of cold winter extremes.
Precipitation	In a warmer world, extreme precipitation events will very likely become more intense and more frequent over most of the mid-latitude land masses and over wet tropical regions by the end of this century. Meanwhile, the risk of drought remains in many parts of the world with substantial increases projected in the Mediterranean, Central and South Americas, southern Africa, and Australia.

Sources: Hong Kong Observatory (n.d.); IPCC (2013).

different phenomena, as air pollutants and greenhouse gases may involve different substances (see Table 2.5). The excessive atmospheric CO_2, the biggest climate change contributor, is emitted from human activities such as fossil fuel combustion for transport and commercial industry. Other GHGs, such as methane and nitrous oxide, are also emitted from inefficient use of these fuels. These gases are not only contributing to global warming but also form air pollutants, such as **ozone**, by interacting with other volatile organic pollutants. Since the 1950s, the atmospheric GHGs and air pollutants concentrations have been rising (see Figure 2.8).

Air pollution, climate change, and public health

Climate change and air pollution interaction influences human health outcomes in a complex manner. Increased amount of air pollutants can aggravate global

Table 2.5 Major air pollutants and greenhouse gases

Air pollutants	Greenhouse gases (GHGs)
PM (particulate matter)	CO_2 (carbon dioxide)
O_3 (ozone)	CH_4 (methane)
NO_2 (nitrogen dioxide)	N_2O (nitrous oxide)
SO_2 (sulphur dioxide)	Fluorinated gases (hydrofluorocarbon)

Source: IPCC (2013).

Note
Concentration units are part per million (ppm) and part per billion (ppb).

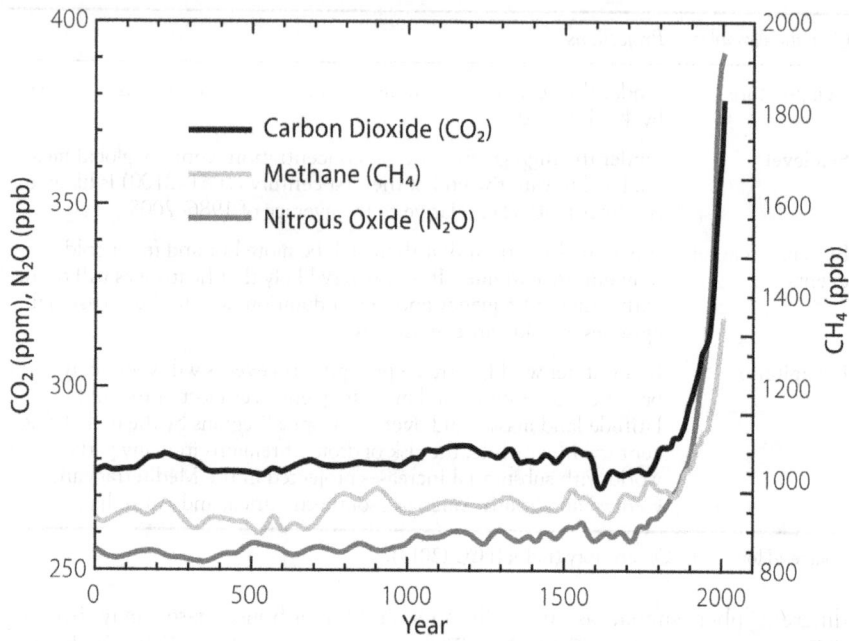

Figure 2.8 Concentrations of greenhouse gases from 0 to 2005.

Source: Adapted from Forster et al. (2007, FAQ 2.1, Figure 1).

warming as air pollutants trap heat and enhance the greenhouse effect. More-over, changes in weather and climate might affect air quality through altering pollutant levels, such as ozone, fine particles, and allergens. Warmer temperatures may enhance photochemical reactions to synthesise ozone and result in **increasing ground ozone production** (IPCC, 2007a). Excessive heat may increase **particulate matter (PM)** levels by encouraging more chemical synthesis or increasing demand for air conditioning. **More allergens** might result from changes in pollen production and distribution range. Tackling both air pollution and climate change in an integrated manner will benefit air quality because many actions mitigating GHG emissions can also reduce the air pollutants (Brasseur, 2009) (see Knowledge Box 2.1).

Changes in air quality may increase certain health risks, e.g. developing or aggravating respiratory diseases (e.g. chronic obstructive pulmonary diseases) (see Table 2.6). WHO (2014) reported that approximately 7 million deaths in 2012, i.e. one in eight of total global deaths, is attributable to air pollution exposure and such trends are expected to increase with the current global air pollution patterns. Therefore, reducing GHG and air pollutant emission does not only protect the environment, but also protects the public from relevant health risks.

Table 2.6 Potential health effects of air pollutants

Pollutants	Health risks
Ozone (O$_3$)	• premature mortality, medication use, hospital admissions • aggravating cardiovascular and respiratory disease, e.g. asthma
Particulate matters, e.g. PM$_{2.5}$	• risk of premature mortality, acute respiratory infections (WHO, 2014) aggravating cardiovascular and respiratory disease • risk of developing chronic lung disease in children
Allergens, e.g. pollen	• risk of allergic response, e.g. inflammation of airways

Sources: Environmental Protection UK (n.d.); WHO (2014).

Knowledge Box 2.1 Ozone and particulate matter

Ozone is a product of chemical reaction between NOx and VOC that are emitted from human activities. Ozone protects humans from harmful ultraviolet radiation however high ozone concentrations could cause adverse health impact.

Particulate matter (PM) is a mixture of solid particles and liquid droplets, including dust, pollen, soot, soil, and smoke. PM varies in size, composition, and origin. PM$_{10}$ refers to particles with a diameter smaller than 10 μm and PM$_{2.5}$ to particles with a diameter smaller than 2.5 μm. PM may be sourced from natural processes, such as forest fires, and from human activities.

Sources: Environmental Protection Agency (n.d.a, n.d.b)

Climate change and health

Climate change affects many aspects of the global living environment. Its health impact may be categorised into four main areas, namely, temperature changes, rainfall changes, sea-level rises, and more extreme weather-related events or disasters. Climate change might also be expressed in the form of an abrupt abnormality or event in a location/context (e.g. snowing in the midst of summer). **Direct health impacts** include deaths and injuries caused by damages and illness from extreme weather events. **Indirect health impacts** may arise from the disruption of interaction between climate change and human systems. Changes in ecosystems, disruption to livelihoods and communities (e.g. malnutrition and mental health illness), economies, and social structure (e.g. migration and conflict) may influence normal living environment (Watts et al., 2015; WHO, 2014). The breakdown of lifeline infrastructure may affect the maintenance of basic health and well-being. Figure 2.9 illustrates the way health effects may alter with various social dynamics.

Health impacts of climate change may manifest differently among regions and population subgroups. Depending on the underlying vulnerabilities and

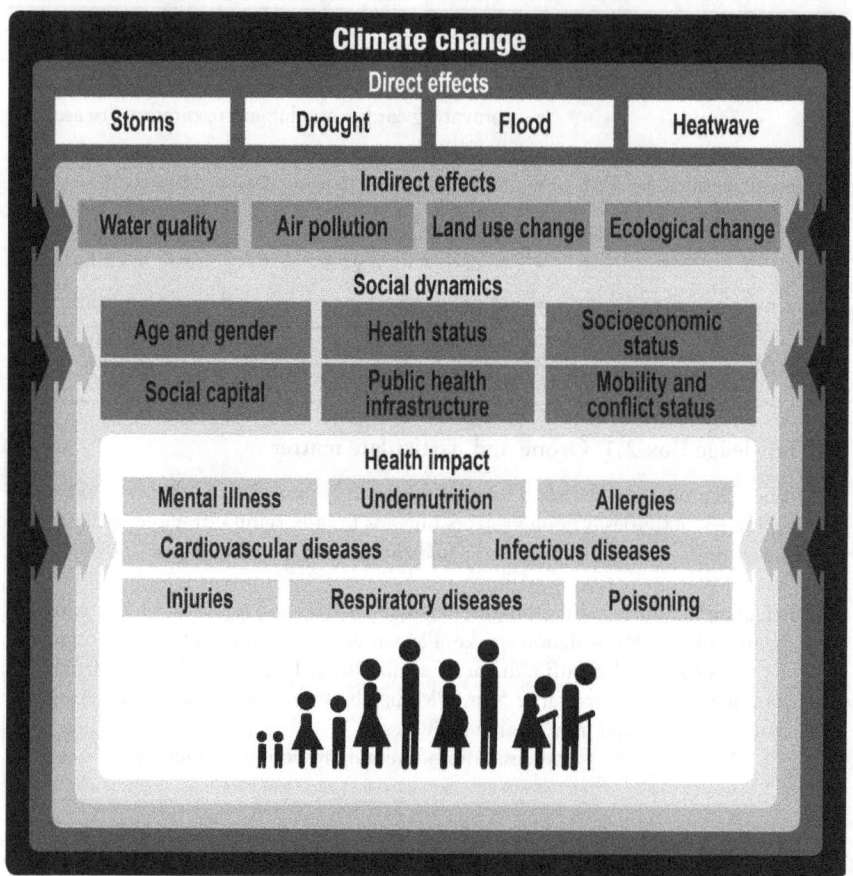

Figure 2.9 Direct and indirect impacts of climate change on health.

Source: Adapted from Watts et al. (2015, Figure 2).

coping capacities, vulnerable demographic subgroups in a country (such as people of extremes of age, the poor, those with pre-existing medical conditions, and people living in a context of human insecurity) will be most affected. Table 2.7 shows the possible health outcomes as predicted by the current climate scenario.

Impacts of climate change on diseases

Climate change may alter the disease burden. It may increase incidences of communicable diseases by creating favourite conditions for pathogens or by changing their habitable ranges. It might also intensify pre-existing conditions

Table 2.7 Possible health impacts of climate change with confidence ratings

Effect	Exposure affected by climate change	Changes in environment and ecosystem	Potential health outcomes	Confidence rating*
Direct	• Frequency and intensity of temperature and precipitation extremes	• Excessive heat • Increased ozone and other pollutants	• Mortality and morbidity • Cardiovascular/respiratory disease • Mental health issues	Very high
	• Number of cold days and nights	• Warmer winter	• Cold-related mortality and morbidity	Low
Indirect through ecosystem	• Temperature and humidity • Altered precipitation patterns • Sea level and temperature of sea/freshwater	• Changes in biology and transmission of pathogens • Lack of safe water and food • Contaminated freshwater with flood water	• Mortality and morbidity from food- and water-borne diseases	Very high
	• Temperature and humidity • Altered precipitation patterns	• Parasite replication • Prolonged transmission seasons • Changing distribution of disease vectors	• Mortality and morbidity from vector-borne disease	Medium
	• Temperature and humidity • Altered precipitation patterns	• Change in pollen production	• Mortality and morbidity from respiratory diseases	Likely
Indirect through human systems	• Temperature • Altered precipitation patterns	• Food production in tropics • Food insecurity due to reduced supply and higher prices	• Mortality and morbidity from under nutrition particularly in poor regions	High

Sources: De Blois et al. (2015); IPCC (2014); WHO (2018).

Note
* The confidence rating corresponds to confidence level in the evidence for potential health impacts from IPCC (2014).

or extend the incidences of non-communicable diseases by exacerbating unfavourable health determinants, e.g. air pollution may exacerbate asthma (Interagency Working Group on Climate Change and Health, 2010). Tables 2.8a and 2.8b describe the potential implication of how the diseases burden might be affected by climate change (see Chapter 3).

Table 2.8a Health impacts of climate change on communicable diseases

Water-borne diseases	• Increase the incidence of water contamination with pathogens and chemicals due to changes in water temperature, precipitation, and coastal ecosystem
Food-borne diseases	• Food can be contaminated by chemical contaminants (e.g. seafood) and pesticides (e.g. crops), and through mishandling of food under changing environment • Increase in diarrhoeal disease and malnutrition
Vector-borne diseases	• Altered transmission and distribution patterns of vector-borne diseases due to expansions in vector habitable ranges, shortening of pathogen incubation periods, and population displacement
Contact-borne disease	• Increase risk of influence and viral-based contact-borne diseases in extreme temperature • Decrease body immunity • Increase flu

Table 2.8b Health impacts of climate change on non-communicable diseases

Respiratory and allergic diseases, e.g. asthma	• Increased exposure to aeroallergens, e.g. pollen and moulds due to altered growing seasons in response to increased temperature and precipitation • Air pollution • Dust, e.g. sand dust from droughts
Cancer	• Raised cancer risk from increased exposure to ultraviolet (UV) radiation
Cardiovascular disease	• Increased mortality and morbidity due to heat stress and air pollution
Human developmental effects	• Through malnutrition due to reduced food supplies during the prenatal period and early childhood • Through exposure to toxic contaminants and biotoxins due to extreme weather events: increased pesticide use for food production, and increases in harmful algal blooms in sea
Mental health and stress-related disorders	• Increased risk of mental illness such as depression and Post-Traumatic Stress Disorder (PTSD) following climate-related disasters, due to population displacement, damage to property, loss of loved ones, and chronic stress
Injury/accidents	• Failing of infrastructure

Source: Interagency Working Group on Climate Change and Health (2010).

Impacts of climate change on health systems

By disrupting healthcare infrastructure and delivery systems, climate change can put stress on existing public health systems. A health system's resilience to climate change-related disasters determines an individual's and a community's coping capacity and so it is important to build strong public health systems. Table 2.9 discuss the direct and indirect climate change impacts on public health systems.

Human and economic costs of climate change-related disasters

Protecting people's health from climate and disaster risk is clearly a social, economic, and political necessity. Disasters between 2005 and 2014 caused 700,000 deaths and affected a total of 1.7 billion people with economic losses of US$1.4 trillion (United Nations Office for Disaster Risk Reduction [UNISDR], 2015). In 2015 alone, 92% of the recorded disasters were climate-related and caused large-scale economic losses, as well as short- and long-term population displacement (UNISDR, 2016). Climate change is expected to cause approximately 250,000 additional deaths per year between 2030 and 2050 from malnutrition, malaria, diarrhoea, and heat stress (WHO, 2014).

Climate change impact on major determinants of health and human survival

Climate change, biodiversity losses, reduced fresh water availability, and land degradation all affect various determinants of health. Although the precise consequences of climate change are impossible to project, a reasonable understanding of potential risks can be surmised from currently available data as shown in Table 2.10. While there may be geographic location-specific benefits from climate change (such as reduced winter mortality in colder regions and higher latitudes), current scientific evidence shows that overall health impacts of climate change are expected to be negative.

Table 2.9 Direct and indirect climate change impacts on public health systems

Direct impacts	• Overwhelmed hospital capacity for service provision due to increased demands • Reduced capacity due to destruction of public health facilities
Indirect impacts	• Destruction of major lifeline infrastructure (e.g. water, electricity, and refrigerators) in climate change-related disasters will reduce the supply of water, electricity, and refrigerating facilities • Lack of healthcare workers due to injuries or temporary displacement • Lack of medical resources and equipment due to disrupted supply chains

Table 2.10 Potential health impacts of changes in determinants of health

Health determinants	Projected changes	Health risks
Air	• Rise in global mean temperature • Frequency and intensity of heatwaves • Air quality due to worsening air pollution	• Mortality and morbidity due to excessive heat and air pollution
Water	• Availability and quality of fresh water • People living in water basin increases to 3–6 billion by 2050 due to population growth and migration • Frequencies of drought by 2090	• Risk of reduced access to safe drinking water and lacks sanitation • Diarrhoeal disease risk due to lack of safe water • Risk of collective violence
Food	• Crop production due to increasing temperatures and precipitation in some African countries by 2020	• Food insecurity, malnutrition • Altering disease patterns, e.g. malaria and diarrhoea
Shelter	• Risk of coastal flooding due to sea-level rise	• Morbidity and mortality due to population displacement
Freedom from diseases	• Changes in infectious disease distribution range due to altered temperature and precipitation patterns	• Malaria risk in Africa by 90 million by 2030 • Dengue risk by 2 billion by 2080

Sources: IPCC (2013); WHO (2009).

Measuring health impacts of climate change

There are many **uncertainties** of climate change and health. It is difficult to quantify precisely about the health risks associated with various agents of climate change. Some major reasons include: (i) uncertainty over future climate; (ii) uncertainty regarding the impacts of climate change on health; (iii) regional variations in the magnitude of impacts; and (iv) difficulties in predicting the level of human adaptation to climate change. Understanding of the basic principles of public health may prevent negative health consequences and protect community. Identifying the potential health impacts of climate change may prevent adverse health impacts. Climate change and health research may support evidence-based policy to address health challenges induced by climate change. Key objectives may include: to improve understanding of current climate-related health risks; to estimate the likely magnitude of the health impacts; to guide policies for reducing health risks; to provide evidence and incentives to prioritise climate change and health issues among other competing issues; and to provide estimates of the benefits of a health-protective strategy (WHO, 2009).

Health impacts of climate change need to be quantified and measured to assess the human impact of climate change. Environmental health research can increase the understanding of the potential health risks resulted from climate change and identify the most effective preventive and response interventions. **Health outcomes** refer to various types of impacts, such as numbers of events (deaths, hospital admission rates) and some outcomes are easy to quantify (e.g. mortality rates and hospital admission rates). For example, an impact of a heat-wave could be investigated by exploring the relationship between temperature and mortality rate. However, there are many unquantifiable health outcomes. For instance, it is challenging to quantify to what extent the changes in air pollutant level would attribute to respiratory diseases. WHO listed some key examples of quantifiable and currently unquantifiable health outcomes attributable to climate change (see Tables 2.11a and 2.11b).

Methods in climate change and health studies

There are two main types of studies for the investigation of the relationships between weather variables and health outcomes. These include empirical data-based studies, or scenario-based studies (see Figure 2.10). Empirical data-based studies mainly focus on pattern learning from recent and currently observable impacts, for example, flooding and morbidity. Scenario-based studies aim to estimate future risks and are used to create mathematical models to predict future climate change and health risks. Thus, scenario-based studies are often used for estimating future risks (refer also to Chapters 5 and 6).

Table 2.11a Quantifiable health outcomes of climate change

Climate-related risk	Health outcome	Incidence/prevalence
Food and water-borne disease	Diarrhoeal episodes	Incidence
Vector-borne disease	Malaria cases	Incidence
Natural disasters	Fatal injuries	Incidence
Malnutrition	Non-availability of recommended daily calorie intake	Prevalence

Table 2.11b Unquantifiable health outcomes of climate change

- **Changes in air pollution and aeroallergen level**
- **Ozone concentration in different climate**
- **Changes in transmission of other vector-borne diseases**
- **Impacts of drought**
- **Famine**
- **Population displacement**

Source: Hales, Edwards, and Kovats (2003).

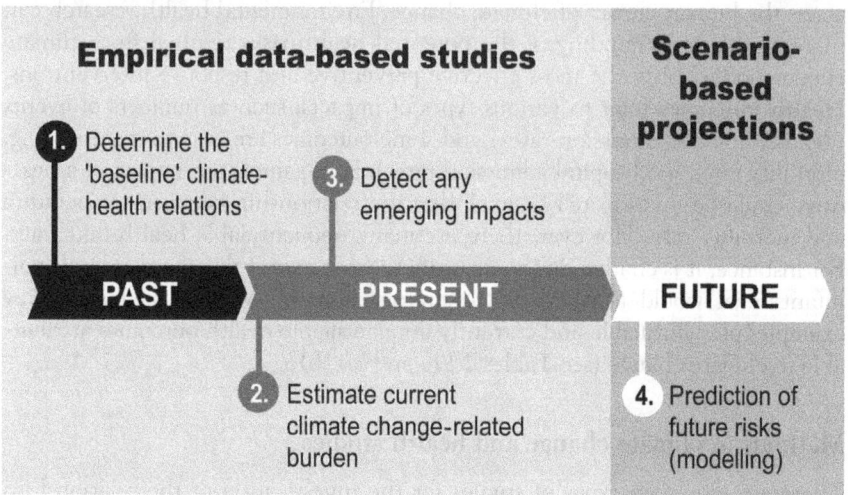

Figure 2.10 Roles of empirical data-based vs scenario-based studies.
Source: Adapted from WHO (2009, Figure 2).

Conclusion

This chapter introduces the key concepts and principles in health, public health, and basic climate change science. In the next chapter, climate change impact on health and diseases will be discussed.

References

Acheson, D. (1988). *Public health in England: The report of the Committee of Inquiry into the Future Development to the Public Health Function.* London, United Kingdom: Her Majesty's Stationery Office.

Anderson, K., & Bows, A. (2011). Beyond "dangerous" climate change: Emission scenarios for a new world. *Philosophical Transactions of the Royal Society A: Mathematical, Physical and Engineering Sciences, 369*(1934), 20–44. doi:10.1098/rsta.2010.0290.

Bindoff, N. L., Willebrand, J., Artale, V., Cazenave, A., Gregory, J., Gulev, S., ... Unnikrishnan, A. (2007). Observations: Oceanic climate change and sea level. In S. Solomon, D. Qin, M. Manning, Z. Chen, M. Marquis, K. B. Averyt, ... H. L. Miller (Eds.), *Climate change 2007: The physical science basis: Contribution of Working Group I to the Fourth Assessment Report of the Intergovernmental Panel on Climate Change.* Cambridge, United Kingdom and New York, NY: Cambridge University Press.

Brasseur, G. P. (2009). Implications of climate change for air quality. *World Meteorological Organization Bulletin, 58*(1), 10.

Chan, E. Y. Y. (2017). *Public health humanitarian responses to natural disasters.* London: Routledge.

Dahlgren, G., & Whitehead, M. (1991). *Policies and strategies to promote social equity in health* (Working Paper). Retrieved from the website of the Institute for Further Studies,

Stockholm, Sweden: www.iffs.se/media/1326/20080109110739filmZ8UVQv2wQFSh MRF6cuT.pdf.

De Blois, J., Kjellstrom, T., Agewall, S., Ezekowitz, J. A., Armstrong, P. W., & Atar, D. (2015). The effects of climate change on cardiac health. *Cardiology, 131*(4), 209–217.

Environmental Protection Agency. (n.d.a). Ozone pollution [online]. Retrieved from www.epa.gov/ozone-pollution.

Environmental Protection Agency. (n.d.b). Particulate matter (PM) basics [online]. Retrieved from www.epa.gov/pm-pollution/particulate-matter-pm-basics#PM.

Environmental Protection UK. (n.d.). Air pollution and health [online]. Retrieved from www.environmental-protection.org.uk/policy-areas/air-quality/about-air-pollution/air-pollution-and-health/.

Forster, P., Ramaswamy, V., Artaxo, P., Berntsen, T., Betts, R., Fahey, D. W., … Van Dorland, R. (2007). Changes in atmospheric constituents and in radiative forcing. In S. Solomon, D. Qin, M. Manning, Z. Chen, M. Marquis, K. B. Averyt, M. Tignor, & H. L. Miller (Eds.), *Climate change 2007: The physical science basis. Contribution of Working Group I to the Fourth Assessment Report of the Intergovernmental Panel on Climate Change.* Cambridge, United Kingdom and New York, NY: Cambridge University Press.

Frumkin, H., Hess, J., Luber, G., Malilay, J., & McGeehin, M. (2008). Climate change: The public health response. *American Journal of Public Health, 98*(3). Retrieved from www.ncbi.nlm.nih.gov/pmc/articles/PMC2253589/pdf/0980435.pdf.

Griffiths, S., Jewell, T., & Donnelly, P. (2005). Public health in practice: The three domains of public health. *Public Health, 119*(10), 907–913.

Guha-Sapir, D., Hoyois, Ph., Wallemacq, P., & Below, R. (2016). Annual disaster review 2016: The numbers and trends. Brussels, Belgium: Centre for Research on the Epidemiology of Disasters (CRED), Université catholique de Louvain. Retrieved from https://reliefweb.int/sites/reliefweb.int/files/resources/adsr_2016.pdf.

Hales, S., Edwards, S. J., & Kovats, R. S. (2003). Impacts on health of climate extremes. In A. J. McMichael, D. H. Campbell-Lendrum, C. F. Corvalán, K. L. Ebi, A. K. Githeko, J. D. Scheraga, & A. Woodward (Eds.), *Climate change and human health* (pp. 79–102). Geneva, Switzerland: World Health Organization.

Hong Kong Observatory. (n.d.). Climate change. Retrieved from www.hko.gov.hk/climate_change/climate_change_e.htm.

Interagency Working Group on Climate Change and Health. (2010). *A human health perspective on climate change: A report outlining the research needs on the human health effects of climate change.* Retrieved from the website of National Institute of Environmental Health Sciences, National Institutes of Health: www.niehs.nih.gov/health/materials/a_human_health_perspective_on_climate_change_full_report_508.pdf.

Intergovernmental Panel on Climate Change [IPCC]. (2007a). *Climate change 2007: Mitigation: Contribution of Working Group III to the Fourth Assessment Report of the Intergovernmental Panel on Climate Change.* Cambridge, United Kingdom and New York, NY: Cambridge University Press.

Intergovernmental Panel on Climate Change [IPCC]. (2007b). *Climate change 2007: Synthesis report. Contribution of Working Groups I, II and III to the Fourth Assessment Report of the Intergovernmental Panel on Climate Change* [Core Writing Team, Pachauri, R. K. and Reisinger, A. (Eds.)]. Geneva, Switzerland: IPCC.

Intergovernmental Panel on Climate Change [IPCC]. (2007c). Summary for policymakers. In M. L. Parry, O. F. Canziani, J. P. Palutikof, P. J. van der Linden, & C. E. Hanson (Eds.), *Climate change 2007: Impacts, adaptation and vulnerability: Contribution* of Working Group II to the Fourth Assessment Report of the Intergovernmental Panel on Climate Change. Cambridge, United Kingdom: Cambridge University Press.

Intergovernmental Panel on Climate Change [IPCC]. (2013). Summary for policy-makers. In T. F. Stocker, D. Qin, G.-K. Plattner, M. Tignor, S. K. Allen, J. Boschung, A. Nauels, Y. Xia, V. Bex, & P. M. Midgley (Eds.), *Climate change 2013: The physical science basis: Contribution of Working Group I to the Fifth Assessment Report of the Intergovernmental Panel on Climate Change.* Cambridge, United Kingdom and New York, NY: Cambridge University Press.

Intergovernmental Panel on Climate Change [IPCC]. (2014). *Climate change 2014: Impacts, adaptation, and vulnerability: Part A: Global and sectoral aspects: Contribution of Working Group II to the Fifth Assessment Report of the Intergovernmental Panel on Climate Change.* Cambridge, United Kingdom and New York, NY: Cambridge University Press.

Le Treut, H., Somerville, R., Cubasch, U., Ding, Y., Mauritzen, C., Mokssit, A., Peterson, T., & Prather, M. (2007). Historical overview of climate change. In S. Solomon, D. Qin, M. Manning, Z. Chen, M. Marquis, K. B. Averyt, M. Tignor, & H. L. Miller (Eds.), *Climate change 2007: The physical science basis. Contribution of Working Group I to the Fourth Assessment Report of the Intergovernmental Panel on Climate Change.* Cambridge, United Kingdom and New York, NY: Cambridge University Press.

United Nations Office for Disaster Risk Reduction [UNISDR]. (2015). *The economic and human impact of disasters in the last 10 years.* Retrieved from www.unisdr.org/files/42862_economichumanimpact20052014unisdr.pdf.

United Nations Office for Disaster Risk Reduction [UNISDR]. (2016). *2015 disasters in numbers.* Retrieved from www.unisdr.org/files/47804_2015disastertrendsinfographic.pdf.

Walter, C. (n.d.). Global warming! The enhanced greenhouse effect [online]. Retrieved from the website of Greenfriends Woodlands Project: https://greenfriendswoodlands. wordpress.com/understanding-global-warming/.

Watts, N., Adger, W. N., Agnolucci, P., Blackstock, J., Byass, P., Cai, W., … Costello, A. (2015). Health and climate change: Policy responses to protect public health. *The Lancet, 386*(10006), 1861–1914. doi:10.1016/S0140-6736(15)60854-6.

World Health Organization [WHO]. (n.d.). The determinants of health [online]. Retrieved from www.who.int/hia/evidence/doh/en/#.

World Health Organization [WHO]. (1946). *Preamble to the Constitution of the World Health Organization* as adopted by the International Health Conference, New York 19–22 June 1976; signed on 22 July 1946 by the representatives of 61 States (Official Records of the World Health Organization, no. 2, p. 100) and entered into force on 7 April 1948.

World Health Organization [WHO]. (2009). *Protecting health from climate change: Global research priorities.* Retrieved from http://apps.who.int/iris/bitstream/10665/44133/1/9789241598187_eng.pdf.

World Health Organization [WHO]. (2014). *Burden of disease from household air pollution for 2012.* Retrieved from www.who.int/phe/health_topics/outdoorair/databases/FINAL_HAP_AAP_BoD_24March2014.pdf?ua=1.

World Health Organization [WHO]. (2018). Climate change and health [online]. Retrieved from www.who.int/en/news-room/fact-sheets/detail/climate-change-and-health.

World Meteorological Organization [WMO]. (1992). *International meteorological vocabulary* (WMO-No. 182, 2nd ed.). Geneva, Switzerland.

World Meteorological Organization [WMO]. (2011). *Manual on flood forecasting and warning* (WMO-No. 1072). Retrieved from www.wmo.int/pages/prog/hwrp/publications/flood_forecasting_warning/WMO%201072_en.pdf.

3   Climate change impact on disease and health

Climate change may impose great society burden on public health. Apart from disruptive changes in the living environment and frequencies of climate-related extreme events and disasters, climate change may also alter transmission and distribution patterns of diseases and their manifestation. This chapter provides an overview of potential impacts of climate change on various communicable and non-communicable human diseases.

Communicable diseases

Risks of communicable disease are associated with distribution of pathogens and vectors, as well as improper human behavioural practices. Environmental factors are also important determinants of many disease transmission patterns. Warmer air or sea temperature, increased precipitation, plus human factors such as urban crowding and deforestation, create more favourable conditions for pathogens and vectors (see Table 3.1), leading to the prevalence of water-, food-, and

Table 3.1 Impacts of environmental changes on infectious diseases

Environmental changes	Diseases	Pathway of effect
Urbanisation **Urban crowding**	Cholera	• Sanitation • Hygiene • Water contamination
	Dengue	• *Aedes aegypti* mosquito breeding sites
Deforestation **New habitation**	Malaria	• Vector breeding sites • Immigration of susceptible population
	Visceral leishmaniasis	• Contact with sandflies
Ocean warming	Red tide	• Toxic algal blooms
Increased precipitation	Rift Valley fever	• Pools for mosquito breeding
	Hantavirus pulmonary syndrome	• Rodent food, habitat

Source: Adapted from Patz et al. (2003, Table 6.1).

vector-borne diseases. The following sections describe the various communicable diseases and their currently known associations with climate change.

Water-borne diseases

Access to clean water is essential for health. However, availability and accessibility of adequate quality and quantity of water depends on complex interactions in climate systems. Climate change-related events, such as floods, droughts, excessive precipitation, rises in temperature and sea level, influence water availability, quality, and accessibility. Water shortage may increase water-borne disease risks. About a third of the world's population are facing moderate to high water stress.

Water-borne diseases are infections caused by pathogens that can be spread by contaminated water via drinking, food consumption, recreational use, as well as suboptimal hygiene practices (Centers for Disease Control and Prevention [CDC], n.d.). Table 3.2 summarises the likely patterns associated with water-borne diseases.

Impacts of climate change on water-borne diseases

Changes in weather patterns may increase water-borne disease incidences in various ways. **Excessive precipitation** increases water runoff, which potentially

Table 3.2 Common water-borne diseases

Pathogen(s)		Disease	Transmission	Symptoms
Bacterial	*Vibrio cholerae*	Cholera	Water/food	Watery diarrhoea, vomiting, leg cramps
	Salmonella typhi	Typhoid	Water/food	Fever, headache, nausea, reduced appetite
Parasitic	*Entamoeba histolytica*	Amoebic dysentery	Water/food	Diarrhoea, stomach pain, cramps
	Cryptosporidium	Cryptosporidiosis	Water	Stomach cramps, nausea, vomiting, fever, weight loss
	Giardia	Giardiasis	Water/food	Diarrhoea, excess gas, stomach cramps, nausea
Viral	Hepatitis A virus	Hepatitis A	Water/food, shellfish	Fever, fatigue, stomach pain, nausea, dark urine, jaundice
	Calicivirus	Gastroenteritis	Water/food, shellfish	Diarrhoea, vomiting, nausea, cramps, headache, muscle aches, tiredness

Source: CDC (n.d.).

overwhelms water and sewage treatment facilities and contaminates fresh water sources to cause **flooding**. Excessive precipitation may also cause river/urban floods and spread contaminated floodwaters. Cholera outbreaks are associated with flooding combined with population displacement when access to fresh water is compromised. **Rising air temperature** may encourage growth of planktonic species in water sources, which may increase pathogen-induced health incidence in human consumption. **Droughts** reduce water availability, which may limit dilution effects and decrease the water quality by increasing concentrations of effluent pathogens, sediments, and minerals. Water highly concentrated in pollutants may also overwhelm ageing water treatment plants and increase the chances of spreading contaminated water. Changes in **ocean and coastal ecosystems might** alter water pH, nutrient, salinity, and current of seawater, and can affect water availability and quality. Exposure to contaminated seawater increases the risk of fungal skin diseases, eye infections, and respiratory illnesses (National Institute of Environmental Health Sciences, 2010). **Rise in sea temperature** may contribute to the emergence of marine bacterial water-borne infectious diseases, **Vibrio infections**, in Northern Europe (Baker-Austin et al., 2012) (see also Case Box 3.1).

Health risks increase with restricted access to treated water for daily activities. Furthermore, reduced water availability could affect local sewage systems. Even for developed countries with established water treatment infrastructure, urban floods may increase the risks of water-borne disease.

Case Box 3.1 Flooding in Southern Africa, 2015

Excessive heavy rainfalls and severe flooding in January 2015 affected 135,000 in Malawi, Mozambique, Madagascar, and Zimbabwe. The first cholera case was reported in December 2014. With exacerbation of poor water and sanitation caused by flooding, more than 8,000 cholera cases and 60 deaths were reported by April 2015.

Sources: Reliefweb (n.d.; 2015, 17 April); World Health Organization Regional Office for Africa (2015, 3 March)

Food-borne diseases

Along with water, food is another basic component to maintain health. Food may be contaminated at any point in production and distribution. Food-borne diseases may be caused by ingesting food contaminated with infectious agents (such as bacteria, viruses, parasites in uncooked meat or vegetables) and by ingesting chemical or toxic substances, persistent organic pollutants, such as dioxins, and heavy metals (WHO, 2015, December). The most common clinical symptoms associated with food-borne diseases (e.g. vomiting and diarrhoea) are usually self-limiting. Nevertheless, food-borne diseases may also be chronic (e.g. worm infestation) and can cause death (e.g. poisoning). Table 3.3 summarises the typical clinical patterns associated with food-borne diseases.

Table 3.3 Common food-borne pathogens and illnesses

Pathogens		Transmission	Symptoms
Bacteria	*Salmonella*	Eggs, poultry, other animal products	Fever, headache, nausea, vomiting, abdominal pain, diarrhoea
	Campylobacter	Raw milk contaminated raw food	
	Escherichia coli	Unpasteurised milk, undercooked meat, contaminated raw food	
Viruses	Norovirus	From faeces to mouth Contaminated food/ water	Nausea, vomiting, watery diarrhoea, abdominal pain
	Hepatitis A	Raw/undercooked contaminated food	Liver disease
Parasites	Fish-borne trematodes	Food	Diarrhoea
Chemical	Chemical or toxic substances, persistent organic pollutants	Food Water	Acute poisoning or long-term diseases, e.g. cancer

Source: WHO (2015, March, December).

Impacts of climate change on food-borne diseases

Changes in climate and weather patterns may increase food-borne disease risks by altering pathogens' growth, survival, habitable ranges, transmission patterns, and environmental context that the pathogen may thrive. Disease incidences are associated with **ambient temperature**, which may increase as warmer temperatures create more favourable breeding conditions for pathogens. Furthermore, human behaviours, such as eating raw food (e.g. sushi), may increase the risk of pathogen exposure. Activities of pathogen-bearing pests (e.g. flies, cockroaches, and rodents) in the domestic environment may also be altered under higher temperature and humidity. For instance, *Salmonella* infections are common in summer and the incidences rise by 5–10% for each 1°C increase in weekly temperature when the ambient temperature is at least 5°C (Kovats et al., 2004). *Campylobacter* also increases rapidly with raising temperatures and the risk of campylobacteriosis is positively associated with mean weekly temperatures. **Excessive precipitation** and **flooding** may reduce clean drinking water availability and overwhelm water treatment systems. Certain food crops and agricultural soil may also be contaminated by pathogen-bearing floodwater. **Rise in sea temperature** may induce *Vibrio* bacteria production, leading to increased seafood-borne disease risks, such as cholera (National Institute of Environmental Health Sciences, 2010). **Changes in seasonality** such as extended warm weather seasons may increase food-handling mistakes. About 32% of food-borne outbreaks in Europe were found to be associated with "temperature misuse"

(European Centre for Disease Prevention and Control, 2012). For example, it has generally been advocated that raw food should not be left out of refrigeration longer than 2 hours in Europe. However, when air temperature is over 90°F (32.2°C), food safety might be compromised if it was left out of the appropriate-temperature storage (e.g. refrigeration) for only 1 hour.

Case Box 3.2 Heatwaves and salmonellosis in Adelaide, Australia

A study on the relationship between heatwaves and salmonellosis incidences during 1990–2012 in Adelaide, Australia confirms that heatwaves have a significant effect on *Salmonella* cases. Results indicated that some *Salmonella* serotypes and phage types are sensitive to heatwaves and may have up to a two-fold increase when compared with non-heatwave days. Heatwave intensity may have a significant effect on daily counts of overall salmonellosis with a 34% increase in risk of infection.

Source: Milazzo et al. (2016)

Unsafe food poses health threats to everyone. Specifically, infants, young children, pregnant women, the older people, and those with an underlying illness are particularly susceptible to food-borne disease risks. People living in developing countries where food supply is insecure, and in areas without sufficient capacity or public health infrastructure to prevent and treat illness are also vulnerable (see also Case Box 3.2).

Vector-borne diseases

Vector-borne diseases (VBDs) are infectious diseases transmitted by the bite of infected arthropod species, such as mosquitoes, ticks, sandflies, and blackflies. Arthropod species are cold-blooded and sensitive to the local meteorological conditions such as temperature, rainfall, and humidity. Non-climate factors, e.g. habitat destruction and pesticide spraying, contribute to vector proliferation. Nevertheless, climate factors, such as temperature and humidity, play a dominant role in determining: (i) habitat suitability to survive and reproduce, (ii) biting frequency, and (iii) the pathogen's incubation period within the vector organism. For example, there is a minimum temperature for activity, below which it is too cold for vectors to breed. Moreover, higher temperature may increase vectors' metabolism needing more blood, hence increased biting frequencies. VBDs such as malaria and dengue fever are major causes of illness and death globally (e.g. in tropical and subtropical regions). Climate change may increase health risks from VBDs by altering transmission, the geographical habitable range, population, and seasonal activity of various vectors (see Table 3.4).

Table 3.4 Some vector-borne diseases sensitive to climate

Vector	Major diseases
Blackflies	Onchocerciasis
Ixodes ticks	Lyme disease, tick-borne encephalitis
Mosquitoes	Malaria, filariasis, dengue fever, yellow fever, West Nile fever, Zika, chikungunya
Sandflies	Leishmaniasis
Snails (intermediate host)	Schistosomiasis
Tsetse flies	African trypanosomiasis

Source: Adapted from Haines, Kovats, Campbell-Lendrum, and Corvalán (2006).

Impacts of climate change on VBDs

General temperature warming, rising sea level, increasing storm intensity, and changing rainfall patterns (Intergovernmental Panel on Climate Change [IPCC], 2014) may lead to the alteration of infectious disease pattern and re-emergence of some vector-borne diseases. Population growth, urbanisation, change of land use, and environmental context may render population vulnerable to disease risks. Case Box 3.3 is an example of how climate change may affect the transmission of malaria.

Observed and predicted climate change impact on malaria

Malaria is caused by the *Plasmodium* parasite and transmitted via the bites of infected vectors, the female *Anopheles* mosquitoes. In the human body, the parasites multiply initially in the liver, then circulate in the blood (inside the red blood cells). Human infection may cause fever, headache, and vomiting between 10 and 15 days after the bite. Some severe forms of malaria, if left untreated, may result in death. Key interventions for malaria include treatment with artemisinin-based combination therapies (ACTs), insecticidal net use, and indoor insecticide spraying.

Malaria has been a leading mortality and morbidity cause in developing countries, especially in Africa. In 2015, malaria caused 214 million cases and 438,000 deaths. Around 90% of all malaria deaths happened in sub-Saharan Africa and 70% among children under five. About 3.2 billion people are at risk worldwide. Although active intervention since 2000 has decreased global malaria incidence and mortality rates by 37% and 60%, respectively (WHO, 2016), malaria still contributes to a significant burden of preventable death in the at-risk developing context.

The breeding of *Anopheles* mosquitoes is highly dependent on weather variables, i.e. **temperature, rainfall**, and **humidity**. Its survival is limited to areas with ambient temperatures between 16 and 40°C. Optimal transmission temperature is around 28–30°C. Higher temperatures increase the vector's metabolic rate, hence more frequent blood meals. Moreover, higher temperatures speed up parasite growth in the body of mosquito, which make vectors more infective. Furthermore, the early onset of the rainy season has been associated with increased malaria incidence (Thomson et al., 2006). Humidity also determines the lifespan of mosquitoes (Chaves & Koenraadt, 2010) and hence transmission capacity. Table 3.5 describes the climate change impact on malaria incidence.

Case Box 3.3 Highland malaria outbreaks in East Africa

Plasmodium falciparum (*Pf*) malaria in Africa is transmitted primarily by the *Anopheles gambiae* mosquito, and the malaria species distribute widely at tropical latitudes where temperatures exceed 16–19°C. Large malaria outbreaks were however recorded during the 1990s in the East African Highlands (in eastern Zimbabwe) at an altitude of more than 1,600 m. Historically, this geographic area was free of malaria transmission because of low temperature on sporogony for parasite development, low human density, and effective control. With the changes in precipitation patterns, warming temperatures, and increased human activities due to movement of people from lowlands to highlands, studies found malaria was emerging in the highlands and may put millions of people at risk of the disease burden.

Source: Levy and Sidel (2015, pp. 137–138)

Assessing the future impact of climate change requires a good understanding of countries' capacity to control the disease. The risk for VBDs is much higher in low and lower middle-income countries where people have the least access to effective services for prevention, diagnosis, and treatment. Particularly in poor tropical countries, VBDs place a major public health burden on the poorest and marginalised subgroups. Climate change may likely exacerbate VBD risks in developed countries by widening the geographic distributions of VBDs such as dengue fever, Lyme disease, and tick-borne encephalitis. For example, disruption of health systems helped resurge malaria in Eastern Europe. Increased international travel and trade has become the means to carry new vector species into new regions, e.g. the West Nile virus case in the United States in 1999.

Table 3.5 Climate change impacts on malaria incidence

Vectors	• Higher temperatures and precipitation may increase mosquito population and geographical range • Decreased distribution where it becomes too dry for mosquitoes • Decline in biodiversity may reduce the predators hence increase in vector populations
Pathogens	• Change in incubation period of pathogens
Host	• Increased population density and migration due to urbanisation • Presence of control programmes • Change in land use

Noticeably, without effective treatment, dengue fever presents a major global VBD risk with its prevalence across the world.

Non-communicable diseases

Non-communicable diseases (NCDs) are diseases that do not transmit from person to person. They tend to progress slowly and their health impact on the individual varies and may last permanently. Since the 20th century, with change of lifestyle and nutritional status, the prevalence of NCD is rapidly growing worldwide. As of 2015, NCDs kill 38 million people each year (63% of total annual deaths), 28 million of which are in low- to middle-income countries. Globally, cardiovascular diseases account for 17.5 million deaths, followed by cancers (8.2 million), respiratory diseases (4 million), and diabetes (1.5 million) per year; together this represents 82% of all NCD death. A number of behavioural risk factors, such as tobacco, alcohol, physical inactivity, and unhealthy diet, can increase the risk of NCDs. Whilst some risk factors are non-modifiable, such as age and sex, some behavioural and environmental factors are modifiable. Reducing the modifiable risk factors (e.g. by quitting smoking) may decrease risk of developing NCDs. Despite many scientific uncertainties, climate change does increase environmental risk factors that may exacerbate certain NCD risks. According to WHO (2014), 24% of the morbidity burden and 23% of all deaths are caused by environmental factors, such as reduced food production, water scarcity, or air pollution.

Climate change impacts on non-communicable diseases

Direct and indirect impacts of climate change on non-communicable diseases are summarised in Table 3.6. Four major global NCDs, namely respiratory diseases, cardiovascular diseases, cancers, and mental health disorders are discussed in the next sections. Many of the reported impacts are associated with the changes in the environment. Case Box 3.4 discusses how air quality may be affected by climate change.

Respiratory and allergic diseases

Globally, major respiratory and allergic diseases that contribute to major burdens of health include asthma, allergic rhinitis (hay fever), and chronic obstructive pulmonary disease (COPD). **Asthma** is a chronic inflammation of the air passages in the lungs. The main risk factors for developing asthma are inhaled substances, pollutants, and particles that trigger allergic reactions. An estimated 235 million people, particularly of those in extremes of age, suffer from the consequences of its clinical impact worldwide (WHO, 2017, August). **Allergic rhinitis** (hay fever) is an inflammation of the nose lining due to inhalation of allergens. Allergic rhinitis can be triggered by outdoor allergens (e.g. mould or trees, grass and weed pollens) or indoor allergens (e.g. animal dander or house dust mites) (WHO, n.d.). **Chronic obstructive pulmonary disease**

Table 3.6 Direct and indirect impacts of climate change on non-communicable diseases (NCDs)

Impact	Climate change-related events	Pathways	NCD outcomes
Direct	Extreme heat	Heat stress	Cardiovascular diseases Respiratory diseases
	Warmer temperatures Drought Changes in seasonality	Higher level of ozone and other pollutants	Respiratory diseases Cardiovascular diseases
		Increased pollen production and changes in distribution	Respiratory and allergic diseases
	Stratospheric ozone depletion	Increased ultraviolet radiation exposure	Cancer Cataract
	Flooding Heavy precipitation	Being hit by an object	Injuries
Indirect	Drought Flooding	Reduced food production Damaged households Population displacement	Poor general health Malnutrition Mental health
	Extreme weather events Flooding Cyclones Bushfires	Traumatic experience Economic hardship Loss of loved ones	Mental health

Source: Adapted from Friel et al. (2011, Table 1).

Case Box 3.4 Impacts of climate change on air quality

By Amos P. K. Tai

Air pollution is one of the most pressing public health concerns today. As the severity of air pollution is strongly sensitive to weather conditions, it is expected that climate change, alongside changes in emissions and other factors, could substantially modify air quality, with significant ramifications for human health. For instance, Fu and Tai (2015) and Fu, Tai, and Liao (2016) examined the effects of historical climate change on air quality in East Asia using numerical model experiments and long-term observations, and found that warming over 1980–2010 has led to substantial increases in summertime ozone (O_3) by 2–10 ppbv and fine particulate matter ($PM_{2.5}$) by 6–8 μg m^{-3} in China, but a decrease in wintertime $PM_{2.5}$ by 4–12 μg m^{-3} in the same regions. The enhanced O_3 levels are mostly attributable to more prevalent air stagnation, enhanced photochemistry, and higher vegetation emissions of volatile organic compounds associated with higher temperatures, and are estimated to have caused ~6,000 more premature deaths annually over 1980–2010. These changes are projected to continue over the next century, further worsening ozone air quality worldwide by 1–10 ppbv by the mid-21st century relative to the present day (e.g. Tai, Mickley, Heald, and Wu, 2013). Climate-induced changes in $PM_{2.5}$ reflect an even more complex array of meteorological, hydrological, and chemical factors (e.g. Leung et al., 2018). Future projections from different models do not even agree on the sign of $PM_{2.5}$ changes following climate change, reflecting the long-standing challenge to understand and predict aerosol–climate interactions.

(COPD) is a lung disease with persistent blockage of airflow from the lungs. Risk factors for COPD are tobacco, indoor/outdoor air pollution, occupational dusts, and chemicals (WHO, 2017, December).

Climate change-related events are found to be associated with the increased risks of mortality and morbidity of respiratory and allergic diseases (D'Amato, Cecchi, D'Amato, & Annesi-Maesano, 2014). Risk of respiratory and allergic diseases are related to reduced outdoor air quality as climate change may: (i) increase concentrations of air pollutants, such as ozone, particulate matters, and dust; (ii) alter production pattern and allergenicity of allergens, e.g. pollen and mould spores; (iii) increase the dusts in the air; and (iv) increase the frequencies of wildfires and wildfire smoke consists of air pollutants (Friel et al., 2011). They may also exacerbate pre-existing medical conditions and worsen disease outcomes and management (D'Amato et al., 2014).

Increased air pollution

Increased human activities and context of high-density urban living may generate more pollutants (such as ozone, fine particles, and dust) in the ambient air, which may raise the incidence of respiratory illnesses, such as asthma and COPD. Table 3.7 summarises the rationale of how air pollutants may cause respiratory health.

Table 3.7 Impacts of air pollutants on respiratory health

Exposure	Pathways	Respiratory health problems
Increased ground-level ozone	Warmer temperatures enhance chemical ozone production (Metz et al., 2007)	• Respiratory tract irritation • Exacerbation of asthma • COPD
Greater fine particle emissions	Increased energy demand for air conditioning capacity, transport and industry	• Acute respiratory infections • Premature mortality (WHO, 2006)
Dust	Longer and severe drought dries soil and increases forest fire risks (Friel, Hanning, Isaak, Prowse, & Miller, 2010)	• Respiratory tract irritation • COPD

Source: Adapted from D'Amato et al. (2014).

Adverse health impact of air pollutants is more apparent with high temperatures. In a multi-city study in Italy, for every 1°C rise in maximum apparent temperature above the city specific threshold, the estimated overall change in all-cause mortality was 3.1% in the Mediterranean region and 1.8% in the north-continental region, with a two to three times greater effect on respiratory mortality (6.7 and 6.1%, respectively) (Ayres et al., 2009; D'Amato et al., 2015; Stafoggia et al., 2008). A heatwave in August 2003 in Europe caused approximately 40,000 additional deaths (Ayres et al., 2009; D'Amato et al., 2014). During the heatwave, ground-level ozone concentrations were above air-quality standards (180 μg/m³) in many monitoring stations in central France and south-western Germany. About one-third of the deaths were attributable to excessive ozone concentrations (Hodzic et al., 2007).

Changes in allergens

Aeroallergens, such as pollen and moulds, are produced from organisms such as weeds, grasses, trees, and fungus. Mucosal contact with allergens on the eyes, nose, or inhalation into the lungs may trigger allergic responses, such as allergic rhinitis (hay fever) and asthma. Changes in numbers of frosty days, temperatures, and carbon dioxide (CO_2) concentration may affect the atmospheric pollen concentration. For example, (i) higher CO_2 level induces more pollen production due to a fertilising effect on plant growth; (ii) warmer temperature may affect time and duration of pollen season (e.g. high temperature is associated with an earlier onset of the spring pollen season in the Northern Hemisphere (D'Amato et al., 2007)); and (iii) these changes may introduce pollen allergens in the new geographical areas (Reid & Gamble, 2009). Higher pollen concentrations and longer pollen seasons may also exacerbate allergic rhinitis, particularly in people with existing problems. Furthermore, the prevalence of allergic illness by exposing new populations to new allergens may be increased (IPCC, 2007).

The most susceptible population groups for respiratory and allergic diseases exacerbated by climate change are those suffering from chronic respiratory diseases, people with pre-existing medical conditions such as asthma and cardiovascular problems, and marginalised population groups such as children and older people (Friel et al., 2011). Higher incidence of respiratory illness is thus expected in the future in the combination of more hot days and higher air pollution.

Cardiovascular and cerebrovascular diseases

Cardiovascular diseases (CVDs) and cerebrovascular diseases are heart and blood vessel disorders. WHO (2017, May) reported that CVDs were the leading global cause of death in 2015, and had contributed to 17.7 million deaths (31% of the total global mortality). Common clinical diseases include hypertension, coronary disease, heart attack, and stroke. Heart attacks and strokes are acute events resulted from blocked blood supply to the heart or the brain and can lead to death. Over three-quarters of CVD deaths occur in low- to middle-income countries.

Impacts of climate change on CVDs

Climate change may directly or indirectly increase CVD risks through three main pathways: (i) increase of air pollution, (ii) physiological exposure to extreme temperatures, and (iii) changes to dietary options (Friel et al., 2011).

Air pollution

Increased exposure to air pollutants may increase CVD-related clinical manifestation through hospitalisation and deaths that may be triggered by inducing physiological stress to cause heart attacks, strokes, and irregular heart rhythms, particularly in people with pre-existing medical conditions (Gold & Samet, 2013).

Extreme temperatures

Hot and cold weather extremes may increase physiological overloading of the cardiovascular and respiratory systems. Excessive heat exposure is linked with higher cardiac episodes due to increase in core body temperature, heart rate, sweating, and dehydration. When extreme heat is combined with high pollution, the CVD risk in susceptible populations may be increased (D'Amato et al., 2014). Seemingly contradictory, global warming may reduce winter CVD mortality, but the overall global net effect of climate change on CVDs is more likely to be negative. With more intense and longer duration of heatwaves due to climate change, deaths and hospitalisation of CVD patients are expected to increase (De Blois et al., 2015).

Changes to dietary options and living styles

Environmental impact of climate change may change agricultural practices and outcomes. As a result, it might alter dietary options and lifestyle (e.g. exercises and activities), which might increase the risks of CVD. Indigenous communities may be forced to adopt their traditional living, hunting, and eating patterns in response to many environmental changes (Friel et al., 2011). For example, the Inuit communities in the Arctic region had to change their traditional lifestyle and livelihood due to the loss of sea-ice and permafrost. This adjustment has reduced physical mobility and increased reliance on imported energy-dense processed food and is increasing the risk of obesity, diabetes, and CVDs (Dixon, Donati, Pike, & Hattersley, 2009).

Age, habits, and genetics may also contribute to higher health risks, e.g. smoking, family history of hypertension, or people over 65 years old (Gold & Samet, 2013). People with history of heart attacks, strokes, and with pre-existing cardiac diseases, e.g. angina or irregular heart rhythm, and people who perform heavy physical labour are thus more vulnerable and sensitive to climate change (De Blois et al., 2015).

Cancer

Cancer is a group of diseases characterised by the rapid growth of abnormal cells, which invade healthy cells in other organs. It is a leading cause of death worldwide, accounting for 8.8 million deaths in 2015 (WHO, 2018, February). A normal cell becomes a tumour cell through multistage transformation due to the interaction of various risk factors: *personal* (age, tobacco use, overweight, alcohol use); *chemical* (asbestos, smoking); *biological* (infections from certain viruses); and *environmental* (increased exposure to ultraviolet (UV) radiation). Between 30 and 50% of cancer deaths could be prevented by modifying key risk factors (WHO, 2018, February).

Impacts of climate change on cancers

Stratospheric ozone is an ozone layer in the stratosphere and protects humans from the sun's ultraviolet rays (UV). This natural protective shield has been gradually depleted by man-made chemicals, such as chlorofluorocarbons (CFCs), allowing more UV radiation to the earth surface. Small doses of UV radiation may help the body produce vitamin D. Excessive but short-term exposure can cause minor health effects such as sunburn. However, long-term UV exposure can damage the skin and eyes and may cause skin cancers, cataracts, and immune system suppression (WHO, 1994, 2006) (see Case Box 3.5).

The relationship among ozone depletion, climate change, and skin cancer risk is complex. Climate change can alter UV radiation level at the earth's surface and increase the skin cancer risks in at least three ways (Arblaster et al., 2014; World Meteorological Organization, n.d.): (i) Although climate change is not the cause of stratospheric ozone depletion, warming temperature may slow down the recovery of the ozone layer. (ii) Altered precipitation patterns and cloud coverage may change the UV level. UV levels are highest under cloudless skies. Thick clouds may reduce UV level, while thin clouds may augment UV levels because of scattering. (iii) Warmer climate may change behavioural patterns, e.g. increased outdoor activities.

Case Box 3.5 Montreal Protocol

Concerns over stratospheric ozone depletion and its health impacts led to the enforcement of the Montreal Protocol (United Nations, 1987). Since then the production of man-made chemicals has substantially declined and the long-term recovery of the ozone layer to pre-1970s levels is expected by 2050.

Case Box 3.6 Warming temperature and skin cancer incidence

The potential impact of air temperature on sun-induced non-melanoma skin cancer incidence was investigated in the 10 regions in the United States. It was found that there is a 5.5% per °C increase for squamous cell carcinoma and 2.9% increase for basal cell carcinoma. This study indicated that higher air temperature enhanced UV radiation-induced carcinogenesis, thus global warming may escalate the risk of non-melanoma skin cancers.

Source: van der Leun, Piacentini, and de Gruijl (2008)

Skin cancer and human behaviour

Skin cancer is correlated to age and skin colour. The greater melanin level in dark skin helps protect against UV radiation, hence the risk of skin cancer is higher for whites than for dark-skinned people (see Case Box 3.6).

Human behaviour may also be a risk factor associated with skin cancer. For example, under high UV levels, in combination with warmer temperature and increased outdoor lifestyle, the associated skin cancer risk in Australia remains high despite many preventative measures. Annually around 450,000 Australians suffer from skin cancer and UV radiation from sunlight may be responsible in over 95% of cases. Hence, many measures to improve sun protection behaviour, such as use of sunscreen and wearing protective clothing and avoiding sun around noon, have been promoted since 1988. These efforts helped reduce sunburn and melanoma incidence among younger people in Victoria (Makin, 2011).

Mental health

The WHO (1946) definition of health includes mental health and emphasises the importance of positive mental health and well-being (Berry, Bowen, &

Kjellstrom, 2010). **Mental health** is defined as "a state of well-being in which an individual realises his or her own abilities, can cope with the normal stresses of life, can work productively and is able to make a contribution to her or his community" (WHO, 2018, March). **Mental well-being** often refers to life satisfaction, a sense of belonging and support, and self-esteem. **Mental illness** refers to a diagnosable mental condition that affects an individual's cognitive, emotional, or social abilities. Mental disorders include depression, anxiety, and schizophrenia. Many factors, such as socio-economic, biological, and environmental, can be stressors to one's life and affect one's mental health state acutely or chronically. Mental health disorders (WHO, 2018, March) are the global leading cause of disability. Mental disorders are risk factors for other diseases such as HIV, cardiovascular disease, and diabetes. The incidence rate of mental disorder doubles after natural disasters.

Impacts of climate change on mental health

Most existing evidence-related health impacts of climate change tend to focus on physical health. Limited consideration has been paid to identify potential impact on mental health (Berry et al., 2010). However, recent climate change events highlighted the substantial impacts of mental illness on society and economy, hence increasing needs to address the mental health effects of natural disasters.

Types of mental illness arising from climate change-related events

Climate change-related extreme events may alter social, economic, and environmental determinants of mental health, including destruction of houses or loss of loved ones, increased competition for limited natural resources, and long-term stress on displaced population. All of these stressors could cause psychological effects, such as anxiety, post-traumatic stress, depression, interpersonal and societal conflict, persistent grief, and child behavioural and developmental problems and decline in academic performance.

Figure 3.1 illustrates the causative pathways between climate change and mental health.

As summarised in Table 3.8, climate change may influence mental health directly or indirectly (Berry, 2009). Onset and types of psychological impacts may be different. For example, populations exposed to extreme weather events may experience acute to sub-acute mental health consequences during and after the event (Kjellstrom, 2009). Many social and economic stressors cumulate gradually and could induce chronic stress, which could also increase the risk of physical illness. For example, disrupted food supply, and disruption in landscapes and community could affect mental health by losing the sense of belonging and connectedness in the home communities (Berry et al., 2010) (see Case Box 3.7).

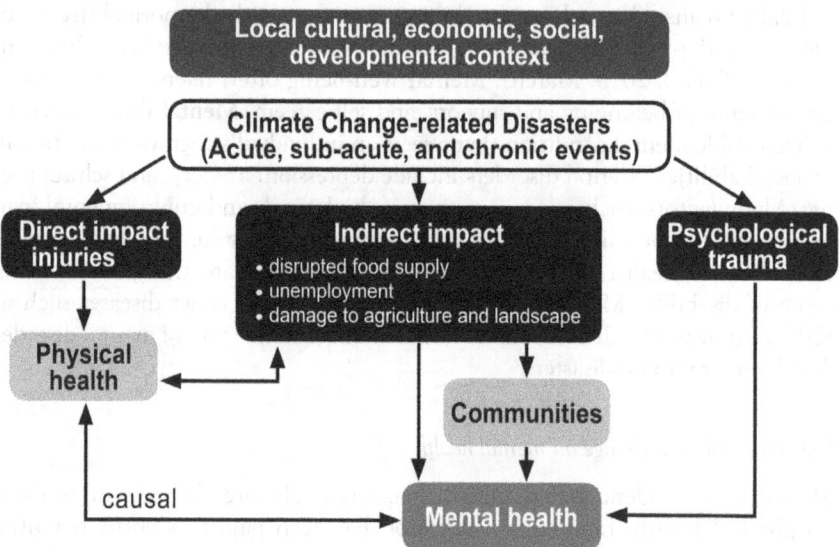

Figure 3.1 Pathways linking climate change and mental health.
Source: Adapted from Berry et al. (2010, p. 125).

Vulnerable populations

People with good access to social support tend to have higher mental resilience thus mental health problems can be minimised or avoided. In contrast, for people who lost or do not have access to resources, social and economic stressors caused by disasters are likely to have cumulative effects on mental well-being. (i) **Individuals who experienced direct damage**: Mental disorders tend to increase during and after emergencies (WHO, 2017, April; 2018, March). WHO estimated 10–15% of the affected population may suffer serious psychological problems after Typhoon Haiyan in the Philippines. People may experience temporary but acute distress at the beginning, which could potentially develop into chronic problems. (ii) **People with compromised access to infrastructure and institutions**: Vulnerability is associated with time extension after a disaster. Two years after Hurricane Katrina, only a third of childcare centres and schools were re-open and a major mental health hospital had not been replaced. These situations may prolong displacement and community fragmentation. (iii) **Individuals with pre-existing physical and mental health disorders**: They are at greater risk of mental illness. Pre-existing physical conditions, e.g. cardiovascular disease, could be contributing risk factors for developing serious mental illness. Likewise, pre-existing mental health conditions triple the risk of any-cause mortality during a heatwave (Bouchama, Dehbi, Mohamed, Matthies, Shoukri, & Menne, 2007). (iv) **Displaced population**: People who are forced to leave their houses and communities tend to lose

Table 3.8 Impacts of climate change on mental health

Impact	Onset and weather events		Risk factors	Health outcomes
Direct	Acute Immediate	Floods Cyclones Fires Tsunamis	Increased exposure to PTSD precursors, e.g. danger, injury, death Reduced agricultural land Repeated crop production Lower profits Lack of social support Geographic displacement due to damage or loss of property Stressful recovery efforts	PTSD Anxiety disorders Depression Somatic complaints Sleep difficulties Sexual dysfunction Social avoidance Drug or alcohol abuse
		Extreme heat	Excessive core body temperature	Increased aggression Suicidal rates (Cohn, Rotton, Peterson, & Tarr, 2004)
	Sub-acute Chronic	Drought	Reduced water availability Permanent/temporary relocation from home land (Haq, Kovats, Reid, & Satterthwaite, 2007) Loss of home, social networks (McMichael, McMichael, Berry, & Bowen, 2009) Loss of farming jobs	Trauma Depression Chronic stress Suicide especially in farmers Social isolation
		Prolonged extreme heat	Excessive core body temperature Dehydration Reduced ability to work and create income	Reduced physical and mental task activity (Kjellstrom, Holmer, & Lemke, 2009)

continued

Table 3.8 Continued

Impact	Types of causal pathways	Risk factors
Indirect	Impacts via physical health	Physical health state having a great impact on mental health, particularly among vulnerable populations, such as older people (Katz, 1996) Positive association between obesity and depression, panic disorders
	Impacts via physical environment	Environmental risk factors caused by climate change, i.e. water scarcity, food insecurity, air pollution, and changes in seasonality, affecting mental health, e.g. prolonged droughts over spring are associated with declined life satisfaction due to reduced agricultural productivity
	Impacts via social environment	Temporary displacement and job loss will create socio-economic difficulties, e.g. lack of social networks and extended families Conflict between displaced and host communities
	Impacts via adaptation and mitigation	For example, while enhancing active mode of transport may help reduce GHG emission, one may have to spend more time on commuting to work, which may reduce the time available to engage family and friends and thus reduce social connectedness (Berry, 2009).

Source: Adapted from Berry et al. (2010).

the sense of connectedness with families, social networks, communities, and cultures (Lundberg, 1998). Population displacement can also increase tensions and conflicts between displaced and host communities, resulting in psychological distress, social isolation, and depression. Moreover, people in refugee camps showed an increased prevalence of domestic violence, suicide, substance abuse, and depression. (v) **Marginalised population**: Older people, children, and the poor are more vulnerable to poor health outcomes due to limited resources and coping capacities. More than one-third of adult and child disaster victims may suffer from PTSD and from increased risks of substance abuse, anxiety, depression, adjustment disorders, interpersonal problems, suicide, vocational difficulties, long-term physiological changes, and subsequent physical health problems (Norris, Friedman, & Watson, 2002). (vi) **People in regions with ongoing conflict**: Due to scarcity of resources, crop failures, economic losses, and population displacement, an increase in violence, conflict, and instability may be triggered, which may have serious implications on mental health consequences (Lundberg, 1998). Regions with ongoing unrest, poverty, unequal access to resources, weak institutions, food insecurity, and poor health are at the greatest risk. In Africa, a year-long drought increases the risk of civil war the next year by 50% (Burke, Miguel, Satyanath, Dykema, & Lobell, 2009).

Injuries

Injuries constitute about 10% of annual global death (5.8 million people). There are two major categories of injuries, namely **intentional injuries** like those violence-related (e.g. suicide, homicide, and war); and **unintentional injuries** like traffic accidents. Nearly one-third of the 5.8 million annual deaths from injuries are the result of violence, while almost one-quarter is the result of road traffic crashes. Drowning causes approximately half a million deaths annually, specifically for children. Nearly all of these deaths are in low- and middle-income countries, especially in Western Pacific. Other major causes of death from injuries are falls, drowning, burns, and poisoning. Injury is one of the direct NCD outcomes of the climate change-related events such as flooding and heavy precipitation. Climate change may alter the frequency, timing, intensity, and duration of the **extreme weather events**. Droughts, hurricanes, storms, and floods could cost numerous human lives and create huge economic losses. With the disaster impact on mental health increased, higher suicide rates were reported after floods (Roberts & Hillman, 2005).

Increased global temperatures will also lead to increased evaporation of surface water and some regions will experience more frequent and severe droughts. The lack of access to essential resources like water is one of the risk factors of national or regional conflicts. The **water shortage** problem could result in more violence and conflicts among the states.

Case Box 3.7 Psychosocial impacts of flooding: a case-control study

In addition to poor physical health outcomes, flooding can exert significant impacts on social and mental health problems that may continue over an extended period of time. A case-control study was conducted to investigate the effects of flooding on Post-Traumatic Stress Disorder (PTSD) in Spain and identify risk factors for PTSD. A "flood-affected" case group (N = 70) was randomly selected from a population affected by a flood in 2012 from an area of 20,000 inhabitants. The "non-flood-affected" control group (N = 41) was selected from a nearby region of 30,000 inhabitants 30 km away. General health and traumatic experience (TQ) scores were compared between the two groups. The case group was found to have a significantly higher TQ score (5.39) than the control group (1.8). The study found age to be a risk factor for increasing TQ scores and older people were more likely to develop PTSD post flooding. People who suffered economical losses also scored significantly greater TQ scores than those who did not (2.94).

Source: Pena-Andreu et al. (2013)

Temperature changes and health

Extreme weather may affect human health and bring public health problems on different levels. Extreme temperature events, such as heatwaves and cold spells (commonly referred to as cold waves), may increase the incidence rate of diseases (see Case Box 3.8). This will affect human health, increase the service burden of the medical system and infrastructure, and increase the demand on social services and welfare (see Case Box 3.10). Figure 3.2 illustrates the potential impact of extreme temperature on human health and well-being.

Impact on health of heatwave

According to the definition given by the World Meteorological Organization (WMO), heatwave is a period of abnormally hot weather. A heatwave occurs in a district invaded by hot air or when its temperature persistently and significantly increases for days or even weeks. It is expected that heatwaves will become more frequent and stronger and last a longer time, which poses a threat to public health in the following ways (IPCC, 2012):

Respiratory tract diseases: As the amount of particulates increases in the air, air pollution may increase the incidence rate of respiratory tract diseases. Strong UV may also increase the intensity of ozone at ground level and may cause damage to the lung or lead to trauma or chronic obstructive pulmonary disease.

Infectious diseases: As the temperature increases, infectious disease patterns change. Some cold regions become warmer and the habitat range of mosquitoes may expand towards high latitude regions. Risk of infectious diseases will be

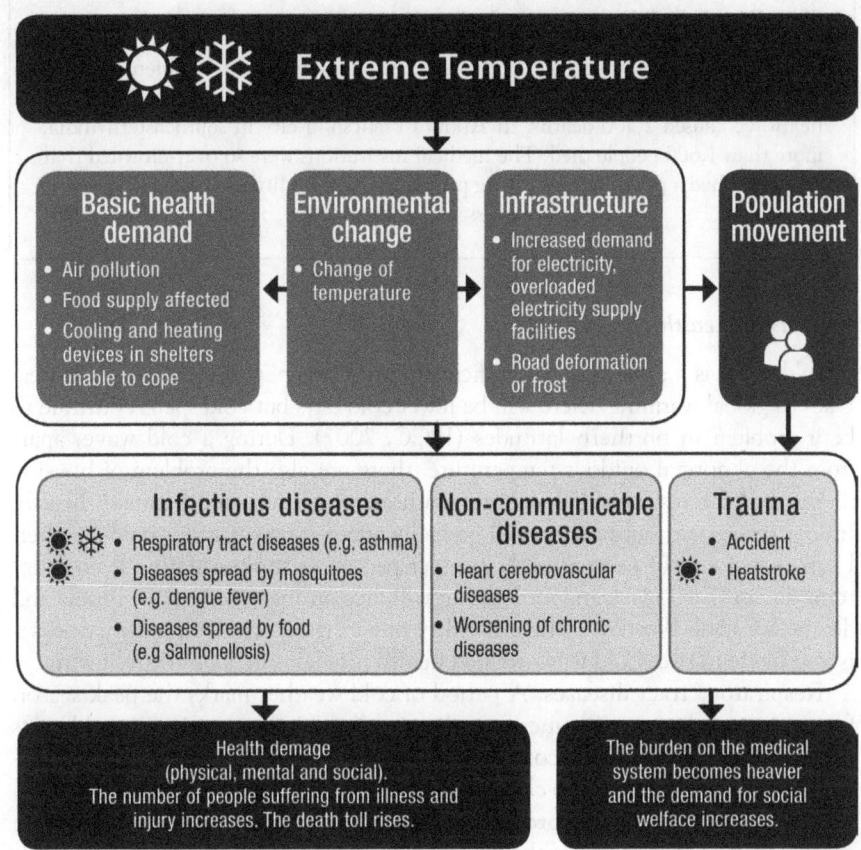

Figure 3.2 Pathways linking extreme temperature and human health.

increased. Common examples of such infectious diseases include intestinal pathogenic bacteria infection (spreading via drinking water), salmonellosis (spreading through eating contaminated food), and dengue fever, malaria, and West Nile virus (spread by mosquitoes). In addition, high temperatures hasten water evaporation and sharply decrease the amount of fresh water, which leads to drought. Inappropriate water storage may breed the mosquitoes and increase the risk of infectious diseases.

Non-communicable diseases: Hot weather may also cause cardiovascular and cerebrovascular disease, or the functions of other organs may deteriorate due to over-heating.

Case Box 3.8 A heatwave in India

In May 2015, India was struck by persistent fatal heatwave with ambient temperature in some Indian cities reported to have reached 48°C. By June 2015, this heatwave caused 2,500 deaths. In Andhra Pradesh, a city in southeastern India, more than 1,600 people died. The medical institutions were so over-crowded that they launched a public appeal asking people to go out as little as possible.

Sources: Associated Press (2015, 31 May); Burton (2015)

Impacts on health of cold spell

A cold wave is a sudden and significant drop of temperature over a wide area. Dues to global warming, there will be fewer cold days but cold spells continue to be a problem in northern latitudes (IPCC, 2007). During a cold wave, apart from the abnormal outdoor temperature, there are also the problem of housing design and the resulting indoor temperatures, which also affect human health. Indoor spaces without heating will be badly affected by persistent cold weather. High-risk groups of people (such as older people or those suffering from long-term diseases) who lack indoor heating will face an increased risk of illness and death (see Case Box 3.9). The morbidity rate of those with respiratory diseases is also likely to rise. Cold wave-related health problems include the following:

Respiratory tract diseases: A period of cold weather marks the peak season for respiratory diseases as it increases the activity of influenza viruses and boosts their transmission. Besides, cold and dry air may directly stimulate the respiratory tract, which may lead to chronic diseases.

Cardiovascular and cerebrovascular diseases: Cold weather can narrow the capillaries near the surface of the skin and cause an increase in blood pressure. It can also cause dilated cardiomyopathy, large amount of blood platelets, and an increase in blood viscosity. These may lead to cardiovascular and cerebrovascular diseases.

Unintentional injuries: In cold weather, human blood vessels become narrow, and the blood circulation comparatively less smooth, which leads to muscle stiffness. Such stiffness can cause sports injuries.

Case Box 3.9 Cold spell in Hong Kong

On 22 January 2016, an extremely cold spell hit Hong Kong. Hong Kong Observatory reported a record-low temperature of 3.1°C in the city on 24 January, which was the lowest temperature for the previous six decades. The temperature on Tai Mo Shan, the city's highest peak, dropped to –6°C. There was ice on Tai Mo Shan and Kowloon Peak. More than 100 people were trapped in the mountainous areas. The Fire Services Department and the Hong Kong Police Force had to dispatch teams to rescue citizens and divert traffic flow. The Education Bureau also had to announce school closure for kindergartens, special schools for children with physical or intellectual disabilities, and primary schools. Home Affairs Department also had to open 17 temporary cold shelters in different districts and provided resources (e.g. blankets) to the needy.

Source: Chan, Huang, Mark, and Guo (2017)

Case Box 3.10 The relationship between temperature and public health

Collaborating Centre for Oxford and CUHK for Disaster and Medical Humanitarian Response (CCOUC) published a number of studies about temperature and public health since 2012. Among them, two specific studies have supported policy changes in Hong Kong. One study examined the relationship between hot temperature and the death toll in Hong Kong. It shows that the death toll increases 1.8% for every 1°C above 28.2°C (Chan, Goggins, Kim, & Griffiths, 2012). The second related study revealed the relationship between the temperature in Hong Kong and the number of hospitalised inpatients from 1998 to 2009. Results indicate that during June to September, the number of inpatients increased 4.5% for 1°C above 29°C; during November to March, when the temperature was between 8.2°C and 26.9°C, the amount of inpatients increased 1.4% for a 1°C drop (Chan, Goggins, Yue, & Lee, 2013). The major reason for the rise in both the number of inpatients and the death toll was the increase in the number of people suffering from respiratory tract diseases and infectious diseases.

These studies enabled the use of evidence to improve planning of emergency service preparedness and response.

Sources: Chan et al. (2012, 2013)

Rainfall changes and health

Rainfall increase

Increases in the total annual rainfall and periods of heavy rain may both cause problems to living environment and ecological system and aggravate the risks of water-related diseases. Heavy rain can also cause secondary natural hazards, including flooding and landslips, which may affect safety and well-being of a population. Figure 3.3 and Table 3.9 show how increase in rainfall might affect health and well-being (see Case Box 3.11).

Heavy rain may flood underlying water runways and sewage systems and as a result pollute drinking water and cause intestinal diseases. Water-borne diseases may spread through the consumption of food and water, such as dysentery, giardiasis, cryptosporidiosis, hepatitis A, cholera, and typhoid fever. Stagnant water may enable excessive breeding of disease vectors such as mosquitoes, bacteria, and fungus, which may lead to diseases spread by mosquitoes, such as Japanese encephalitis, malaria, and dengue fever.

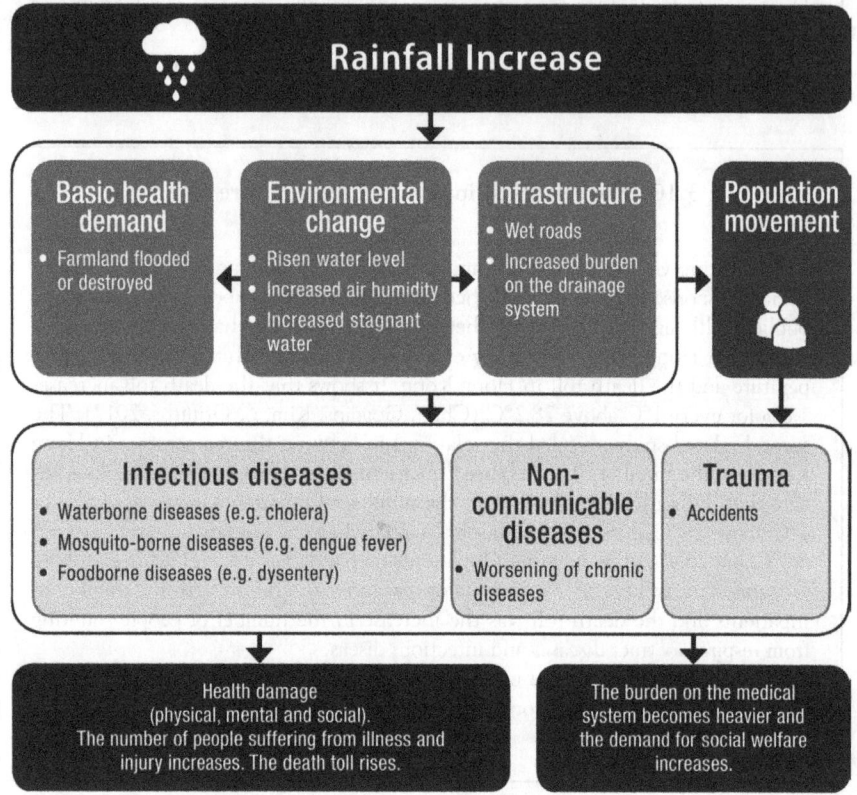

Figure 3.3 Pathways linking increased rainfall and human health.

Case Box 3.11 Heavy rain and its impact in Hong Kong

On 30 March 2014, Hong Kong experienced heavy rain. During the heavy precipitation event, the Drainage Services Department received 29 severe flooding reports throughout the city. By the evening, heavy rain rapidly became extremely heavy. Hong Kong Observatory had to issue Yellow, Red, and Black Rainstorm Warnings consecutively within 1 hour and major Landslip Warnings. The downpour led to flight delays and traffic congestion. Flooding was reported for the major underground metro stations of Kowloon Tong and Wong Tai Sin. Two big malls in the city (Festival Walk in Kowloon Tong and Trend Plaza in Tuen Mun) were drenched as the heavy rain crashed through their ceilings and poured in like a waterfall. Local food production was affected, many vegetable fields were submerged, and major economic losses by local farmers were reported.

Sources: Hong Kong Observatory (2015, 23 March); Kao (2014, 31 March)

Table 3.9 Impacts of rainfall increase on human well-being

Rainfall increase			
Basic health demand	Environmental change	Infrastructure	Population movement
• Farmland flooded or destroyed	• Risen water level • Increased air humidity • Increased stagnant water	• Wet roads • Increased burden on the drainage system	
Infectious diseases		Non-communicable diseases	Trauma
• Infectious diseases spread by water (e.g. cholera) • Infectious diseases spread by mosquitoes (e.g. dengue fever) • Infectious diseases spread through contaminated food (e.g. dysentery)		• Existing long-term diseases worsen	• Accidents
Health damage (physical, mental, and social) Increased number of people suffering from illness and injury Higher death toll		Heavier burden on the medical system and increased demand for social welfare	

Major health impacts of flooding

Flooding can affect human health in different ways, e.g. polluting the water source, interrupting the health system, and forcing mass migration (see Table 3.10; see also Case Box 3.12). The following are some of the major health problems flooding brings about.

Physical harm and injuries: Most casualties caused by flooding are due to drowning, electrical shock, and trauma, and the speed, height, and volume of floodwater can directly affect the mortality. For example, flash floods are much more dangerous than other kinds of flooding. In general, people who drown at home are mostly older people. Flooding-related trauma includes contusions and laceration. In addition, if hospitals and clinics are damaged by flooding, patients will not be able to visit doctors and receive timely treatment.

Impaired mental health: The victims of flooding may suffer from mental health problems like anxiety, depression, and sleep disorders brought about by experiencing the damage from floods such as witnessing houses collapsing, suffering the loss of their properties and livelihoods, and being forced to move.

Infectious diseases: The water treatment facilities and public health facilities in developed countries are more resilient comparatively and they are therefore less likely to have outbreaks of infectious diseases. In developing countries, however, the outbreak of infectious diseases after disasters is more common due to the unprotected weak underlying water treatment and public health systems. Drinking water source may be easily polluted by floodwater after disasters, thus

Table 3.10 Impacts of flooding on human well-being

Flooding			
Basic health demand	Environmental change	Infrastructure	Population movement
• Fresh water polluted • Food supply affected • Living conditions affected	• The land flooded	• Water and electricity supply facilities damaged • Transportation and telecommunication systems malfunction	
Infectious diseases		Non-communicable diseases	Trauma
• Infectious diseases spread by water (e.g. cholera) • Infectious diseases spread by mosquitoes (e.g. malaria) • Infectious diseases spread by contact (e.g. skin diseases) • Parasitic diseases (e.g. schistosomiasis)		• Existing long-term diseases worsen	• Accidents (e.g. drowning, food poisoning) • Conflict
Health damage (physical, mental, and social)		Heavier burden on medical system, heavier and increased demand for social welfare	
The number of people who suffer from death, illness, and injury increased			

the risk of diseases spread by water like cholera, leptospirosis, and hepatitis A increases. In addition, although the initial deluge washes away mosquito eggs, the stagnant water left after flooding becomes a hotbed of breeding mosquitoes and the incidence rate of diseases spread by the insect (such as dengue fever and malaria). There is also data that shows that respiratory tract, skin, and eye infection cases increase after flooding.

Shortage of food and malnutrition: Crops are submerged and the food supply may affect and lead to food insecurity.

Case Box 3.12 Flooding in Myanmar

In August 2015, flooding occurred in Myanmar due to persistent heavy rain. More than 100 people died and over 1 million people were affected. The western regions were inundated and suffered from the heaviest damage with some areas covered by a few metres of stagnant water. The roads, bridges, and houses in the disaster areas were severely damaged, more than 500,000 hectares of crops were destroyed, and there was a serious threat to the safety of food and drinking water.

Source: FloodList (2015, 22 October)

Rainfall decrease: drought

Decrease of water access might affect hygiene and well-being. Figure 3.4 and Table 3.11 show how drought or water shortage might affect health (see also Case Box 3.13).

Major health impacts of drought

Water is the source of life, but from 1994 to 2013, there were more than a billion people suffering from drought. Drought causes crops failure, a shortage of drinking water, and large-scale outbreaks of infectious diseases. It can also have a long-term effect on the environment, the social economy, and health (Centre for Research on the Epidemiology of Disasters, 2015). Table 3.11 outlines the various health well-being impacts of drought. Key health problems arising from drought include:

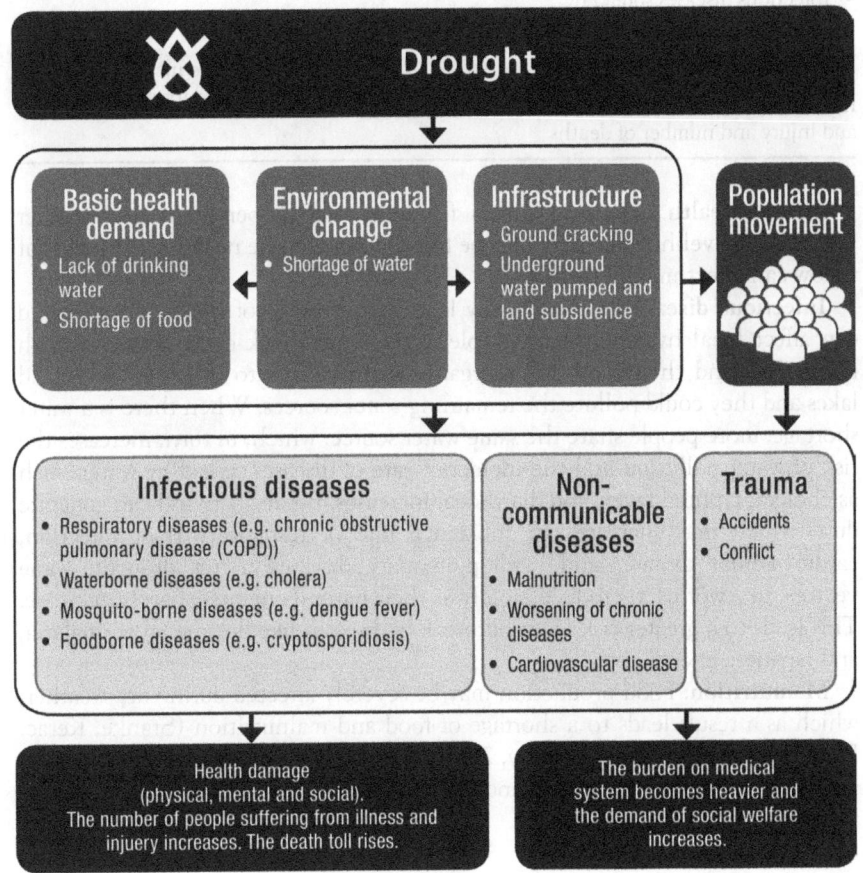

Figure 3.4 Pathways linking drought and human health.

Table 3.11 Impacts of drought on human well-being

Drought			
Basic health demand	Environmental change	Infrastructure	Population movement
• Lack of drinking water • Shortage of food	• Shortage of water	• Ground cracking • Underground water pumped and land subsidence	
Infectious diseases		Non-communicable diseases	Trauma
• Respiratory diseases (e.g. chronic obstructive pulmonary disease (COPD)) • Infectious diseases spread by water (e.g. cholera) • Infectious diseases spread by mosquitoes (e.g. dengue fever) • Infectious diseases spread by food (e.g. cryptosporidiosis)		• Malnutrition • Existing long-term diseases worsen • Cardiovascular disease	• Accidents • Conflict
Health damage (physical, mental, and social) Increased number of people suffering illness and injury and number of deaths		Heavier burden on the medical system and increased demand for social welfare	

Mental health damage: Farmers feel desperate as persistent dry weather affects their livelihood or they may be forced to move; the negative feelings that follow can affect mental health.

Infectious diseases: Drought may lead to a shortage of water resources and can affect local hygiene. For example, citizens may lack clean water to wash themselves and their food. Microorganisms thrive due to dried-up rivers and lakes and they could pollute the remaining water sources. When there is a water shortage, more people share the same water source, which, in turn, increases the risk of water pollution and the incidence rate of diseases spread by water, such as cholera, typhoid fever, and diarrhoea, increases. Besides, dry soil can generate dust, which may increase the incidence rate of respiratory tract infection, cardiovascular disease, and cardiopulmonary diseases. After drought, some vectors, like worms, reproduce rapidly as their natural enemies sharply decrease. This leads to a greater risk of an outbreak of diseases like dengue fever, malaria, and Japanese encephalitis.

Malnutrition: Food production may be severely affected during dry weather, which as a result leads to a shortage of food and malnutrition (Stanke, Kerac, Prudhomme, Medlock, & Murray, 2013). The effect is particularly significant in agriculture-based, marginalised, and poverty-stricken communities.

Case Box 3.13 Drought in Vietnam

During the dry season from November 2015 to April 2016, the middle and southern regions of Vietnam suffered from persistent and severe drought. The Mekong Delta is the worst affected with the heaviest damage, and the farmers living in the delta region have lost their livelihood. Affected by the strong El Niño, 39 out of 63 provinces in Vietnam suffered from a shortage of water and the storage of fresh water in lakes decreased. The water level of Mekong Delta reached its lowest point since 1926 with residents nearby facing a shortage of both domestic and agricultural water. The Mekong Delta also suffered from the intrusion of seawater as the sea level rose. The soil was severely salinised and crop production decreased sharply with more than 1.75 million people affected.

Sources: Daiss (2016, 25 May); Reliefweb (2016, 14 April)

Sea-level rise and health

Climate change affects average weather conditions and alters the climate system. Sea-level rise may affect habitat and livelihood of population living around the coastal area. The impact would bring long-term socio-economic as well as health challenges. It is predicted that climate change will cause further **sea-level rises** of between 18 and 59 cm by 2100 (IPCC, 2007). People living close to the sea are particularly at risk during storms or cyclones. Figure 3.5 describes the potential health impact of sea-level rise.

The major health impacts of sea-level rise

As the phenomenon of sea-level rise is a slow process, the impact is often neglected and forgotten by population living beyond the affected coastal areas and delta regions. Table 3.12 shows the impact of sea-level rise on human well-being. Sea-level rise may contribute to the following health problems.

Disease burden: The drainage system in cities may be flooded by seawater intrusion. Fresh water may be polluted, which can lead to a water shortage. The outbreak of diseases might result.

Population migration: Populations may be forced to migrate when their residences and homes are destroyed by floodwater. Floods cause casualties and deaths (see Case Box 3.14).

Food insecurity: Seawater may cause salinisation and pollute wetlands. Ecology may be altered and fishes, birds, and plants thus lose their habitats. It may also cause human food shortages and food insecurity, ultimately, malnutrition, or lead to conflicts over scarce resources.

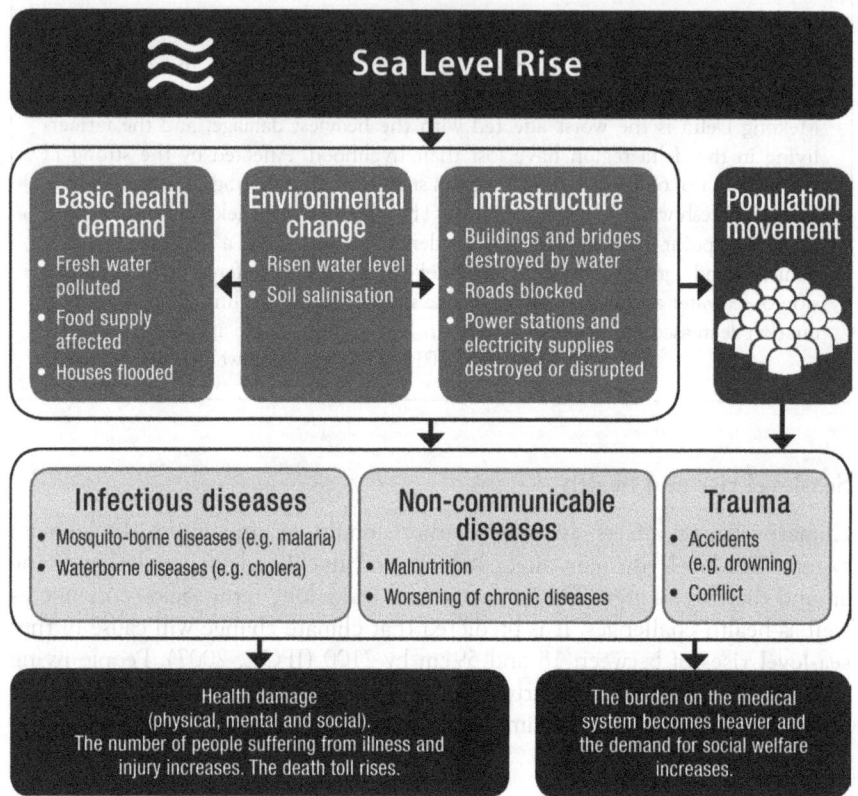

Figure 3.5 Pathways linking sea-level rise and human health.

Case Box 3.14 Sea-level rise and Tuvalu

Tuvalu, a tiny Western Pacific island nation, was the first country to announce the nationwide relocation of its population because of rising sea levels. Located in Oceania, its landmass is only 1.8 metres above the mean sea level on average, and 4 metres at the maximum. According to satellite images, the sea level around Tuvalu has been rising 5 mm per year since 1993 and disasters have been more frequent. It is estimated that the sea level will rise above more than half of the country's land by 2050. Since 2002, the Tuvaluans have been moving to New Zealand due to climate change.

Sources: Australian Bureau of Meteorology, and Commonwealth Scientific and Industrial Research Organisation (2011); Australian Government (2012, August); Bedford and Bedford (2010)

Table 3.12 Impacts of sea-level rise on human well-being

Sea-level rise			
Basic health demand	Environmental change	Infrastructure	Population movement
• Fresh water polluted • Food supply affected • Houses flooded	• Water-level rise • Soil salinisation	• Buildings and bridges destroyed by water • Roads blocked • Power stations and electricity supplies destroyed or disrupted	
Infectious diseases		Non-communicable diseases	Trauma
• Infectious diseases spread by mosquitoes (e.g. malaria) • Infectious diseases spread by water (e.g. cholera)		• Malnutrition • Existing long-term diseases worsen	• Accidents (e.g. drowning) • Conflict
Health damage (physical, mental, and social) Increased number of people suffering from death, illness, and injury		Heavier burden for the medical system and higher demand for social welfare	

Conclusion

Climate change may alter disease burden and transmission patterns. It lays a great burden on public health by changing the patterns and incidences of various communicable and non-communicable diseases. Changes in temperature and precipitation patterns have impacts on the transmission and distribution of the vector-borne diseases. Temperature and rainfall have increased bacterial and viral water-borne diseases and food-borne toxins. For the coming decades, urgent scientific evidence will be needed to understand the change of epidemiological patterns in order to enhance disease surveillance and to upgrade capacity to protect community from the public health risks and potential health implications. It is necessary to learn more about the underlying complex causal relationships and apply this information to predict future impacts.

References

Arblaster, J. M., Gillett, N. P., Calvo, N., Forster, P. M., Polvani, L. M., Son, S.-W., … Young, P. J. (2014). Stratospheric ozone changes and climate. In *Scientific assessment of ozone depletion: 2014*. Geneva, Switzerland: World Meteorological Organization. Retrieved from www.esrl.noaa.gov/csd/assessments/ozone/2014/chapters/chapter4_2014OzoneAssessment.pdf.

Associated Press. (2015, 31 May). Rain brings little relief to southern India as heatwave death toll nears 2,200 [online]. *Guardian*. Retrieved from www.theguardian.com/weather/2015/may/31/southern-india-heatwave-death-toll-nears-2200-rain-brings-little-relief.

Australian Bureau of Meteorology, & Commonwealth Scientific and Industrial Research Organisation. (2011). *Climate change in the Pacific: Scientific assessment and new research* (Volume 2: Country reports). Retrieved from www.pacificclimatechangescience.org/wp-content/uploads/2013/09/Volume-2-country-reports.pdf.

Australian Government. (2012, August). *Tuvalu annual program performance report 2011.* Retrieved from https://dfat.gov.au/about-us/publications/Documents/tuvalu-appr-2011.pdf.

Ayres, J. G., Forsberg, B., Annesi-Maesano, I, Dey, R, Ebi, K. L. & Helms, P. J., … Forastiere, F. (2009). Climate change and respiratory disease: European Respiratory Society position statement. *European Respiratory Journal, 34*(2), 295–302. doi:10.1183/09031936.00003409.

Baker-Austin, C., Trinanes, J. A., Taylor, N. G., Hartnell, R., Siitonen, A., & Martinez-Urtaza, J. (2012). Emerging Vibrio risk at high latitudes in response to ocean warming. *Nature Climate Change, 3*(1), 73–77.

Bedford, R., & Bedford, C. (2010). International migration and climate change: A post-Copenhagen perspective on options for Kiribati and Tuvalu. In B. Burson (Ed.), *Climate change and migration: South Pacific perspectives* (pp. 89–134). Wellington, New Zealand: Institute of Policy Studies, Victoria University of Wellington. doi:10.13140/RG.2.1.2910.2166.

Berry, H. (2009). Pearl in the oyster: Climate change as a mental health opportunity. *Australasian Psychiatry, 17*(6), 453–456.

Berry, H. L., Bowen, K., & Kjellstrom, T. (2010). Climate change and mental health: A causal pathways framework. *International Journal of Public Health, 55*(2), 123–132.

Bouchama, A., Dehbi, M., Mohamed, G., Matthies, F., Shoukri, M., & Menne, B. (2007). Prognostic factors in heat wave related deaths: A meta-analysis. *Archives of Internal Medicine, 167*(20), 2170–2176.

Burke, M., Miguel, E., Satyanath, S., Dykema, J., & Lobell, D. B. (2009). Warming increases the risk of civil war in Africa. *Proceedings of the National Academy of Sciences of the United States of America, 106*(49), 20670–20674. doi:10.1073/pnas.0907998106.

Burton, C. (2015). India's deadly heatwave nears end as monsoon arrives [online]. *The Weather Network.* Retrieved from www.theweathernetwork.com/uk/news/articles/indias-deadly-heatwave-nears-end-as-monsoon-arrives/52420/.

Centers for Disease Control and Prevention [CDC]. (n.d.). A-Z index of water-related topics [online]. Retrieved from www.cdc.gov/healthywater/disease/az.html.

Centre for Research on the Epidemiology of Disasters. (2015). The human cost of natural disasters 2015: A global perspective. Retrieved from http://reliefweb.int/sites/reliefweb.int/files/resources/PAND_report.pdf.

Chan, E. Y. Y., Goggins, W. B., Kim, J. J., & Griffiths, S. M. (2012). A study of intracity variation of temperature-related mortality and socioeconomic status among the Chinese population in Hong Kong. *Journal of Epidemiology and Community Health, 66*(4), 322–327.

Chan, E. Y. Y., Goggins, W. B., Kim, J. J., Griffiths, S. M., & Ma, T. K. (2011). Help-seeking behavior during elevated temperature in Chinese population. *Journal of Urban Health, 88*(4), 637–650.

Chan, E. Y. Y., Goggins, W. B., Yue, S. K., & Lee, P. Y. (2013). Hospital admissions as a function of temperature, other weather phenomena and pollution levels in an urban setting in China. *Bulletin of World Health Organization, 91*(8), 576–584. doi: 10.2471/BLT.12.113035.

Chan, E. Y. Y., Huang, Z., Mark, C. K. M., & Guo, C. (2017). Weather information acquisition and health significance during extreme cold weather in a subtropical city: A cross-sectional survey in Hong Kong. *International Journal of Disaster Risk Science*, 8(2), 134–144. doi:10.1007/s13753-017-0127-8.

Chaves, L. F., & Koenraadt, C. J. (2010). Climate change and highland malaria: Fresh air for a hot debate. *The Quarterly Review of Biology*, 85(1), 27–55.

Cohn, E., Rotton, J., Peterson, A., & Tarr, D. (2004). Temperature, city size, and the southern subculture of violence: Support for social escape/avoidance (SEA) theory. *Journal of Applied Social Psychology*, 34, 1652–1674.

Daiss, T. (2016, 25 May). Why Vietnam is running dry, worst drought in nearly 100 years. *Forbes*. Retrieved from www.forbes.com/sites/timdaiss/2016/05/25/why-vietnam-is-running-dry-worst-drought-in-nearly-100-years/#4e0a83a974b3.

D'Amato, G., Cecchi, L., Bonini, S., Nunes, C., Annesi-Maesano, I., Behrendt, H., ... Van Cauwenberge, P. (2007). Allergenic pollen and pollen allergy in Europe. *Allergy*, 62(9), 976–990.

D'Amato, G., Cecchi, L., D'Amato, M., & Annesi-Maesano, I. (2014). Climate change and respiratory diseases. *European Respiratory Review*, 23(132), 161–169.

D'Amato, G., Vitale, C., De Martino, A., Giovanni, V., Maurizia, L., Antonio, M., ... D'Amato, M. (2015). Effects on asthma and respiratory allergy of climate change and air pollution. *Multidisciplinary Respiratory Medicine*, 39(1), 10–39. doi:10.1186/s40248-015-0036-x.

De Blois, J., Kjellstrom, T., Agewall, S., Ezekowitz, J. A., Armstrong, P. W., & Atar, D. (2015). The effects of climate change on cardiac health. *Cardiology*, 131(4), 209–217.

Dixon, J. M., Donati, K. J., Pike, L. L., & Hattersley, L. (2009). Functional foods and urban agriculture: Two responses to climate change-related food insecurity. *New South Wales Public Health Bulletin*, 20(2), 14–18.

European Centre for Disease Prevention and Control. (2012). *Assessing the potential impacts of climate change on food- and waterborne diseases in Europe*. Stockholm: ECDC. Retrieved from http://foodpoisoningbulletin.com/wp-content/uploads/Climate-change-food-diseases.pdf.

FloodList. (2015, 22 October). UN report—Floods in Myanmar had devastating impact on agriculture [online]. Retrieved from http://floodlist.com/asia/un-myanmar-floods-food-security.

Friel, J. K., Hanning, R. M., Isaak, C. A., Prowse, D., & Miller, A. C. (2010). Canadian infants' nutrient intakes from complementary foods during the first year of life. *BMC Pediatrics*, 10(1), 1.

Friel, S., Bowen, K., Campbell-Lendrum, D., Frumkin, H., McMichael, A. J., & Rasanathan, K. (2011). Climate change, noncommunicable diseases, and development: The relationships and common policy opportunities. *Annual Review of Public Health*, 32, 133–147.

Fu, Y., & Tai, A. P. K. (2015). Impact of climate and land cover changes on tropospheric ozone air quality and public health in East Asia between 1980 and 2010. *Atmospheric Chemistry and Physics*, 15(17), 10093–10106. doi:10.5194/acp-15-10093-2015.

Fu, Y., Tai, A. P. K., & Liao, H. (2016). Impacts of historical climate and land cover changes on fine particulate matter ($PM_{2.5}$) air quality in East Asia between 1980 and 2010. *Atmospheric Chemistry and Physics*, 16(16), 10369–10383. doi:10.5194/acp-16-10369-2016.

Gold, D. R., & Samet, J. M. (2013). Air pollution, climate, and heart disease. *Circulation*, 128(21), e411–e414.

Haines, A., Kovats, R. S., Campbell-Lendrum, D., & Corvalán, C. (2006). Climate change and human health: Impacts, vulnerability and public health. *Public Health*, 120(7), 585–596.

Haq, S., Kovats, S., Reid, H., & Satterthwaite, D. (2007). Editorial: Reducing risks to cities from disasters and climate change. *Environment and Urbanization*, 19(1), 3–15.

Hodzic, A., Madronich, S., Bohn, B., Massie, S., Menut, L., & Wiedinmyer, C. (2007). Wildfire particulate matter in Europe during summer 2003: Meso-scale modeling of smoke emissions, transport and radiative effects. *Atmospheric Chemistry and Physics*, 7(15), 4043–4064.

Hong Kong Observatory. (2015, March 23). The weather of March 2014 [online]. Retrieved from www.weather.gov.hk/wxinfo/pastwx/mws2014/mws201403.htm.

Intergovernmental Panel on Climate Change [IPCC]. (2007). *Climate change 2007: The physical science basis: Contribution of Working Group I to the Fourth Assessment Report of the Intergovernmental Panel on Climate Change*. Cambridge, United Kingdom and New York, NY: Cambridge University Press.

Intergovernmental Panel on Climate Change [IPCC]. (2012). *Managing the risks of extreme events and disasters to advance climate change adaptation: A special report of Working Groups I and II of the Intergovernmental Panel on Climate Change*. Cambridge, United Kingdom and New York, NY: Cambridge University Press.

Intergovernmental Panel on Climate Change [IPCC]. (2014). *Climate change 2014: Impacts, adaptation, and vulnerability: Part A: Global and sectoral aspects: Contribution of Working Group II to the Fifth Assessment Report of the Intergovernmental Panel on Climate Change*. Cambridge, United Kingdom and New York, NY: Cambridge University Press.

Kao, E. (2014, 31 March). Giant hailstones batter Hong Kong as Observatory warns of heavy rain for days to come [online]. *South China Morning Post*. Retrieved from www.scmp.com/news/hong-kong/article/1461200/giant-hailstones-batter-hong-kong-observatory-hoists-black-rainstorm.

Katz, I. R. (1996). On the inseparability of mental and physical health in aged persons: Lessons from depression and medical comorbidity. *American Journal of Geriatric Psychiatry*, 4(1), 1–16.

Kjellstrom, T. (2009). *Climate change exposures, chronic diseases and mental health in urban populations*. Kobe, Japan: World Health Organization Centre for Health Development.

Kjellstrom, T., Holmer, I., & Lemke, B. (2009). Workplace heat stress and health: An increasing challenge for low and middle income countries during climate change. *Global Health Action*, 2(1). doi:10.3402/gha.v2i0.2047.

Kovats, R. S., Edwards, S. J., Hajat, S., Armstrong, B. G., Ebi, K. L., & Menne, B. (2004). The effect of temperature on food poisoning: A time-series analysis of salmonellosis in ten European countries. *Epidemiology and Infection*, 132(3), 443–453.

Leung, D. M., Tai, A. P. K., Mickley, L. J., Moch, J. M., van Donkelaar, A., Shen, L., & Martin, R. V. (2018). Synoptic meteorological modes of variability for fine particulate matter ($PM_{2.5}$) air quality in major metropolitan regions of China. *Atmospheric Chemistry and Physics*, 18(9), 6733–6748. doi:10.5194/acp-18-6733-2018.

Levy, B. S., & Sidel. V. W. (2015). Collective violence. In B. Levy & J. Patz (Eds.), *Climate change and public health*. Oxford, United Kingdom: Oxford University Press.

Lundberg, A. (1998). *The environment and mental health: A guide for clinicians*. Mahwah, NJ: Lawrence Erlbaum Associates.

Makin, J. (2011). Implications of climate change for skin cancer prevention in Australia. *Health Promotion Journal of Australia*, 22(4), 39–41.

McMichael, A. J., McMichael, C., Berry, H., & Bowen, K. J. (2009). Climate change, displacement and health. In J. McAdam (Ed.), *Climate change and displacement: Multi-disciplinary perspectives*. Oxford, United Kingdom: Hart Publishing.

Metz, B., Davidson, O. R., Bosch, P. R., Dave, R., & Meyer, A. (Eds.). (2007). *Climate change 2007: Mitigation of climate change: Contribution of Working Group III to the fourth assessment report of the Intergovernmental Panel on Climate Change*. Cambridge, United Kingdom; New York, NY: Cambridge University Press.

Milazzo, A., Giles, L. C., Zhang, Y., Koehler, A. P., Hiller, J. E., & Bi, P. (2016). Heat-waves differentially affect risk of *Salmonella* serotypes. *Journal of Infection, 73*(3), 231–240. doi: 10.1016/j.jinf.2016.04.034.

National Institute of Environmental Health Sciences. (2010). *Foodborne diseases and nutrition: Health impacts of climate change*. Retrieved from www.niehs.nih.gov/research/programs/geh/climatechange/health_impacts/foodborne_diseases/index.cfm.

Norris, F. H., Friedman, M. J., & Watson, P. J. (2002). 60,000 disaster victims speak: Part II. Summary and implications of the disaster mental health research. *Psychiatry, 65*(3), 240–260.

Patz, J. A., Githeko, A. K., McCarty, J. P., Hussein, S., Confalonieri, U., & de Wet, N. (2003). Climate change and infectious diseases. In A. J. McMichael, D. H. Campbell-Lendrum, C. F. Corvalán, K. L. Ebi, A. K. Githeko, J. D. Scheraga, & A. Woodward (Eds.), *Climate change and human health* (pp. 103–132). Geneva, Switzerland: World Health Organization.

Pena-Andreu, J. M., Gil Aguilar, V., Lucas Borja, P., Lucas Borja, M., Molero Carrasco, J., & Fontalba Navas, A. (2013). *Effects of flooding on mental health: A case-control study* [Working Paper].

Reid, C. E., & Gamble, J. L. (2009). Aeroallergens, allergic disease, and climate change: Impacts and adaptation. *Ecohealth, 6*(3), 458–470.

Reliefweb. (n.d.). Southern Africa: Floods—Jan 2015. Retrieved from https://reliefweb.int/disaster/fl-2015-000006-mwi.

Reliefweb. (2015, 17 April). Mozambique, Malawi, Zimbabwe: Cholera situation (as of 15 April 2015) [online]. Retrieved from https://reliefweb.int/report/mozambique/mozambique-malawi-zimbabwe-cholera-situation-15-april-2015.

Reliefweb. (2016, 14 April). Viet Nam: Drought and saltwater intrusion (Situation Update No. 2 (as of 14 April 2016)). Retrieved from https://reliefweb.int/report/viet-nam/viet-nam-drought-and-saltwater-intrusion-situation-update-no-2-14-april-2016.

Roberts, I., & Hillman, M. (2005). Climate change: The implications for policy on injury control and health promotion. *Injury Prevention, 11*, 326–329.

Stafoggia, M., Forastiere, F., Agostini, D., Caranci, N., de'Donato, F., Demaria, M., ... Perucci, C. A. (2008). Factors affecting in-hospital heat-related mortality: A multi-city case-crossover analysis. *Journal of Epidemiology & Community Health, 62*(3), 209–215.

Stanke, C., Kerac, M., Prudhomme, C., Medlock, J., & Murray, V. (2013). Health effects of drought: A systematic review of the evidence. *PLOS Currents Disasters*, 5 June.

Tai, A. P. K., Mickley, L. J., Heald, C. L., & Wu, S. (2013). Effect of CO_2 inhibition on biogenic isoprene emission: Implications for air quality under 2000 to 2050 changes in climate, vegetation, and land use. *Geophysical Research Letters, 40*(13), 3479–3483. doi:10.1002/grl.50650.

Thomson, M. C., Doblas-Reyes, F. J., Mason, S. J., Hagedorn, R., Connor, S. J., Phindela, T., ... Palmer, T. N. (2006). Malaria early warnings based on seasonal climate forecasts from multi-model ensembles. *Nature, 439*(7076), 576–579.

United Nations. (1987). *Montreal protocol on substances that deplete the ozone layer*. Montreal. 16 September 1987. Retrieved from https://treaties.un.org/doc/Treaties/1989/01/19890101%2003-25%20AM/Ch_XXVII_02_ap.pdf.

van der Leun, J. C., Piacentini, R. D., & de Gruijl, F. R. (2008). Climate change and human skin cancer. *Photochemical & Photobiological Sciences, 7*(6), 730–733. doi:10.1039/b719302e.

World Health Organization [WHO]. (n.d.). Chronic respiratory diseases: Allergic rhinitis and sinusitis [online]. Retrieved from www.who.int/respiratory/other/Rhinitis_sinusitis/en/.

World Health Organization [WHO]. (1946). *Preamble to the Constitution of the World Health Organization* as adopted by the International Health Conference, New York 19–22 June 1976; signed on 22 July 1946 by the representatives of 61 States (Official Records of the World Health Organization, no. 2, p. 100) and entered into force on 7 April 1948.

World Health Organization [WHO]. (1994). *Environmental Health Criteria (EHC) 160: Ultraviolet radiation*. Retrieved from www.who.int/uv/publications/EHC160/en/.

World Health Organization [WHO]. (2006). Health consequences of excessive solar UV radiation [online]. Retrieved from www.who.int/mediacentre/news/notes/2006/np16/en/.

World Health Organization [WHO]. (2014). Burden of disease from household air pollution for 2012 [online]. Retrieved from www.who.int/phe/health_topics/outdoorair/databases/FINAL_HAP_AAP_BoD_24March2014.pdf?ua=1.

World Health Organization [WHO]. (2015, March). *Food safety* (Fact sheet No. 399). Retrieved from www.who.int/campaigns/world-health-day/2015/fact-sheet.pdf.

World Health Organization [WHO]. (2015, December). *WHO estimates of the global burden of foodborne diseases*. Retrieved from www.who.int/foodsafety/publications/foodborne_disease/fergreport/en/.

World Health Organization [WHO]. (2016). Fact sheet: World Malaria Day 2016 [online]. Retrieved from www.who.int/malaria/media/world-malaria-day-2016/en/.

World Health Organization [WHO]. (2017, April). Mental health in emergencies [online]. Retrieved from www.who.int/news-room/fact-sheets/detail/mental-health-in-emergencies.

World Health Organization [WHO]. (2017, May). Cardiovascular diseases (CVDs) [online]. Retrieved from www.who.int/en/news-room/fact-sheets/detail/cardiovascular-diseases-(cvds).

World Health Organization [WHO]. (2017, August). Asthma [online]. Retrieved from www.who.int/en/news-room/fact-sheets/detail/asthma.

World Health Organization [WHO]. (2017, December). Chronic obstructive pulmonary disease (COPD). Retrieved from www.who.int/news-room/fact-sheets/detail/chronic-obstructive-pulmonary-disease-(copd).

World Health Organization [WHO]. (2018, February). Cancer [online]. Retrieved from www.who.int/en/news-room/fact-sheets/detail/cancer.

World Health Organization [WHO]. (2018, March). Mental health: Strengthening our response. Retrieved from www.who.int/en/news-room/fact-sheets/detail/mental-health-strengthening-our-response.

World Health Organization Regional Office for Africa. (2015, 3 March). WHO intensifies support to cholera outbreak in Malawi and Mozambique [online]. Retrieved from www.afro.who.int/news/who-intensifies-support-cholera-outbreak-malawi-and-mozambique.

World Meteorological Organization [WMO]. (n.d.). Global Atmosphere Watch (GAW): UV radiation [online]. Retrieved from www.wmo.int/pages/prog/arep/gaw/UV-radiation.html.

4 Climate change and disasters

This chapter discusses the basic concepts of disasters and health, the relationship between climate change and trends of natural disaster occurrence, as well as population vulnerability towards these mega events.

Disasters and extreme events

Natural hazards are extreme environmental impacting events that might cause large-scale human and economic losses to result in disasters. A **hazard** describes a phenomenon, substance, human activity, or condition that may cause injury, loss of life, property damage, loss of livelihoods and services, social and economic disruption, or long-term environmental damage. Meanwhile, a **disaster** is a serious disruption of the functioning of a community or a society involving human, economic, or environmental losses and impacts, which exceeds the ability of the affected community or society to cope using its own resources (United Nations International Strategy for Disaster Reduction [UNISDR], 2009). Earthquake, heatwave, and tropical cyclone are examples of "natural hazards" that might cause major human impact, but these natural phenomena may only be considered as a "disaster" when causing damages to human lives, health, or systems. Globally, different geographic locations might be affected by their underlying natural hazards. Depending on the socio-demographic characteristics, infrastructure, resilience, and response capacity, the outcome of a disaster might vary considerably and lead to different human impacts as a result.

Natural disaster classification

Disaster may, in principle, be classified into two major subgroups, namely natural and man-made disasters. Whilst man-made disasters are originated from human activities such as technological accidents, transport accidents, and complex emergencies, natural disasters have specific characteristics and may be categorised into six main types according to their root causes. These include:

- **Geophysical:** Events originating from underground and solid earth, e.g. earthquakes and volcanic activities;

- **Meteorological:** Events caused by short-lived/micro-scale atmospheric processes, e.g. storms and extreme temperature;
- **Hydrological:** Events caused by deviations in the normal water cycle and/ or overflow of bodies of water caused by wind, e.g. floods and landslides;
- **Climatological:** Events caused by long-lived/meso- to macro-scale processes, e.g. droughts and wildfires;
- **Biological:** Events caused by the exposure of living organisms to germs and toxic substances, e.g. epidemics and insect infestations; and
- **Extra-terrestrial:** Events caused by asteroids, meteoroids, and comets as they pass near earth or strike the earth, or any changes in interplanetary conditions that affect the earth's magnetosphere, e.g. impacts and space weather.

As hydrological, meteorological, and climatological as well as biological events are interlinked with the dynamics of climate changes, they are often referred to as climate-related disasters (Below, Wirtz, & Guha-Sapir, 2009; Centre for Research on the Epidemiology of Disasters [CRED], n.d.b; Chan, 2017; Integrated Research on Disaster Risk, 2014).

Global disaster trends

For the past few decades, natural disasters have been shown in an overall increasing trend (see Figure 2.7). In addition to an actual increase in frequencies of climate-related disasters, improved global communication and reporting systems have resulted in this overall increasing trend in the number of reported natural disasters. As consistently highlighted by various global reports, climate-related disasters will remain the major contributor to disaster patterns in the 21st century (CRED, n.d.a, 2015).

Figure 4.1 illustrates the worldwide distribution of natural disasters that occurred between 1994 and 2013. The occurrences of natural disasters vary with the underlying geographical hazards. Globally, People's Republic of China and the United States, mainly due to their large landmasses and huge population size, are reported to be the countries with the highest accumulated incidence of natural disasters since 2000.

Climate-related disasters

Epidemiological analysis of global disaster during the past three decades shows that a substantial increase in the number of climate-related hazards, such as storms and floods, may have contributed to the increase in disaster incidence and their related human toll (see Figure 4.2). While the numbers of geophysical hazards and disaster events, such as earthquakes, have remained stable (CRED, 2015), climate-related events, such as floods, storms, and drought, account for 87% of the global disaster events in 2014 (CRED, n.d.a).

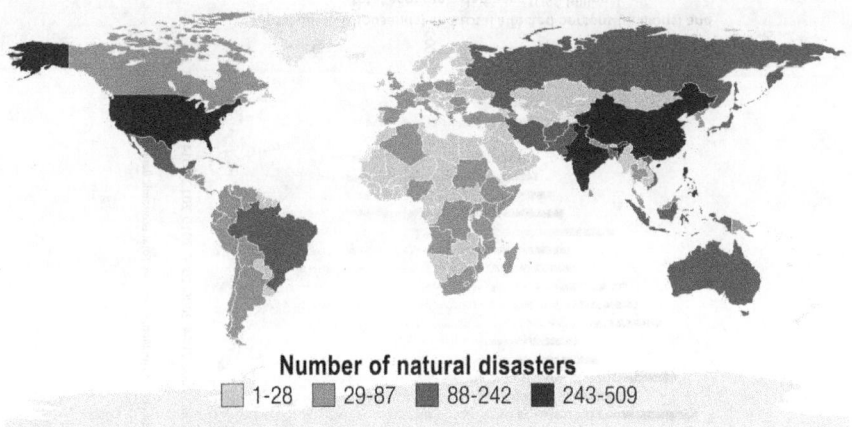

Number of natural disasters
1-28 29-87 88-242 243-509

Figure 4.1 Number of disasters reported per country (1994–2013).
Source: Adapted from CRED (2015).

Disasters in Asia

Asia is the most natural disaster-prone region in the world. Among the 10 most disaster-affected countries in the world between 1994 and 2013, China, the Philippines, India, Indonesia, and Bangladesh have numerous natural hazard events and are the most disaster-prone countries globally. Asia's large landmass contains many river basins, flood plains, mountains, active seismic and volcanic zones, in combination with densely populated cities—all of these topological and human factors posed substantial challenges in climate change-related issues. Asia reported 2,778 disasters between the 1994 and 2013 periods, with 3.8 billion affected people and approximately 841,000 deaths. In 2015, 152 out of 346 natural disasters occurred in Asia (see Figure 4.3), which represented 44% of the total number of global disasters (CRED, 2016).

Projection of natural disasters

As related to projection of future natural disasters, abnormal meteorological phenomena, such as extreme temperature, raining, and flooding events, may significantly affect the occurrences of extreme events and result in major adverse health outcomes in living habitat and environment (IPCC, 2012).

Risk and vulnerability

Urbanisation, population ageing, migration pattern, and technology-dependent modern lifestyles (e.g. dense living context in cities the functioning of which relies on lifeline infrastructure) have increased human

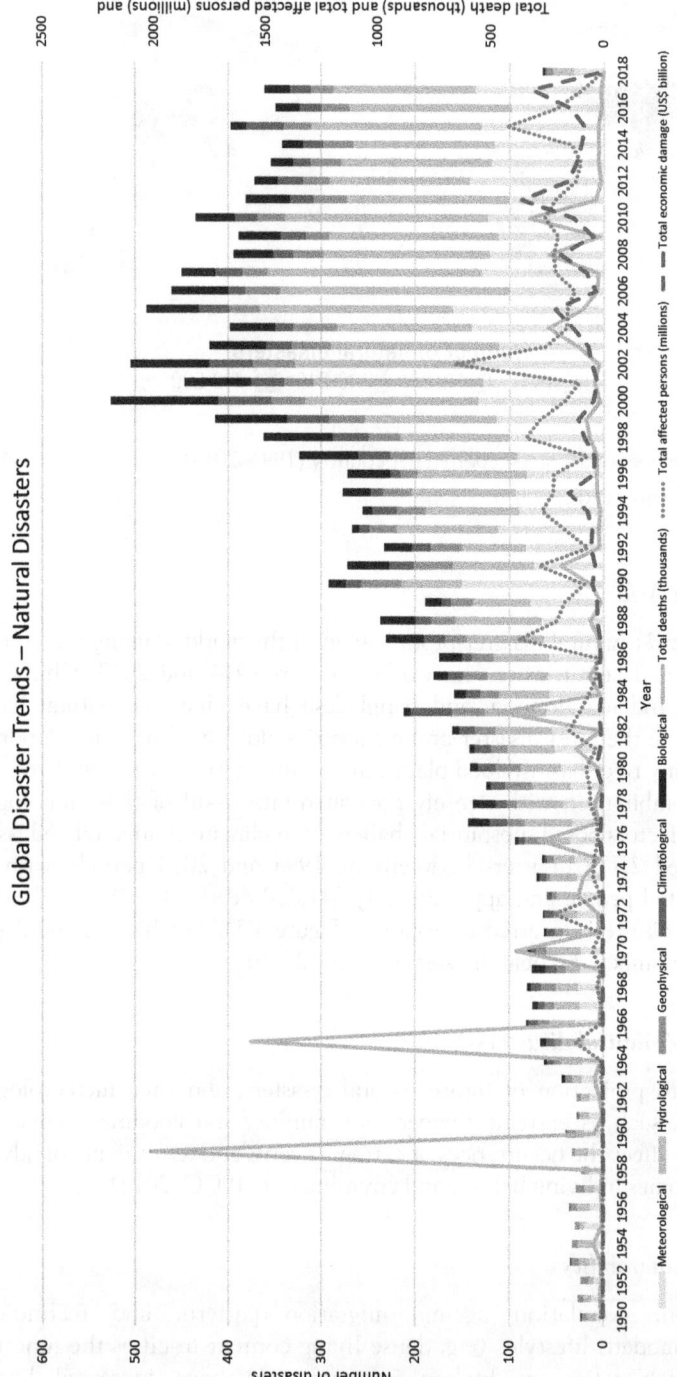

Figure 4.2 Number of climate-related and geophysical disasters (1950–2017).

Source: Adapted from CRED (2015).

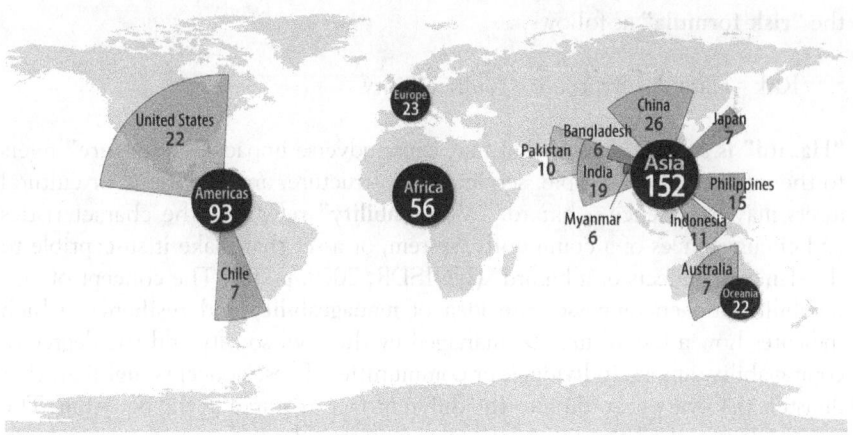

Figure 4.3 Top 10 number of reported disasters by country (2015).
Source: CRED (2016).

vulnerability towards natural hazards and disasters (World Health Organization [WHO] & World Meteorological Organization [WMO], 2012). **"Risk"** is defined as "the probability of harmful consequences, or expected losses (deaths, injuries, property, livelihoods, economic activity disrupted or environment damaged) resulting from interactions between natural or human-induced hazards and vulnerable conditions" (UNISDR, 2009). As illustrated in Figure 4.4, risk of climate-related impacts is determined by the interaction of three factors: climate-related **hazards**, the **vulnerability** and **exposure** of

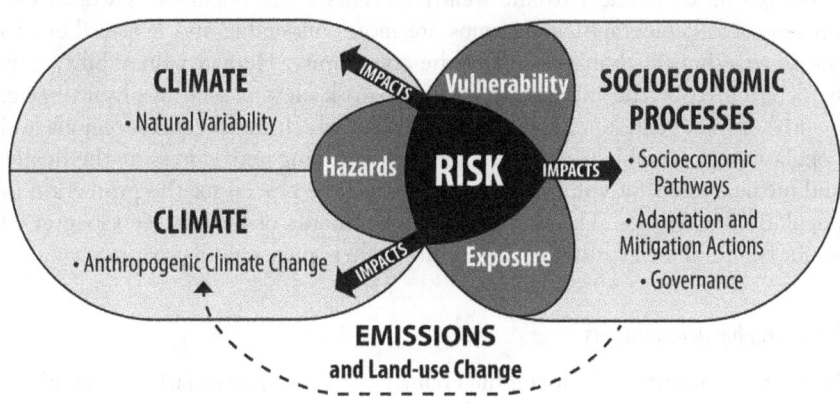

Figure 4.4 Concept of risk.
Source: Adapted from IPCC (2014, Figure SPM.1).

human and natural systems (IPCC, 2014). The concept may be understood in the **"risk formula"** as follows,

Risk = Hazard × Exposure × Vulnerability

"Hazard" is a phenomenon that may cause adverse impacts. **"Exposure"** refers to the extent of how people, services, infrastructure, and economic or cultural assets may experience a hazard. **"Vulnerability"** refers to "the characteristics and circumstances of a community, system, or asset that make it susceptible to the damaging effects of a hazard" (UNISDR, 2009, p. 30). The concept of vulnerability also encompasses the idea of **manageability** and **resilience**, which indicates how a hazard may be managed by the civil society and the degree of coping ability among individuals or communities. These concepts highlight that disasters risks vary according to the different factors stated in the equation. The risks or degree of a hazard's impact on society thus depend on exposure and vulnerability of the affected population. For example, although both developed and developing countries may be bearing similar exposure risk of natural hazards, developing countries may often suffer higher human life losses than developed countries. Yet, the expensive essential infrastructure, systems, and resources in the developed context would render a disaster more "costly" or "expensive" from an economic perspective in a developed country than a developing counterpart.

This concept is applicable to the planning of public health actions to reduce the impacts and to increase community resilience in disaster and extreme climate events. For example, a community may have higher underlying hazard and exposure risks; their vulnerability might be reduced if the coping and response capacity is enhanced.

Who are most vulnerable?

Although disasters and extreme weather events affect populations worldwide, certain socio-demographic subgroups are more vulnerable and less resilient to the adverse impact than the rest of the community. Human vulnerability may be determined by the interaction of various risk factors, such as physical (e.g. health), social, economic, and environmental, which make certain regions and populations vulnerable to natural hazards. Identifying and addressing the health and medical needs of vulnerable subgroups will be crucial for the protection of population subgroups. The concept of determinants of health (see Chapter 2) might be useful for identifying these vulnerable population subgroups.

Demographic determinants

Populations of certain demographic characteristics are particularly vulnerable to disasters. For instance, disasters lay higher health impact burden on the extremes of age. Regarding the burden of malaria and diarrhoea—the climate-related disease burden (refer also to Chapter 3)—285,000 malaria deaths (70%

of all malaria deaths) are found in **children under 5 years of age** in developing countries with high transmission of malaria in 2016 (WHO, 2018); while 499,000 diarrhoeal deaths (38% of all) in 2015 occurred in this age group (Troeger et al., 2017). Regardless of development context, **older people** and **people with pre-existing health problems** would require continuous or extra support/special medical attention following disasters (Chan, in press). Disasters also cause excess mortality and morbidity rate in **women** when compared with men (Chan, 2017). People with **pre-existing mental health problems** are more likely to develop PTSD after a disaster (Norris, Friedman, & Watson, 2002). *Ethnic minority and indigenous groups* also reported to experience increased physical impact (due to limited pre-existing infrastructure, resilience capacity), adverse mental and social health outcomes (e.g. severe PTSTD) due to frequent relocation, lack of social and economic support (Adams & Boscarino, 2005; Chan, 2018). Indigenous people who depend on their physical environment for their livelihoods may lose their traditional ways of life (WHO, 2008) and had less coping capacity during the post-disaster rebuilding process.

Social and economic determinants

People with limited economic means (e.g. people residing in the poorest countries and poor individuals in richer countries) are more vulnerable to extreme weather events and disasters. Due to their underlying socio-economical vulnerability, their access to information, education, employment opportunities, and healthcare are often curtailed. Poorer individuals' survival might depend intimately on the ecosystems, and their climate-sensitive livelihood, such as agriculture-based economy, might have minimum capacity to cope with and adapt to rapid environmental changes. They are more likely to reside in the higher hazard risk environment (due to poverty and the lack of choices), poorly constructed houses, or suboptimal infrastructural support. They are likely to be the most vulnerable to stress and catastrophic events.

Physical/environmental/geographical determinants

Specific climate-related phenomena will differently affect populations living in different geographic context. For example, droughts, floods, and seasonal climatic variability may affect access to water and sanitation. Sub-Saharan Africa is at particular risk of drought, which results in food scarcity due to crop failure and a lack of clean water. At the same time, monsoon rainfall is expected to increase in the Brahmaputra basin of the South Asian region, which may cause up to a seven-fold increase in the number of people affected by flooding annually by 2080. Areas with weak health infrastructure and economic ability will likely be the least able to cope without assistance to prepare and respond.

Extreme weather events

Definition and types of extreme weather events

An **extreme weather event** (EWE) is a rare weather condition, which is significantly different from the average weather patterns over 1 day or a period of time at a particular place (IPCC, 2012). With climate change, many global regions are experiencing increased frequencies in extreme weather events (EWEs). Heatwaves in Europe, severe drought in sub-Saharan Africa and the US, and widespread flooding in Asia were all important EWEs of the past millennium. Defining an EWE as a disaster may vary geographically as critical impact thresholds are locally specific due to regional differences in physiological, behavioural, cultural, and technological contexts. EWEs can be classified based on the disaster grouping system by CRED (see Table 4.1).

Between 1970 and 2012, there were 8,835 EWEs reported worldwide and these events had caused 1.94 million deaths and economic damage of US$2.4 trillion (WMO, 2014). These disasters were linked to weather (heat and cold waves), climate, and water extremes situation (such as droughts, floods, cyclones, and storms).

Human impacts of EWEs

All EWEs may cause direct and indirect health impacts. EWEs may be categorised into three main groups in Table 4.2 as simple extremes, complex extremes, and singular phenomena. These events occur over a longer time period, hence the impacts of which are gradual and harder to examine.

It is challenging to quantify the health impacts of EWEs. First, most human health disorders are multifactorial, therefore attributing direct human health impact to an EWE could be presumptuous. Second, different types of EWEs can be closely interrelated and may occur simultaneously. Hence, it is difficult to pinpoint the effects of an individual event on health. Third, as human context and technology for responding to and coping with the adverse impacts of EWEs

Table 4.1 Disaster groups and types of EWEs

Disaster group	Description	EWE types	Subtypes
Climatological	Caused by meso/macro-scale processes	Extreme temperature	Heatwave/cold wave/drought
Meteorological	Caused by small/medium-scale atmospheric processes	Storms Heavy rain	Tropical/winter storms
Hydrological	Caused by normal water cycle deviations or water overflow	Floods Landslides	River/flash/coastal flood Storm surge Subsidence

Source: Adapted from Guha-Sapir, Below, and Hoyois (n.d.).

Table 4.2 Types of extreme weather events and potential health impacts

Type	Events	Description	Potential impacts on health
i) Simple extremes	High/low temperature Heavy precipitation	Individual local weather above critical level	Mortality and morbidity Risk of damaging crops Fine particles due to raised demand for air conditioning, increasing respiratory diseases Overwhelmed healthcare services
ii) Complex extremes	Tropical cyclones Droughts Floods	Single weather event combined with other climatic events	Reduced crop yields Damage to building foundations Reduced water quantity and quality Unavailability of fresh food and water Long-term mental health impacts, e.g. depression and Post-Traumatic Stress Disorder (PTSD) Risks of infectious disease epidemics, e.g. diarrhoeal illness and malaria
iii) Singular phenomena	Melting glacier Water cycle changes	Predicted global climatic conditions	Coastal erosion and damage to coastal buildings and infrastructure Population displacement

Source: Adapted from IPCC (2001, Table SPM-1).

change rapidly, predicting the future health impacts remains as a major technical challenge scientifically (UNISDR, 2017).

Different types of EWEs

Extreme temperature events

The World Meteorological Organization (WMO) classifies climatological events like heatwaves and cold waves as extreme temperature events. A **heatwave** refers to a prolonged period of excessively hot weather relative to normal climate patterns of a certain region and may be accompanied by high humidity. A **cold wave** can be a prolonged period of excessively cold weather or a sudden advance of very cold air over a large area. Cold waves can immobilise an entire region and can cause damage to agriculture, infrastructure, and property (Below et al., 2009). The Intergovernmental Panel on Climate Change (IPCC) projected

> more frequent hot and fewer cold temperature extremes over most land areas [worldwide] on daily and seasonal timescales as global mean temperatures increase. It is *very likely* that heat waves will occur with a higher frequency and duration. Occasional cold winter extremes will continue to occur.
>
> (IPCC, 2013, p. 20)

Figure 4.5 illustrates how increased mean temperature will lead to changes in the frequency of extreme temperature events.

Health impacts of extreme temperature events

Extreme heat

Increases in average temperatures and frequency of extreme heat events may create greater risks of heat-related illness, ranging from mild discomfort to deaths. Heatwaves are expected to increase in incidence, severity, and duration in many regions. These events pose substantial public health threats (IPCC, 2012). The temperature-health impact pyramid/iceberg (see Figure 4.6) describes the range of symptoms and health outcomes produced by increasing temperatures. It also illustrates the relationship between the severity of health outcomes from heatwaves and the proportion of the population experiencing the outcomes.

As illustrated in this diagram, health outcomes of different severity may affect various proportions of the population.

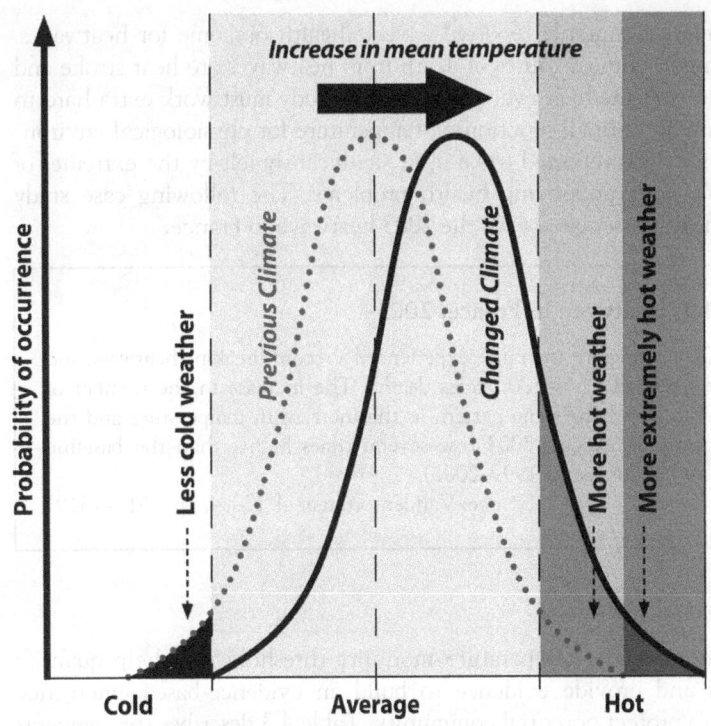

Figure 4.5 Projecting global mean temperature and its impact on heat event frequency.
Source: Solomon et al. (2007, Box TS.5, Figure 1).

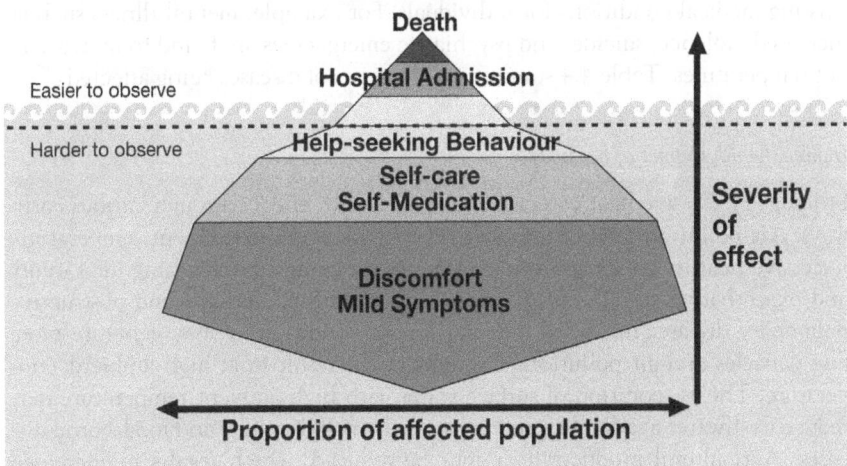

Figure 4.6 Iceberg diagram for heat-related health outcomes.
Source: Adapted from Chan (2017).

Direct health impacts of heatwaves

Death is the most commonly reported adverse health outcome for heatwaves. The most common clinical causes of death from heatwaves are heat stroke and dehydration. In extreme heat events, the human body must work extra hard to maintain within an optimal functioning temperature for physiological environment. The impact was reported to be most significantly felt by the extremes of age and people with underlying health problems. The following case study describes the deaths associated with the 2003 heatwave in France.

Case Box 4.1 Heatwave in France, 2003

In August 2003, all regions in France experienced a record-breaking heatwave and the event was related to 14,800 excess deaths. The increase in the number of excess deaths followed the same pattern as the increase in temperature and the number of deaths in August 2003 rose several times higher than the baseline (mean daily number of deaths 1999–2002).

Source: Vandentorren et al. (2004, pp. 1518–1519)

Temperature–mortality threshold

The identification of the temperature–mortality threshold may help quantify health impact and provide evidence to build an evidence-based emergency response plan to protect potential community. Table 4.3 describes the temperature–mortality threshold and the relative risk of non-cancer-related mortality ±3°C the average daily temperature (28.2°C) threshold in Hong Kong.

Excessive heat may increase the incidence of diseases or aggravate pre-existing medical conditions for individuals. For example, mental illness such as increased violence, suicide, and psychiatric emergencies are found to increase in hot temperatures. Table 4.4 summarises the types of diseases being affected.

Indirect health impact of heatwaves

Prolonged excessive heat can cause indirect health effects through various pathways. **Air pollution** might be exacerbated by increases in ambient temperature. Excessive heat increases ground-level ozone concentrations, causing lung injury and exacerbating respiratory diseases, such as asthma and chronic obstructive pulmonary disease. Increased demand for air conditioning may generate more fine particles and air pollution. **Drought** might result from high ambient temperature. The evaporation of surface water with high ambient temperature may reduce freshwater availability and increase the risk of water- and food-borne diseases. Agricultural productivity might be reduced, which results in increased food prices and food shortages to potentially increase the risk of malnutrition. High ambient temperature might also cause **changes in ecological system** and cause **disease vector migration** (with warming of ambient temperature, the

Table 4.3 Relative risk of non-cancer-related mortality 3°C above and below average daily temperature in Hong Kong

Non-cancer-related death	3.0°C increase above 28.2°C		3.0°C increase below 28.2°C		N#
	Relative risk (95% CI)	p-value	Relative risk (95% CI)	p-value	
Cardiovascular	1.085 (1.014 to 1.162)	0.019**	1.044 (1.137 to 0.959)	0.094	30,054
Stroke	1.108 (0.972 to 1.264)	0.123	1.043 (0.947 to 1.149)	0.392	9623
Respiratory	1.010 (0.959 to 1.064)	0.715	1.002 (0.964 to 1.041)	0.938	8648
Nephritis	1.165 (0.966 to 1.405)	0.110	1.113 (0.968 to 1.280)	0.132	4035
Diabetes	1.093 (0.851 to 1.404)	0.485	0.990 (0.823 to 1.190)	0.911	2411
Septicaemia	1.128 (0.870 to 1.464)	0.363	1.030 (0.848 to 1.251)	0.766	2295
Aortic aneurism	0.859 (0.573 to 1.288)	0.462	0.987 (0.732 to 1.330)	0.930	992
Cirrhosis	0.979 (0.715 to 1.341)	0.894	1.005 (0.795 to 1.272)	0.964	1574
Respiratory infection	1.102 (0.997 to 1.217)	0.057	1.010 (0.937 to 1.089)	0.790	14,479
Other	1.083 (0.978 to 1.199)	0.125	1.009 (0.936 to 1.089)	0.809	13,634

Source: Chan, Goggins, Kim, and Griffiths (2012).

Notes

** = $p < 0.05$

N = 79,069 total non-cancer deaths were included in the analysis. Subgroup totals may not add up due to other or unknown cases.

Table 4.4 Extreme temperature impact on diseases

Communicable diseases	Non-communicable diseases
• Enteric pathogens • Campylobacter • Salmonella • Dengue fever • Malaria • West Nile virus • Respiratory infections	• Respiratory • Renal diseases • Cerebrovascular accidents • Transient ischemic attack • Subarachnoid haemorrhage • Septicaemia

survival of certain vectors might be enhanced and the species might even thrive in areas that might be too cold for its survival previously).

Extreme cold

Although cold days are projected to decrease in frequencies due to global trends in ambient temperature warming in the coming decades, cold spells will continue to be a problem that affects communities in northern latitudes (IPCC, 2007). Even for countries that are well adapted to cold weather context, substantial increases in mortality and morbidity may be expected when lifeline urban infrastructure such as water, electricity, or heating collapse in cold weather. Table 4.5 summarises the potential health impacts of cold-related morbidity. The impact of cold spells might also be significant in the traditional non-cold spell affecting communities as these communities have limited resilience and infrastructure (e.g. central heating) to respond to the emergency impact.

At-risk populations

Impact of extreme heat and cold temperature affects some populations disproportionately. Susceptibility and vulnerability of populations to temperature-related events is determined by many factors, such as: (i) **host factors**, referring to the demography of the exposed population (for example, age, socio-economic

Table 4.5 Health impacts of cold spells

Health impacts	
Respiratory disease	Increase in hospitalisation
Infectious disease	Increase in hospitalisations due to infectious diseases
Cardiovascular disease	For 1°C decrease, 2.1% increase in cardiovascular disease for population in Hong Kong
Intentional injuries	For 1°C decrease, 2.4% increase in intentional injuries (assaults and attempted suicides) for population in Hong Kong

Source: Chan, Goggins, Yue, and Lee (2013).

level, and health status) who may be vulnerable to temperature-related illness; (ii) **geographical factors**, which imply the location of habitats may exacerbate an EWE (for example, as temperatures in urban environments are a few degrees Celsius higher than rural areas, people living in urban areas may be at greater health risk from a prolonged heatwave due to the "*urban heat island*" effect.); and (iii) **adaptive capacity** of the local population to cope and respond.

Heavy precipitation and flooding

Heavy precipitation refers to excessive amount of precipitation experienced in a location, which might be substantially exceeding the average for that location and season in a specific period of time. However, heavy precipitation may not necessarily increase the total amount of annual or monthly precipitation at one location as it could occur as an intense event. Examples of common causes of intense heavy precipitation events include tropical cyclones and snow storms. Direct influence of global warming on changes in precipitation has been observed globally. The water-holding capacity of air increases by approximately 7% per 1°C temperature increase, which means more water vapour in the atmosphere as a result of global warming and thus greater global mean precipitation. Due to climate change, the frequency and intensity of extreme precipitation events is projected to increase (IPCC, 2013).

Flooding is an example of extreme weather events associated with heavy precipitation that might be brought about by climate change. **Flooding** is the effects of a flood, defined as "[o]verflowing by water of the normal confines of a stream or other body of water, or accumulation of water by drainage over areas that are not normally submerged" (WMO, 2011, pp. 1–4). According to the commonly used WMO definition, a **flood** refers to: (i) rise, usually brief, in the water level in a stream (and river, lake, coastal line) to a peak, from which the water level recedes at a slower rate; (ii) relatively high flow as measured by stage height or discharge; and (iii) rising tide. Floods may increase mortality and morbidity through various pathways (such as contaminating fresh water, disrupting the health system, and increasing population displacement). The degree of impacts differs according to population vulnerability and types of flood event.

Globally, flooding is the most common natural hazard. It accounted for 43% of global natural disasters during 1994–2013. In 2014 alone, hydrological disasters accounted for 71% of deaths and 36% of the total number of people affected (CRED, 2015). Flooding alone was responsible for 55% of the total people affected (around 2.4 billion people) by natural disasters from 1994 to 2013. In 2015, 152 floods were recorded and affected 27.5 million people and floods in India alone affected 16.4 million people (UNISDR, 2016).

Risk factors to flooding

Although the main cause of a flood is rainfall, many other factors may also contribute to this hazard.

First of all, **human** factors such as the lack of structural flood control measures like embankments, and obstruction of river water flow due to debris and
wastes are common shortfalls in human urban planning process that might give
rise to the disaster events. Second, **meteorological** factors might also complicate
the flooding risks. Solidified ground surface after a drought might reduce the
soil's ability to quickly absorb excessive rainwater. Excessive precipitation over
a prolonged period may oversaturate the soil and increase overland runoff.
Ambient temperature warming may lead to melting of glacier (the phenomenon
known as "Glacier Lake Outburst Flooding", or GLOF) or causing avalanche.
Last but not least, **topographical** factors might also contribute to the flooding
risks. Topography, vegetation, and landscape around a river influence how
quickly rainwater reaches the channel. A river channel surrounded by steep
slopes is also at higher risk. With a lack of trees and plants to intercept precipitation, when a river bank bursts, the water overflows directly onto the floodplain
(Associated Programme on Flood Management, 2013).

Types of flooding

Floods may be categorised by their intensity, volume, timing of precipitation,
conditions of rivers and their drainage basins. Due to these differences, health
risks and implications for a post-flooding community may vary accordingly. Four
types of floods are summarised in Table 4.6.

Risks of flooding depend on location, spatial distribution, and demographic
fluctuations. It is estimated that by 2030, flooding will affect large numbers of
people in the world, particularly in Asia (Richardson, 2014).

Table 4.6 Types of flood

Flash floods
Sudden flooding over a small area due to severe rainfalls, dam break, or rapid snowmelt.
Flash floods can wash away houses, roads, and bridges and cause mud slides, hence
destructing communities and transport and threat to human life.

Fluvial (river) floods
When the stream channel capacity is overwhelmed by prolonged or intense rainfall, river
water overflows the banks on floodplains. This type of flood may cause temporary
population displacement, deaths, and injuries.

Coastal floods
The coast is flooded by the high sea surge due to severe rainstorm.
Temporary population displacement, deaths, injuries, salinising agricultural soils and
drinking water may result.

Urban floods
Intense rainfall in cities may cause rapid runoff which overwhelms the pumping capacity
of storm drainage systems. This could increase the risk of water-borne pathogens flowing
into drinking water sources due to sewage overflows.

Source: Adapted from WMO (2011).

Health impacts of flooding

Globally, flooding is reported to cause disasters that lead to the highest number of affected people. Figure 4.7 shows how floods might affect various health and human well-being-related outcomes while Table 4.7 summarises various health outcomes due to flooding.

Flood-related mortality and morbidity

Characteristics of flood (speed, depth, and extent of water) are primary risk factors for immediate flood-related deaths. For example, flash floods are more hazardous than slow-onset ones. Of the deaths from drowning, 70% were males; deaths by drowning in homes occurred among older people (Ahern et al., 2005). In addition to mortality, the most important impact of floods was reported to be the various morbidities directly or indirectly arising from floods. Injuries,

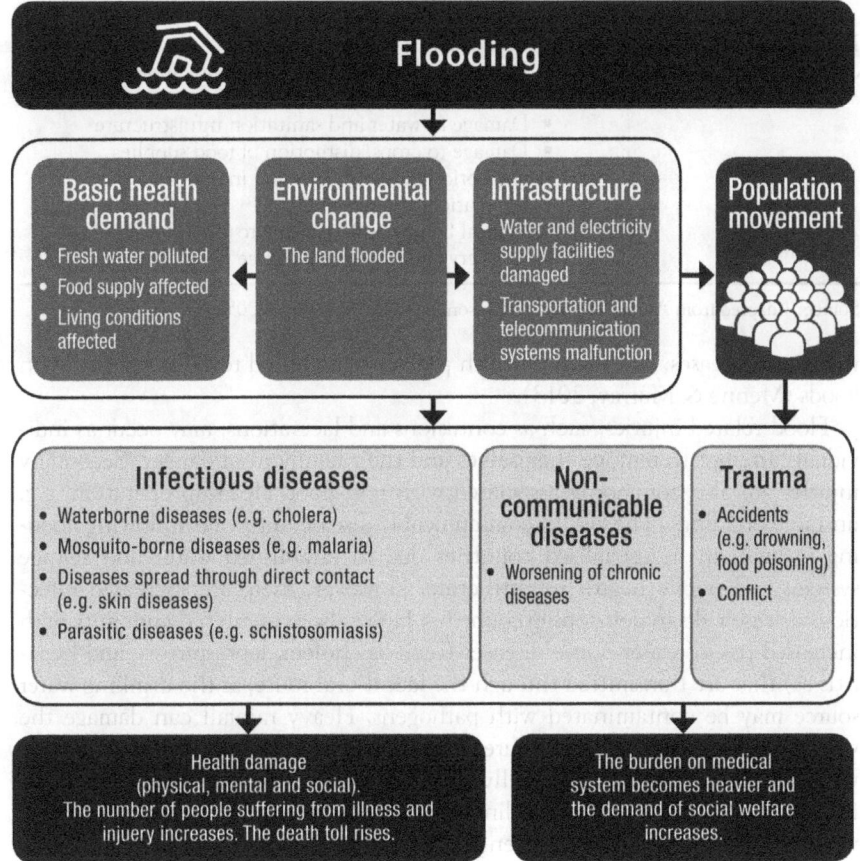

Figure 4.7 Pathways linking flooding and human health.

Table 4.7 Direct and indirect health impacts of flooding

Type of effect	Health impacts
Direct impacts e.g. direct exposure to floodwater	• Drowning and injuries from walking or driving through floodwater, contact with debris in floodwater, falling into hidden manholes, injuries from submerged objects, injuries while trying to move possessions during floods • Building collapse and damage (injuries) • Electrocution • Diarrhoeal, vector- and rodent-borne diseases • Respiratory, skin, and eye infections • Chemical contamination, particularly carbon monoxide poisoning from generators used for pumping and dehumidifying • Water shortages and contamination due to loss of water treatment works and sewage treatment plants • Stress, short- and long-term mental health issues, including the impacts of displacement
Indirect impacts e.g. impacts on other health determinants	• Loss of access to healthcare • Damage to healthcare infrastructure and other vital community facilities • Damage to water and sanitation infrastructure • Damage to crops, disruption of food supplies • Disruption of livelihoods and income • Population displacement • Mental health problems due to length of flood recovery and fear of recurrence

Source: Adapted from Ahern, Kovats, Wilkinson, Few, and Matthies (2005).

infectious diseases, and mental health problems are found to be associated with floods (Menne & Murray, 2013).

Flood-related injuries, such as contusions and lacerations, may occur as individuals attempt to remove themselves and their family from danger. Secondary injuries are also commonly associated with post-flood clean-up operation, e.g. unstable buildings. The risk of communicable disease outbreaks following flooding is small in industrialised countries due to established water and sewage systems and public health infrastructure. However, there are increased infectious disease risks in developing countries. Flood also presents a community with increased risk of water-borne diseases (such as cholera, leptospirosis, and hepatitis A) that are transmitted through the faecal-oral route, as the drinking water source may be contaminated with pathogens. Heavy rainfall can damage the water and sanitation infrastructure, triggering sewage overflows into drinking water. Although floodwater initially washes away mosquito breeding sites, standing water may be a perfect breeding site for mosquitoes to increase the risk of vector-borne disease, such as dengue and malaria. For example, flooding in Costa Rica in 1991 and in the Dominican Republic in 2004 led to malaria outbreaks. Increased incidence of mental health problems was observed directly from the experience of living in the flooded areas and indirectly from geographic displacement, damage to houses and assets, and stress in the restoration process.

The true impact of flooding on health, however, is difficult to estimate as it is challenging to characterise health risks from flooding due to the complexity and multidisciplinary impact (e.g. the pollution of drinking water sources by flooding in addition to its direct impact), insufficient epidemiological data and the lack of follow-up of longer-term health effects from flooding (e.g. the impacts of displacement or delayed recovery).

At-risk populations

People living around flood plains are the most at-risk communities. A study in 2014 estimated that about 2.6% of the world's population (around 177 million people) live in areas that will be prone to chronic flooding in the next 100 years (Climate Central, 2014). Understanding the vulnerability of population subgroups may help guide appropriate solutions to reduce the impact of flooding. Older people, the disabled, children, women, ethnic minorities, and those with low incomes are particularly at risk (Hajat et al., 2003). Additionally, displaced populations often experience compromised access to clean water and sanitation.

Cyclones, floods, and landslides

Strong stormy events such as tropical cyclones/hurricanes/typhoons may lead to disaster events such as flooding, landslides, and infectious disease outbreaks (Chan, 2017). As information in less developed countries is often inaccurate, or inaccessible, the true impact of heavy precipitation events has yet to be accurately quantified. Doocy, Dick, Daniels, and Kirsch (2013) summarise direct health impacts of cyclones in their literature review (see Table 4.8).

Table 4.8 Direct health impacts of cyclones

Health impacts			Risk factors
Mortality	Direct deaths 54%	1. Drowning (59% of direct deaths) 2. Trauma (39% of direct deaths)	Sex: higher mortality risk for men Age: children and older people Residence type Geographic location
	Indirect deaths 43%	Trauma from: Motor vehicle accidents Fires Electrocution	Race Flood level and types Deforestation
Injury	Lacerations, contusions, animal/insect bites, and motor vehicle injuries		Sex: higher risk for men for injury Age: highest among middle-aged adults Location: e.g. storm path, living in a city, and being outdoors

Source: Adapted from Doocy et al. (2013).

Heavy rainfall brought by strong wind events may also cause secondary disasters with its exacerbation of underlying natural hazards, such as outburst lake floods and landslides. These additional events may also carry important health implications for an affected community (see Table 4.9).

At-risk populations

Since the 20th century, populations in Southeast Asia, the Western Pacific, and the Americas were increasingly affected by cyclones, typhoons, and hurricane risks. Vulnerability depends on location, infrastructure, as well as local preparedness and warning systems. Coastal areas are particularly vulnerable to storm surges and heavy rain that may cause coastal flooding or temporary displacement. People near the rivers are also at risk of flash floods. Population vulnerability to cyclones is further increased by population growth, urbanisation, increasing coastal settlement, and global warming (Doocy et al., 2013).

Drought

Water is essential for human survival. A drought is often slow-onset. It usually starts with an extended dry period that leads to reduced water availability. There are three main pathways that lead to drought: (i) a lack of precipitation over a long period; (ii) demand for water supply exceeds the natural water availability during periods of average or below-average precipitation; and (iii) changes in water quality when the available water sources become contaminated (IPCC, 2007). Droughts can lead to serious hydrological imbalances and shortages of water and food, and potentially cause long-term environmental, socio-economic, and health impacts. Between 1994 and 2013, although drought accounted for 5% of disaster events globally, it affected more than 1 billion people. In 2015, which was the hottest year on record, there were 32 major droughts recorded as compared to an annual average of 15 over the previous

Table 4.9 Potential health impacts from floods and landslides from heavy rainfall

Secondary event	Impacts	Health impacts
Floods e.g.Flash flood Coastal flood	Direct	Deaths Injuries
	Indirect	Damages to buildings and infrastructure Loss of crops and livestock Population displacement Contaminating water sources
Landslides Increased water runoff causing sliding of a mass of soil	Direct	Deaths Injuries
	Indirect	Disrupting transport and communications Damages to buildings and infrastructure

decade. A total of 50.5 million people were affected by droughts, well above the 10-year average of 35.4 million (UNISDR, 2016). Table 4.10 describes how droughts may be categorised into three main groups and their potential impact on the community.

Due to the lack of reliable data, insufficient evidence is available for concluding global trends in drought since the 1950s. IPCC projects that an increased risk of drought is likely in currently dry regions, such as the Mediterranean, Southwest USA, and southern Africa, because of decreases in soil moisture by 2100 (IPCC, 2013).

Socio-economic and environmental impacts of drought

Economically, with reduction of crop production, farmers' incomes decline. Furthermore, reduced food availability also increases food market prices. Drought may trigger insect infestations and increase plant diseases, soil erosion, landscape degradation, as well as decrease air quality. For short-term droughts, **natural environments** may often rebound. But in long-term droughts, it often requires a long time for the ecosystems to recover. There are also **social impacts**. Water utilisation rights are often disputed among users. Additionally, when people migrate from a drought-stricken area, increased demand for water may threaten the water security of the host communities, which may lead to complex emergencies, such as civil wars and conflicts.

Health impacts of drought

Drought may cause multiple health impacts through various pathways (see Figure 3.4). Various risk factors determine the degree of health impact of drought. Its effects may manifest slowly and are complex thus it is not easy to understand the true impacts.

Some important health impacts of drought include (Stanke et al., 2013): (i) **Malnutrition**: Reduced food intake and varied nutrient deficiencies due to disrupted food production. Malnutrition from food insecurity is the major health

Table 4.10 Types of drought

Drought type	Used by	Description	Potential impacts
Meteorological	General public	Most common "drought" from prolonged below-average precipitation period	Water shortage
Agricultural	Farmers	Low soil moisture to support crop production	Reduced crop production
Hydrological	Urban planners for managing water supplies	When water reserves in reservoirs fall below average	Water shortage

Source: Adapted from Stanke, Kerac, Prudhomme, Medlock, and Murray (2013).

risk of drought. (ii) **Communicable diseases**: Lack of drinking water and sanitation, malnutrition, and displacement contribute to higher population vulnerability to infectious diseases such as cholera, typhoid fever, diarrhoea, acute respiratory infections, and measles. (iii) **Psychosocial stress and mental health disorders**: Although more studies are required in mental health impacts of drought, drought may create a broad range of stressors and weaken the ability to avoid mental health problems (O'Brien, Sygna, & Haugen, 2014). (iv) **Reduced health service delivery**: Health can be compromised by disrupted local health services due to lack of water supplies or healthcare worker migration. (v) **Migration**: Loss of livelihood and lack of health facilities limits people's access to health services and increases overall morbidity and mortality.

At-risk populations

While a significant proportion can be prevented through safe drinking water and adequate sanitation and hygiene, diarrhoeal disease is the second leading cause of death and a leading cause of malnutrition among children under five years old, causing around 525,000 under-five deaths annually (WHO, 2017). The increased frequency of droughts in the future may intensify disease and health risks. Risk factors that are associated with drought vulnerability include: demographic pressure on the environment; inappropriate land use; food insecurity; socio-economic status of the population; economic systems strictly dependent on agriculture; poor infrastructure, e.g. irrigation, water supply, and sanitation; poor health status of the population before the disaster; time of the year, with the most critical period being before the harvest; absence of warning systems; population displacement; and other concurrent situations: economic crisis, political instability, armed conflict (WHO, 2015).

Sea-level rise

Global mean sea level has been rising gradually throughout the last century. Increased flood risks, salinising water, and land erosion are common problems discussed under sea-level rise. This section will explain the potential health impacts of sea-level rise. Globally, 95% of the ocean's area will experience sea-level rise during this century (IPCC, 2013). In some regions, sea levels may rise more rapidly because changes are affected by the speed of water temperature rise and continental drift.

Current situation and future projection

Global average sea level has risen by 0.19 metre since 1900. By 2100, a further 28–98 cm is expected by the IPCC. This prediction is considered conservative. If sea level rises by 50 cm, the survival of people in coastal cities and islands will be threatened.

Health impacts of sea-level rise

Around 120 million people are affected by coastal floods from cyclones and storm surges every year (IPCC, 2007). As the impact of sea-level rises will only slowly emerge, the problems and associated impact may remain invisible for decades before the real impact is revealed and quantified. Sea-level rise can have significant impacts on livelihoods and food security, particularly in low-lying coastal zones and river deltas through various pathways as summarised in Table 4.11.

At-risk populations

People living in low-lying coastal areas and river deltas are particularly vulnerable to the risk of coastal flooding. People may be forced to abandon their homes permanently. Vulnerability tends to be higher in developing countries that have limited sea defence or other counter-flood measures.

Complex emergencies

Climate change impacts may create environmental stress and new complex emergencies, such as conflicts and wars, around the world, particularly in already fragile states. The World Health Organization (2002) defined a **complex emergency** as: "*Complex emergencies are situation of disrupted livelihoods and threats to life produced by warfare, civil disturbance and large-scale movements of people, in which any emergency response has to be conducted in a difficult political and security environment.*" An internal conflict may evolve into complex emergencies that cause large-scale population displacements, food shortages, and fragile or failing economic, political, and social institutions.

Many cities and countries in the developing world are threatened by the risks of complex emergencies (Robert S. Strauss Center for International Security and Law, n.d.). Four main types of instability are identified as the causal risk: (i) **political instability** (e.g. civil wars, civil unrest, and political transition); (ii) **economic instability** (e.g. increasing income inequality, poverty, and vulnerability); (iii) **environmental instability** (e.g. chronic and recurrent natural disasters, persistent drought, and altered temperature and precipitation patterns); and (iv) **demographic instability** (e.g. urban population growth and internal displacement) (see Knowledge Box 4.1).

Knowledge Box 4.1 Green war hypothesis

Green war hypothesis argues that environmental degradation can increase poverty and insecurity, leading to increasing likelihood of conflict. Unequal distribution of resources as a result of climate change impact will elevate risks of conflicts and complex emergencies.

Source: Homer-Dixon (2001)

Table 4.11 Potential impacts of sea-level rise

Effects		Causal factors		Health risks
		Climate	*Non-climate*	
Inundation **Flood** **Storm surge**	Coastal surge	Wave Storm	Sediment supply Flood management Land use	• Reduced water and food availability due to soil contamination/salination • Loss of habitation for fish, birds, and plants • Population displacement due to building destruction
	Backflush in river	Runoff	Land use	• Reduced water availability—soil contamination
Wetland loss		CO_2 fertilisation	Sediment supply	Loss of habitation for fish, birds, and plants
Erosion		Wave Storm	Sediment supply Topology	Loss of habitant Population displacement
Salt water intrusion	Surface water	Runoff	Land use	High blood pressure
	Ground water	Rainfall	Land use	Cardiovascular diseases
	Soil	Runoff Wave		
Rising water level **Drainage overflow**		Rainfall	Land use	Contaminated drinking water

Source: Adapted from Nicholls (2003).

Impacts of climate change on complex emergencies

Climate alone does not necessarily cause conflicts. However, changes in climate may alter weather, environment, and access to key natural resources, which in turn may fuel economic, social, and political instabilities. These instabilities may increase the likelihood of complex emergencies, e.g. civil wars that can increase population migration, leading to humanitarian disasters, economic disruption, and pose threats to human security (Burke, Hsiang, & Miguel, 2015; Chan, 2017; Levy & Sidel, 2014).

The climate change-related weather and environmental context that may exacerbate the risk of complex emergencies include the following three determinants. First and foremost, as to **temperature warming**, a meta-analysis by Hsiang, Burke, and Miguel (2013) found a strong association between warmer temperature and civil war occurrence in sub-Saharan Africa between 1981 and 2002. Rises in temperature could intensify group conflicts, such as civil wars, by 50% in many parts of the world. Furthermore, a study on the relationship between seasonal temperature changes and increased risk of violence indicated that extended durations of warm weather are associated with an increased risk of civil war. Possible reasons for this association are that temperature change affects both the scarcity of resources and population mobility within countries (Landis, 2014). Second of all, **altered precipitation patterns**, like rainfall shortages and the ensuing drought, are associated with a higher risk of communal conflict. A conflict may occur in communities who have limited availability of alternative coping mechanisms. Increased intensity and duration of droughts and erratic precipitation patterns influence the availability of food, water, and habitable land, which could trigger increased violence against neighbouring communities over scarce resources. A chronic drought situation may increase the number of environmental refugees and enhance the likelihood of complex emergencies with other communities over scarce resources. The impact was also found to be more prominent in regions with high political instability (Fjelde & von Uexkull, 2012). Third, **sea-level rise**, as described above, poses substantial survival challenges to coastal populations worldwide. It is projected that a large number of people will be forced to leave their homes due to submerged land thereby becoming environmental refugees. This situation may spark conflict with other communities, competing over land availability and scarce resources. Additionally, reduced economic development and political instability could aggravate poverty and civil unrest, which fuel frustration, aggression, and violence (Levy & Sidel, 2015).

Health impacts of complex emergencies

Health impacts of complex emergencies are very difficult to identify and quantify due to their chronic and multifaceted nature. Complex emergencies may disrupt livelihoods and increase the size of internally displaced populations (IDPs) in a community and put people at risk of losing economic security and their home temporarily or permanently. Hence, people may experience a reduced access to water, sanitation, shelters, and food. Access to healthcare would also be reduced due to damage to health infrastructure, disrupted supply chains for medicine and medical equipment, and reduced availability of health workers. All these potential disruptions could increase health risks.

General health impact of complex emergencies

During complex emergencies, violent events may occur and lead to **injury**, including physical and sexual violence and death. The health system and life-line infrastructure (e.g. water and sanitation) is damaged. With the lack of health service facilities and disease prevention and control, **infectious diseases** spread easily. Unstable food supply means that people may lack sufficient nutrition and suffer from mild or severe **malnutrition**. Adverse **mental health outcomes** are consistently reported in published literature. In addition to direct injury and trauma, affected populations frequently suffer from loss of possessions, being forced to leave their homes, and having to separate from their family and friends. The lack of social support and suffering from different trauma can lead to mental health problems. Table 4.12 summarises the key health impacts on population who might be affected by complex emergencies.

Table 4.12 Potential health impacts of complex emergencies

Health outcomes	Potential causes	Examples
Increased mortality	Physical trauma Communicable diseases Mortality from preventable diseases due to reduced/lack of access to healthcare	War injuries Physical and sexual violence Malaria, diarrhoeal diseases Asthma, diabetes, emergency surgery, maternal and neonatal mortality
Increased morbidity	Injuries from physical trauma Infectious diseases due to • disrupted water and sanitation systems • compromised water and sanitation in displaced population • disruption of public health programmes Malnutrition Morbidity due to lack of access to healthcare Mental disorders	War injuries Physical and sexual violence Water-, food-, and vector-borne diseases (e.g. cholera, dysentery, malaria) Sexually transmitted diseases (e.g. HIV) Vaccine preventable diseases (e.g. measles) Acute and chronic malnutrition Lack of long-term care (e.g. cancer, diabetes, HIV) Aggression, violence Anxiety, depression, post-traumatic stress disorders

Sources: Adapted from Howard, Sondorp, and Ter Veen (2012); Krug, Dahlberg, Mercy, Zwi, and Lozano (2002).

At-risk populations

In general, complex emergencies increase health risks for all members of society. However, politically, socially, and economically marginalised groups are normally the most vulnerable. Pregnant women, children, older people, those who are chronically ill or disabled, internally displaced or refugee populations face additional risks to their security and health. Furthermore, climate change-related events may aggravate social inequalities and widen the gap between the rich and the poor. Socio-economic structures before complex emergencies also determine population vulnerability. For example, a drought may reduce water availability and since the poor cannot afford to get safe drinking water, they become even more vulnerable to climate change. Health impacts of sea-level rise and climate-induced complex emergencies are difficult to identify and quantify because of the slow progress and complex causative pathways to adverse health outcomes. Therefore, it is key to anticipate long-term impacts by strengthening adaptation plans to reduce human exposure to health risk.

Conclusion

Climate change has created numerous extreme weather events and disasters that have led to a broad range of direct, indirect, or even long-term health outcomes. Due to the complexities and uncertainties, precise health impact predictions of these extreme events are difficult. However, the effects of climate change impact on the well-being of population and its living environment are non-negligible globally.

References

Adams, R. E., & Boscarino, J. A. (2005). Stress and well-being in the aftermath of the World Trade Center attack: The continuing effects of a communitywide disaster. *Journal of Community Psychology, 33*(2), 175–190.

Ahern, M., Kovats, R. S., Wilkinson, P., Few, R., & Matthies, F. (2005). Global health impacts of floods: Epidemiologic evidence. *Epidemiologic Reviews, 27*(1), 36–46.

Associated Programme on Flood Management. (2013). What human factors contribute to flooding [online]? Retrieved from www.floodmanagement.info/what-human-factors-contribute-to-flooding/.

Below, R., Wirtz, A., & Guha-Sapir, D. (2009). *Disaster category classification and peril terminology for operational purposes* (Working Paper No. 264). Brussels, Belgium: Centre for Research on the Epidemiology of Disasters (CRED), & Germany: Munich Reinsurance (Munich RE). Retrieved from http://cred.be/sites/default/files/DisCatClass_264.pdf.

Burke, M., Hsiang, S. M., & Miguel, E. (2015). Climate and conflict. *Annual Review of Economics, 7*, 577–617.

Centre for Research on the Epidemiology of Disasters [CRED]. (n.d.a). EM-DAT: The emergency events database [online]. Retrieved from www.emdat.be/emdat_db/.

Centre for Research on the Epidemiology of Disasters [CRED]. (n.d.b). EM-DAT: The international disaster database: General classification [online]. Retrieved from www.emdat.be/classification.

Centre for Research on the Epidemiology of Disasters [CRED]. (2015). *The human cost of natural disasters 2015: A global perspective.* Brussels, Belgium: Author.

Centre for Research on the Epidemiology of Disasters. [CRED] (2016). *2015 disasters in numbers.* Retrieved from http://cred.be/sites/default/files/2015_DisastersInNumbers.pdf.

Chan, E. Y. Y. (2017). *Public health humanitarian responses to natural disasters.* London: Routledge.

Chan, E. Y. Y. (2018). *Building bottom-up health and disaster risk reduction programmes.* Oxford, United Kingdom: Oxford University Press.

Chan, E. Y. Y. (in press). *Disaster public health and older people.* London: Routledge.

Chan, E. Y. Y., Goggins, W. B., Kim, J. J., & Griffiths, S. M. (2012). A study of intracity variation of temperature-related mortality and socioeconomic status among the Chinese population in Hong Kong. *Journal of Epidemiology and Community Health, 66*(4), 322–327.

Chan, E. Y. Y., Goggins, W. B., Yue, S. K., & Lee, P. Y. (2013). Hospital admissions as a function of temperature, other weather phenomena and pollution levels in an urban setting in China. *Bulletin of World Health Organization, 91*(8), 576–584. doi:10.2471/BLT.12.113035.

Climate Central. (2014). New analysis shows global exposure to sea level rise. Retrieved from www.climatecentral.org/news/new-analysis-global-exposure-to-sea-level-rise-flooding-18066.

Doocy, S., Dick, A., Daniels, A., & Kirsch, T. D. (2013). The human impact of tropical cyclones: A historical review of events 1980–2009 and systematic literature review. *PLOS Currents Disasters,* 16 April.

Fjelde, H., & von Uexkull, N. (2012). Climate triggers: Rainfall anomalies, vulnerability and communal conflict in sub-Saharan Africa. *Political Geography, 31*(7), 444–453.

Guha-Sapir, D., Below, R., & Hoyois, P. (n.d.). EM-DAT: The CRED/OFDA International Disaster Database [Internet]. Brussels, Belgium: Centre for Research on the Epidemiology of Disasters (CRED), Université Catholique de Louvain. Retrieved from www.emdat.be.

Hajat, S., Ebi, K. L., Kovats, R. S., Menne, B., Edwards, S., & Haines, A. (2003). The human health consequences of flooding in Europe: A review of the evidence. *Applied Environmental Science and Public Health, 1,* 13–21.

Homer-Dixon, T. (2001). *Environment, scarcity, and violence.* Princeton, NJ: Princeton University Press.

Howard, N., Sondorp, E., & Ter Veen, A. (2012). *Conflict and health.* England: Open University Press.

Hsiang, S. M., Burke, M., & Miguel, E. (2013). Quantifying the influence of climate on human conflict. *Science, 341*(6151), 1235367.

Integrated Research on Disaster Risk. (2014). *Peril classification and hazard glossary* (IRDR DATA Publication No. 1). Beijing: Integrated Research on Disaster Risk. Retrieved from www.irdrinternational.org/wp-content/uploads/2014/04/IRDR_DATA-Project-Report-No.-1.pdf.

Intergovernmental Panel on Climate Change [IPCC]. (2001). Summary for policymakers. In J. J. McCarthy, O. F. Canziani, N. A. Leary, D. J. Dokken, & K. S. White (Eds.), *Climate change 2001: Impacts, adaptation, and vulnerability: Contribution of Working Group II to the Third Assessment Report of the Intergovernmental Panel on Climate Change.* Cambridge, United Kingdom: Cambridge University Press.

Intergovernmental Panel on Climate Change [IPCC]. (2007). *Climate change 2007: The physical science basis: Contribution of Working Group I to the Fourth Assessment Report of* the *Intergovernmental Panel on Climate Change*. Cambridge, United Kingdom and New York, NY: Cambridge University Press.

Intergovernmental Panel on Climate Change [IPCC]. (2012). *Managing the risks of extreme events and disasters to advance climate change adaptation: A special report of Working Groups I and II of the Intergovernmental Panel on Climate Change.* Cambridge, United Kingdom and New York, NY: Cambridge University Press.

Intergovernmental Panel on Climate Change [IPCC]. (2013). Summary for policy-makers. In T. F. Stocker, D. Qin, G.-K. Plattner, M. Tignor, S. K. Allen, J. Boschung, A. Nauels, Y. Xia, V. Bex, & P. M. Midgley (Eds.), *Climate change 2013: The physical science basis: Contribution of Working Group I to the Fifth Assessment Report of the Inter-governmental Panel on Climate Change.* Cambridge, United Kingdom and New York, NY: Cambridge University Press.

Intergovernmental Panel on Climate Change [IPCC]. (2014). Summary for policy-makers. In C. B. Field, V. R. Barros, D. J. Dokken, K. J. Mach, M. D. Mastrandrea, T. E. Bilir, ... L. L. White (Eds.), *Climate change 2014: Impacts, adaptation, and vulner-ability: Part A: Global and sectoral aspects: Contribution of Working Group II to the Fifth Assessment Report of the Intergovernmental Panel on Climate Change.* Cambridge, United Kingdom and New York, NY: Cambridge University Press.

Krug, E. G., Dahlberg, L. L., Mercy, J. A., Zwi, A. B., & Lozano, R. (2002). *World report on violence and health.* Geneva, Switzerland: World Health Organization. Retrieved from http://apps.who.int/iris/bitstream/10665/42495/1/9241545615_eng.pdf.

Landis, S. T. (2014). Temperature seasonality and violent conflict: The inconsistencies of a warming planet. *Journal of Peace Research, 51*(5), 603–618.

Levy, B. S., & Sidel, V. W. (2014). Collective violence caused by climate change and how it threatens health and human rights. *Health and Human Rights Journal, 16*(1), 32–40.

Levy, B. S., & Sidel. V. W. (2015). Collective violence. In B. Levy & J. Patz (Eds.), *Climate change and public health.* Oxford, United Kingdom: Oxford University Press.

Menne, B., & Murray, V. (2013). *Floods in the WHO European region: Health effects and their prevention.* Retrieved from www.euro.who.int/__data/assets/pdf_file/0020/189020/e96853.pdf.

Nicholls, R. J. (2003). *Case study on sea-level rise impacts.* Retrieved from http://search.oecd.org/environment/cc/2483213.pdf.

Norris, F. H., Friedman, M. J., & Watson, P. J. (2002). 60,000 disaster victims speak: Part II. Summary and implications of the disaster mental health research. *Psychiatry, 65*(3), 240–260.

O'Brien, K., Sygna, L., & Haugen, J. E. (2014). Vulnerable or resilient? A multi-scale assessment of climate impacts and vulnerable in Norway. *Climate Change, 64*(1–2), 193–225.

Richardson, K. (2014). *Human dynamics of climate change: Technical report.* Retrieved from the website of Met Office, United Kingdom: www.metoffice.gov.uk/binaries/content/assets/mohippo/pdf/climate/hdcc_technical_report.pdf.

Robert S. Strauss Center for International Security and Law. (n.d.). *Complex emergencies.* Retrieved from www.strausscenter.org/ccaps-research/about.html.

Solomon, S., Qin, D., Manning, M., Alley, R. B., Berntsen, T., Bindoff, N. L., ... Wratt, D. (2007). Technical summary. In S. Solomon, D. Qin, M. Manning, Z. Chen, M. Marquis, K. B. Averyt, ... H. L. Miller (Eds.), *Climate change 2007: The physical science basis: Contribution of Working Group I to the Fourth Assessment Report of the Intergovern-mental Panel on Climate Change.* Cambridge, United Kingdom and New York, NY: Cambridge University Press.

Stanke, C., Kerac, M., Prudhomme, C., Medlock, J., & Murray, V. (2013). Health effects of drought: A systematic review of the evidence. *PLOS Currents Disasters*, 5 June.

Troeger, C., Forouzanfar, M., Rao, P. C., Khalil, I., Brown, A., Reiner, R. C., Jr.,... Mokdad, A. H. (2017). Estimates of global, regional, and national morbidity, mortality, and aetiologies of diarrhoeal diseases: A systematic analysis for the Global Burden of Disease Study 2015. *The Lancet: Infectious Diseases*, *17*(9), 909–948.

United Nations International Strategy for Disaster Reduction [UNISDR]. (2009). 2009 UNISDR terminology on disaster risk reduction. Retrieved from www.unisdr.org/files/7817_UNISDRTerminologyEnglish.pdf.

United Nations Office for Disaster Risk Reduction [UNISDR]. (2016). *The human cost of the hottest year on record: Climate change and El Nino drove disasters worldwide in 2015*. Retrieved from www.unisdr.org/archive/47791.

United Nations Office for Disaster Risk Reduction. (2017). *UNISDR annual report 2016*. Retrieved from www.unisdr.org/files/52253_unisdr2016annualreport.pdf.

Vandentorren, S., Suzan, F., Medina, S., Pascal, M., Maulpoix, A., Cohen, J. C., & Ledrans, M. (2004). Mortality in 13 French cities during the August 2003 heat wave. *American Journal of Public Health*, *94*(9), 1518–1520.

World Health Organization [WHO]. (2002). *Complex emergencies*. Retrieved from www.who.int/environmental_health_emergencies/complex_emergencies/en/.

World Health Organization [WHO]. (2008). *Protecting health from climate change: World Health Day 2008*. Switzerland: Author.

World Health Organization [WHO]. (2015). *Drought: Technical hazard sheet: Natural disaster profiles*. Retrieved from www.who.int/hac/techguidance/ems/drought/en/.

World Health Organization [WHO]. (2017). Diarrhoeal disease [online]. Retrieved from www.who.int/news-room/fact-sheets/detail/diarrhoeal-disease.

World Health Organization [WHO]. (2018). Malaria [online]. Retrieved from www.who.int/news-room/fact-sheets/detail/malaria

World Health Organization, & World Meteorological Organization. (2012). *Atlas of health and climate*. Retrieved from www.who.int/globalchange/publications/atlas/report/en/.

World Meteorological Organization [WMO]. (2011). *Manual on flood forecasting and warning*. Retrieved from www.wmo.int/pages/prog/hwrp/publications/flood_forecasting_warning/WMO%201072_en.pdf.

World Meteorological Organization. (2014). *Atlas of mortality and economic losses from weather, climate and water extremes (1970–2012)*. Retrieved from www.wmo.int/amcomet/sites/default/files/field/doc/events/atlas_of_mortality_and_econ_losses_en.pdf.

5 Research Methodology I
Climate and health outcome modelling

William B. Goggins III and Emily Ying Yang Chan

Chapters 5 and 6 discuss the main research methodologies that were used to examine human health outcomes and the approaches to model the impact of meteorological variables (such as temperature, rainfall, and humidity), the behavioural determinants, and implications of climate-related events for the health of the population in the subtropical metropolis of Hong Kong.

Climate and health outcome modelling

The study of the health effects of climate change poses many methodological challenges to scientists and epidemiologists (McMichael et al., 2004). Epidemiologists perform studies for individuals. Their approach uses exposure status, namely exposed and unexposed groups, as the unit of analysis. Conclusions of epidemiological studies often involve inferring future consequences from past observations. For example, the observation that individuals who smoke tobacco are far more likely to develop lung cancer leads to the inference that individuals who smoke now or in the future will have increased risk of lung cancer.

For climate change, future projections based on past observations of the health impact of climate change are currently impracticable due to the relatively small climate changes that have occurred so far (relative to expected much larger changes in the future), the lack of long-term data on health outcomes in many locations, and the presence of many potential confounding variables that also influence long-term rates on health outcomes (McMichael et al., 2004). For instance, although all-cause age-adjusted mortality rates have been declining in most locations for many decades, the decrease in mortality is unrelated to climatic changes.

Most existing research examines how meteorological variables may be associated with health-related outcomes, e.g. mortality or hospitalisation, or some sort of intermediary, e.g. associations between temperature and rainfall with *Anopheles* biting rates and duration of *Plasmodium* life cycles, due to their importance in malaria transmission (Detinova, Bertram, & World Health Organization, 1962; Martens et al., 1999; Parham & Michael, 2010). Process-based models use explicit knowledge of well-studied causal relationships to simulate dynamic processes underlying disease spread (Ebi & Rocklov, 2014) and are often used in the study of vector-borne diseases. Parham and Michael (2010) modelled the basic reproduction number, R_0, as a function of mosquito abundance (dependent on temperature and rainfall) and mortality rate (dependent on temperature), mosquito biting rate (dependent on temperature), the proportion of infected mosquitoes who become infectious (dependent on temperature), and other non-climate dependent parameters, and used this model to predict the future distribution of malaria R_0 in Tanzania under climate change scenarios.

Mathematical models for infectious diseases may also be empirical (data-driven). For instance, Chong, Goggins, Zee, and Wang (2015) fit an extended, Susceptible-Infected-Recovered (SIR) model, with four compartments, S-I-R-Dead (D), to weekly meteorological and influenza mortality data in Hong Kong from 2002 to 2009, employing a deterministic system of differential equations describing the rates of subject movements between the S, I, R, and D compartments. They found that lower temperature and more rainfall were positively associated with transmission rates during most epidemics. Process-based models may also be validated using empirical data. For example, Bannister-Tyrrell et al. (2013) employed a process-based dengue simulation model (DENSiM) that uses information on temperature, humidity, and rainfall, along with virologic, epidemiologic, and demographic factors to simulate vector populations and viral transmission, and to further simulate the dengue outbreaks in Cairns, Australia, and then correlated modelled and observed dengue infections from 1992 to 2009.

Context

In Hong Kong, similar to other metropolises of most developed countries, chronic diseases (including cancer, cardiovascular diseases, chronic respiratory diseases, diabetes, and chronic liver and kidney diseases) are the leading causes of mortality and hospitalisation post millennium. Published research examining associations between meteorological variables and mortality/morbidity for these outcomes is data-driven and statistical, with short-term time-series models being particularly prevalent. The methods used for studies relating meteorological variables to (usually) daily mortality or hospitalisation counts were largely borrowed from those used for time-series studies of associations between daily pollutant levels and these outcomes, which were commonly employed in the 1990s, while methodological refinements have been made. Bhaskaran, Gasparrini, Hajat, Smeeth, and Armstrong (2013) provided a general review on the use of time-series regression studies in environmental epidemiology and the methodological complications that differentiate these models from ordinary regression models, including the often non-linear and delayed associations between health outcomes and meteorological variables, the need to control for seasonal patterns and long-term trends, possible residual serial autocorrelation in the outcomes and confounding by other time-varying factors. The complications involved in modelling short-term associations between weather and health outcomes are basically the same as those for studies of those between pollutants and health outcomes, and in fact, pollutants are generally included as potential confounders in studies of weather and health, and vice versa. The issue of non-linearity is generally more important for meteorological studies though, as pollutant associations are usually at least monotonic, whereas the associations between temperature and health outcomes are usually U-shaped.

Statistical methods

As daily (or weekly) deaths or hospitalisations are count outcomes, Poisson regression is the most commonly employed approach. As outcomes in such studies tend to be over-dispersed, variance greater than the mean (Bhaskaran et al., 2013), some adjustment to the Poisson results is necessary, or negative binomial regression may be used. Some autocorrelation in outcomes is also usually present, which violates the independence assumption of Poisson regression. However, after controlling for long-term trends, seasonality, and time-varying meteorological and pollutant variables, this autocorrelation will be much reduced (Bhaskaran et al., 2013). Nonetheless residual autocorrelation should be checked as part of the model-fitting data, particularly for infectious disease outcomes.

Bhaskaran et al. (2013) outlined three commonly used approaches for controlling for trend and seasonality, including the time-stratified approach, which involves using indicator variables to denote different blocks of time (e.g. a 10-year time series could have $10*12 = 120$ strata, or if separate terms were used for trend and season, separate indicator variables for the 12 months and 10 years could be used for season and trend, respectively). This approach however involves the use of many parameters and also assumes jumps in outcome risks between strata (Bhaskaran et al., 2013). In a second approach, Fourier terms (i.e. pairs of sine and cosine functions) can also be used to model season and trend, and this approach was commonly used in early time-series studies in environmental epidemiology. However, this approach is mathematically complex and less flexible (Bhaskaran et al., 2013).

The third approach outlined in Bhaskaran et al. (2013) is the use of flexible spline functions. This approach has been the most popular since the development of the R package mgcv for generalised additive model fitting (Wood, 2006). Most studies have used a single function with many degrees of freedom (df) to control both trend and season. For example, Gasparrini et al. (2015) employed a single natural cubic B-spline with 8 df per year of study in a multi-country study of associations between temperature and mortality. CUHK's studies (e.g. Goggins & Chan, 2017; Goggins, Chan, Ng, Ren, & Chen, 2012; Goggins, Yang, Hokama, Law, & Chan, 2015) have generally used separate terms for season, day of year, with maximum df = 6, and trend, day of study (e.g. day of decade), with the maximum df varying from study to study but usually between 5 and 10. The reason for using two separate terms is the concern that some of the temperature effect may be "absorbed" by the seasonal term, i.e. overadjustment, especially for cold temperature effects, which often have very long delays of up to 4 weeks. One consequence of using separate terms is that the seasonal effect is forced to follow the same pattern from year to year. Bhaskaran et al. (2013) pointed out that this restriction also applies when Fourier terms are used and that this is a drawback as the timing of winter peaks in mortality may change from year to year. Control for season in studies of weather effects is a complex issue as often meteorological variables are so highly correlated with season. Ideally, the seasonal term would capture health effects of factors other than weather that vary with season (e.g. diet or virus circulation) and thus could be confounders for weather-health associations, but virus circulation could also be influenced by weather and thus could also be considered a mediator. The CUHK research team has often performed sensitivity analyses and found little difference in the meteorology results between models with a single term for day of study or separate terms for both day of study and day of year. This is an issue that deserves further study.

Lagged effects

The consideration of delayed (lagged) effects is also important and lagged effects for temperature, particularly for cold temperature, tend to be longer than those for pollutants. Various methods have been tried to handle this, for example, (i) fitting lagged terms one at a time in models, which has the drawback of giving estimates for each lag, which are biased due to the lack of control for the other lags (Bhaskaran et al., 2013), and (ii) including separate terms for each lag term in the same model. This latter approach is referred to as an unconstrained distributed lag model and, as pointed out by Schwartz (2000) in the context of air pollution studies, the coefficients for individual lags are quite unstable due to collinearity between the highly correlated daily values of pollutants. This problem is even more serious for ambient temperature as lagged effects are longer and the correlation between adjacent days are likely higher. Figure 5.1 shows the autocorrelation of successive measures of daily ambient temperature in Hong Kong from 2000 to 2009. Correlation between adjacent days is very high, r = 0.959, and remains quite high for subsequent days as well.

Figure 5.2 shows the results of a generalised additive model with 9 separate terms for mean daily temperature (i.e. same day, lag 1,... lag 8) included together in a model for daily non-cancer mortality in Hong Kong during 2000–2009. The confidence intervals for most terms are quite wide and the RR estimates are difficult to interpret. For this reason, constrained distributed lag models are generally used. One approach, which was used in Chan, Goggins, Kim, and Griffiths (2012) and others (e.g. Carder et al., 2005), is to take the average over groups of lags rather than adding all of the individual terms into the model. For example, in Chan et al. (2012), lag 0 and lag 1 mean temperature were entered into the model individually along with means of lags 2–7 and 8–14. This method reduces the number of terms in the model while allowing effects lagged up to 14 days (in this example) to be considered. However, it assumes that the effects of individual lags within each grouping are identical.

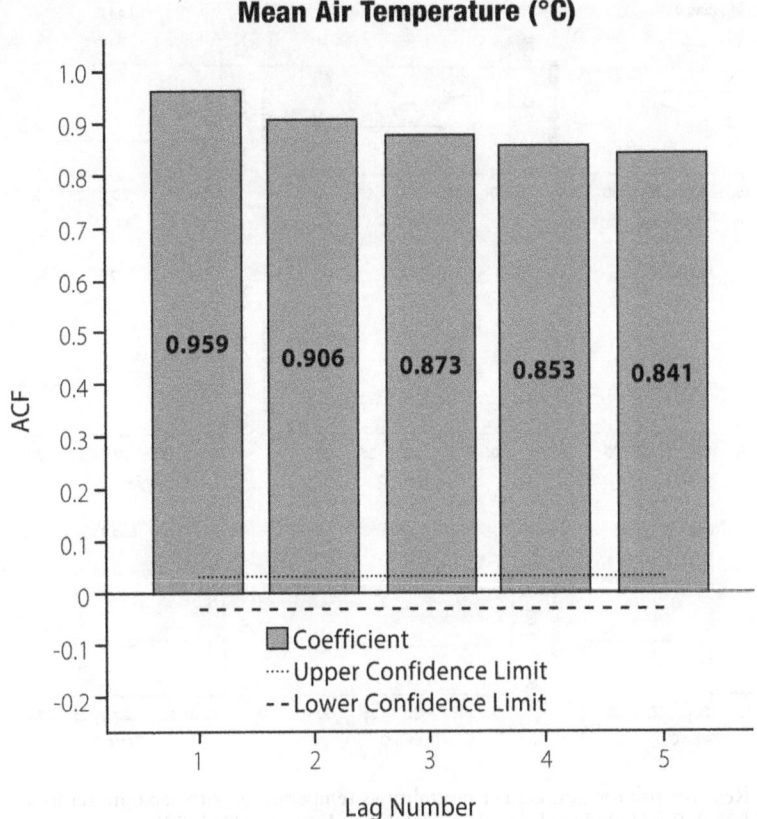

Figure 5.1 Autocorrelation of daily mean daily temperatures in Hong Kong (2000–2009).

The development of the dlnm package in the R statistical software (Gasparrini, 2011) has led to expanded use of the more flexible distributed lag non-linear models (DLNM) in these types of analyses. The dlnm package allows the use of cross-basis functions to model the bi-dimensional space consisting of predictor and lag effects, which can both then be modelled with splines (Gasparrini, 2011). Figure 5.3 shows the results of a DLNM with basis splines used to model both outcome-temperature and outcome lag associations, fit to daily non-cancer mortality in Hong Kong during 2000–2009. Plot (a) shows the cumulative association to lag 8; note the relatively narrow confidence intervals. Plot (b) shows the same-day association controlling for, but not including, the effect of lags 1–7 mean temperatures. Note that the immediate temperature–mortality association is positive and linear and very different from the longer-term associations. Plot (c) shows the RR for non-cancer mortality for 12°C versus 27.5°C by individual lag. Note that the cold temperature effect is protective at lag 0, which is consistent with plot (b), but becomes harmful at longer lags, peaking at lags 2–3 and

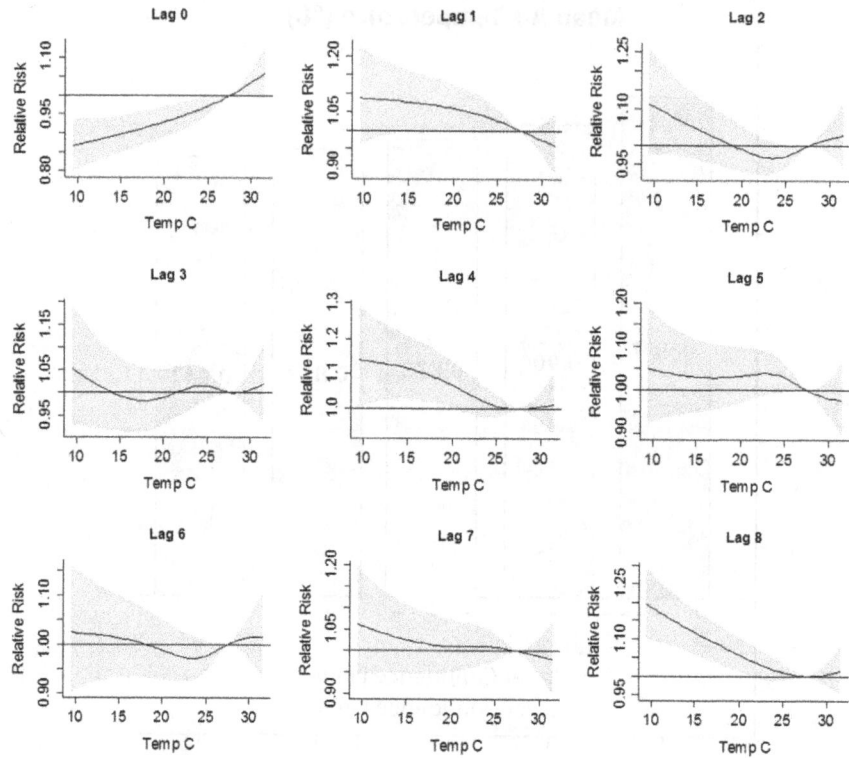

Figure 5.2 Relative risk for non-cancer mortality vs temperature, with separate terms for lags 0–8 included in the same model, Hong Kong (2000–2009).

again at lag 8. The large lag 8 effect is probably due to the correlation of lag 8 temperature with lags 9, 10, ..., which also have harmful associations with mortality. Plot (d) shows the cumulative association by lag that keeps rising, consistent with RR >1.0 across the lags in plot (c). Plot (e) shows the RR for non-cancer mortality for 30.5°C versus 27.5°C by individual lag. The harmful association with high temperature persists out to lag 4 but peaks on the same day. Plot (f) shows the cumulative association by lag that plateaus at lag = 4.

The choice of inclusion criteria

Another issue that arises in studies examining associations between weather and mortality/morbidity is the inclusion criteria for the outcomes. It is common in these studies to examine mortality including all causes except for deaths due to external causes (McMichael et al., 2008) although some studies use all-cause mortality (Gasparrini et al., 2015) and others may focus on mortality from a particular cause such as cardiovascular deaths (Yu et al., 2011) or perform

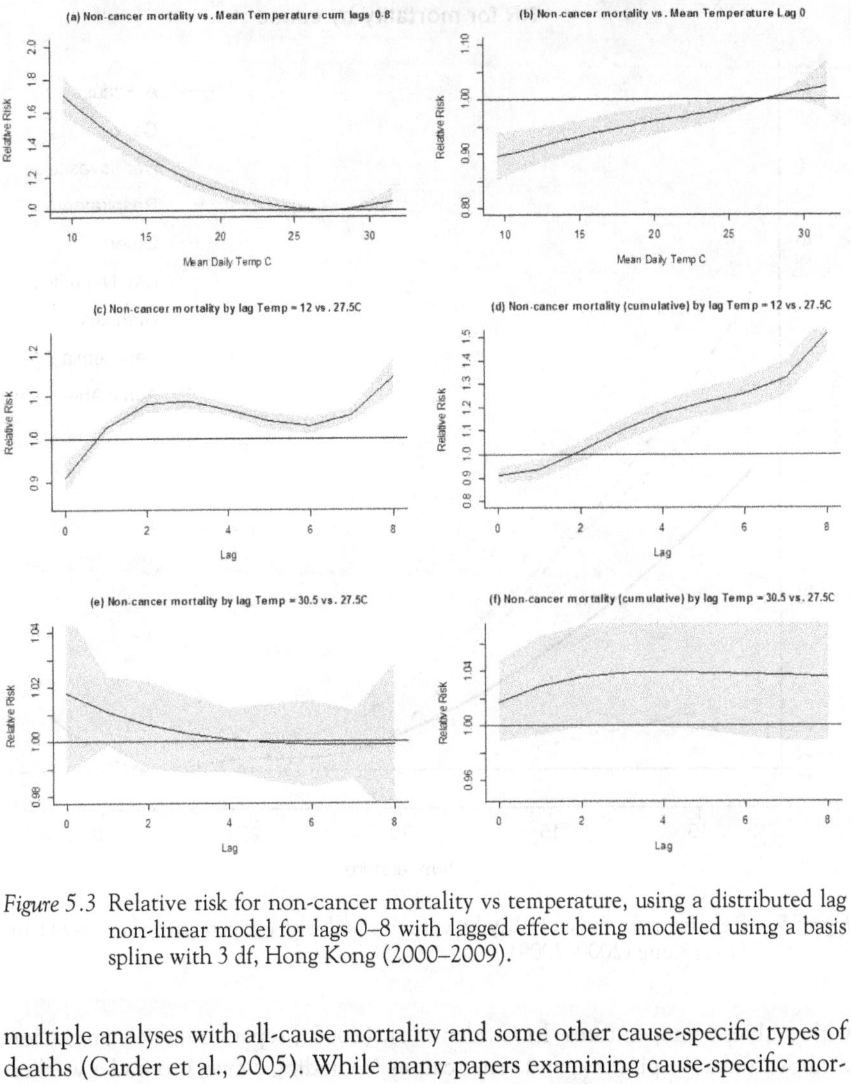

Figure 5.3 Relative risk for non-cancer mortality vs temperature, using a distributed lag non-linear model for lags 0–8 with lagged effect being modelled using a basis spline with 3 df, Hong Kong (2000–2009).

multiple analyses with all-cause mortality and some other cause-specific types of deaths (Carder et al., 2005). While many papers examining cause-specific mortality focus on cardiovascular and/or respiratory mortality, in papers examining temperature–mortality associations in Hong Kong (Chan et al., 2012; Goggins, Chan, Yang, & Chong, 2013) the CUHK team chose to examine several common causes of death separately including, in addition to cardiovascular and respiratory, cancer, diabetes, nephritis, and septicaemia, finding that deaths from most common causes, except cancer, were sensitive to ambient temperature. Figure 5.4 shows relative risks for mortality for various causes versus ambient temperatures (lag 0–21) in Hong Kong during 2000–2009. The response curve for "Others" is quite similar to those for cardiovascular and respiratory diseases while cancer mortality shows a substantially weaker association

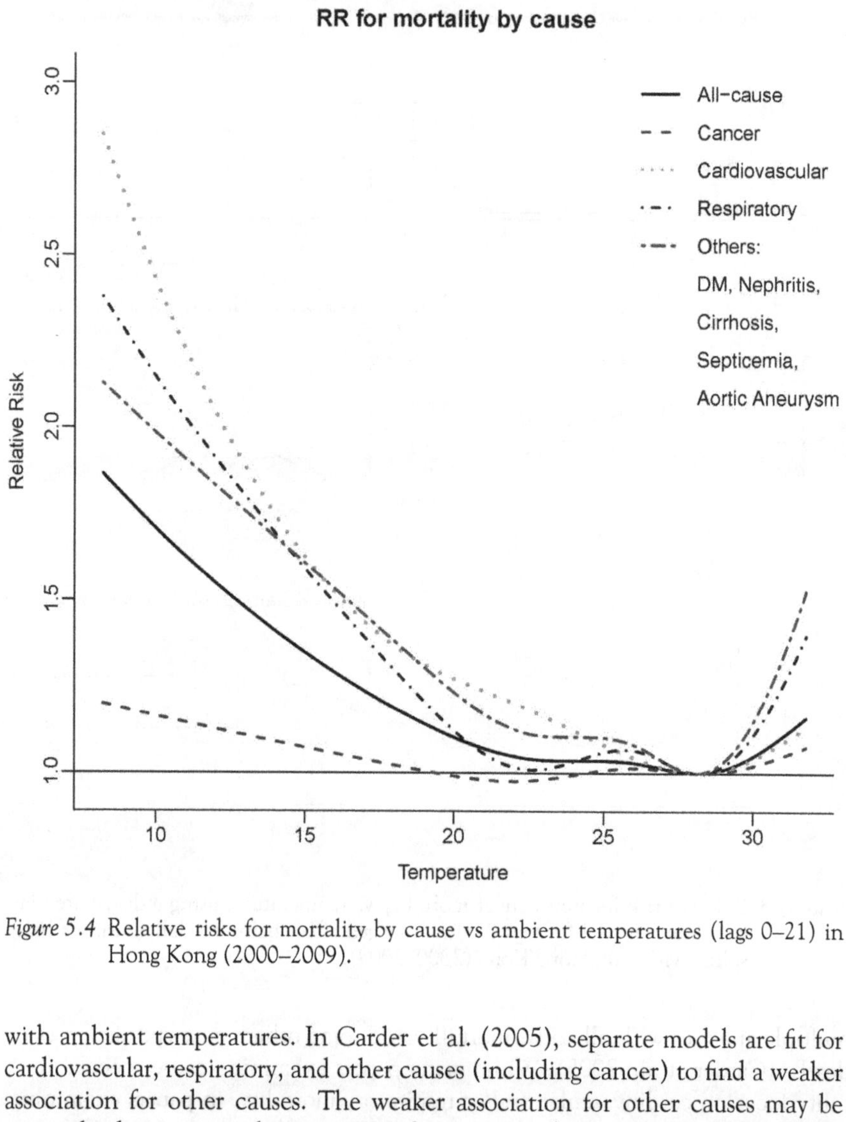

RR for mortality by cause

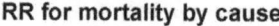

Figure 5.4 Relative risks for mortality by cause vs ambient temperatures (lags 0–21) in Hong Kong (2000–2009).

with ambient temperatures. In Carder et al. (2005), separate models are fit for cardiovascular, respiratory, and other causes (including cancer) to find a weaker association for other causes. The weaker association for other causes may be primarily due to a weak association for cancer, which is generally the most common causes of death other than cardiovascular disease in most developed countries. Researchers should consider examining causes of death other than cardiovascular and respiratory diseases and cancer when doing subgroup analyses, and/or considering looking at "non-cancer" causes of death separately.

The results of models used to characterise the short-term association between temperature and mortality have been used to project long-term mortality changes under climate change scenarios. Some studies, including those from Quebec, Canada (Doyon, Belanger, & Gosselin, 2008), the United Kingdom

(Hajat, Vardoulakis, Heaviside, & Eggen, 2014), Korea (Lee & Kim, 2016), and New York City (Li, Horton, & Kinney, 2013) have projected net increases in mortality, i.e. increases in heat-related mortality greater than decreases in cold-related mortality. A study projecting net temperature-related mortality for Europe (Ballester, Robine, Herrmann, & Rodo, 2011) found that overall temperature-related mortality would decrease during the first half of the 21st century, but start to increase in the second half when increases in heat-related mortality start to outweigh decreases in cold-related mortality. A study from Australia (Guo et al., 2016) projected net increases in mortality for Brisbane and Sydney, but decreases for Melbourne. A recent systematic review (Sanderson, Arbuthnott, Kovats, Hajat, & Falloon, 2017) found that many of the existing studies on this topic had several limitations including not considering future demographic changes, only projecting future changes in heat-related mortality but not considering potential reductions in cold-related mortality, and not performing projections under the mitigation scenario (RCP 2.6). A recent study using data from multiple continents, countries, and cities (Gasparrini et al., 2017) projected overall net increases in mortality but with considerable variation depending on location and degree of warming. That study's results indicated that temperature areas including Northern Europe, East Asia, and Australia are projected to have little or no net change in mortality, while warmer areas, especially Southeast Asia, are projected to experience large net increases.

Other variables

As associations between temperature and health have been found to be heavily dependent on local climatic conditions, conducting such studies in areas with varying climates is important. Previous studies have not taken into account potential effects of potentially increasing urban heat island effects and the differences in the effects of temperature on mortality due to different causes. While adaptation to future climatic conditions is impossible to predict, future research should consider the projected demographic changes, cause of death, and urbanisation.

Conclusion

This chapter has provided a brief overview of methodological challenges in the study of weather, climate change, and health outcomes, with specific reference to temperature and health studies in the urban context. As interest in this field has grown substantially only recently, there is a great deal of work left to be done and a great deal of uncertainty surrounding current predictions of the future health consequences of climate change. Although most existing studies examine direct effects of climate on health, indirect effects are also likely to be substantial, including potential adverse health effects due to flooding and possible disruptions to agriculture and transportation.

References

Ballester, J., Robine, J. M., Herrmann, R., & Rodo, X. (2011). Long-term projections and acclimatization scenarios of temperature-related mortality in Europe. *Nature Communications*, 2, 358.

Bannister-Tyrrell, M., Williams, C., Ritchie, S. A., Rau, G., Lindesay, J., Mercer, G., & Harley, D. (2013). Weather-driven variation in dengue activity in Australia examined using a process-based modeling approach. *American Journal of Tropical Medicine and Hygiene*, 88(1), 65–72. doi:10.4269/ajtmh.2012.11-0451.

Bhaskaran, K., Gasparrini, A., Hajat, S., Smeeth, L., & Armstrong, B. (2013). Time series regression studies in environmental epidemiology. *International Journal of Epidemiology*, 42(4), 1187–1195. doi:10.1093/ije/dyt092.

Carder, M., McNamee, R., Beverland, I., Elton, R., Cohen, G. R., Boyd, J., & Agius, R. M. (2005). The lagged effect of cold temperature and wind chill on cardiorespiratory mortality in Scotland. *Occupational and Environmental Medicine*, 62(10), 702–710. doi:10.1136/oem.2004.016394.

Chan, E. Y. Y., Goggins, W. B., Kim, J. J., & Griffiths, S. M. (2012). A study of intracity variation of temperature-related mortality and socioeconomic status among the Chinese population in Hong Kong. *Journal of Epidemiology and Community Health*, 66(4), 322–327.

Chong, K. C., Goggins, W., Zee, B. C., & Wang, M. H. (2015). Identifying meteorological drivers for the seasonal variations of influenza infections in a subtropical city— Hong Kong. *International Journal of Environmental Research and Public Health*, 12(2), 1560–1576. doi:10.3390/ijerph120201560.

Detinova, T. S., Bertram, D. S., & World Health Organization. (1962). *Age-grouping methods in diptera of medical importance, with special reference to some vectors of malaria/T. S. Detinova; [with] an Annex on the ovary and ovarioles of mosquitos (with glossary) by D. S. Bertram* (World Health Organization Monograph Series No. 47). Geneva, Switzerland: World Health Organization. Retrieved from www.who.int/iris/handle/10665/41724.

Doyon, B., Belanger, D., & Gosselin, P. (2008). The potential impact of climate change on annual and seasonal mortality for three cities in Quebec, Canada. *International Journal of Health Geographics*, 7, 23.

Ebi, K. L., & Rocklov, J. (2014). Climate change and health modeling: Horses for courses. *Global Health Action*, 7, 24154. doi:10.3402/gha.v7.24154.

Gasparrini, A. (2011). Distributed lag linear and non-linear models in R: The package dlnm. *Journal of Statistical Software*, 43(8), 1–20.

Gasparrini, A., Guo, Y., Hashizume, M., Lavigne, E., Zanobetti, A., Schwartz, J., ... Armstrong, B. (2015). Mortality risk attributable to high and low ambient temperature: A multicountry observational study. *The Lancet*, 386(9991), 369–375. doi:10.1016/S0140-6736(14)62114-0.

Gasparrini, A., Guo, Y., Sera, F., Vicedo-Cabrera, A. M., Huber, V., Tong, S., ... Armstrong, B. (2017). Projections of temperature-related excess mortality under climate change scenarios. *Lancet Planet Health*, 1(9), e360–e367. doi:10.1016/S2542-5196(17)30156-0.

Goggins, W. B., & Chan, E. Y. (2017). A study of the short-term associations between hospital admissions and mortality from heart failure and meteorological variables in Hong Kong: Weather and heart failure in Hong Kong. *International Journal of Cardiology*, 228, 537–542.

Goggins, W. B., Chan, E. Y., Ng, E., Ren, C., & Chen, L. (2012). Effect modification of the association between short-term meteorological factors and mortality by urban heat islands in Hong Kong. *PLOS One, 7*(6), e38551. doi:10.1371/journal.pone.0038551.

Goggins, W. B., Chan, E. Y. Y., Yang, C., & Chong, M. (2013). Associations between mortality and meteorological and pollutant variables during the cool season in two Asian cities with sub-tropical climates: Hong Kong and Taipei. *Environmental Health, 12*(1), 59. doi:10.1186/1476-069X-12-59.

Goggins, W. B., Yang, C. Y., Hokama, T., Law, L. S. K., & Chan, E. Y. (2015). Using annual data to estimate the public health impact of extreme temperatures. *American Journal of Epidemiology, 182*, 80–87.

Guo, Y., Li, S., Liu, D. L., Chen, D., Williams, G., & Tong, S. (2016). Projecting future temperature-related mortality in three largest Australian cities. *Environmental Pollution, 208*, 66–73.

Hajat, S., Vardoulakis, S., Heaviside, C., & Eggen, B. (2014). Climate change effects on human health: Projections of temperature-related mortality for the UK during the 2020s, 2050s, and 2080s. *Journal of Epidemiology and Community Health, 68*, 641–648.

Lee, J. Y., & Kim, H. (2016). Projection of future temperature-related mortality due to climate and demographic changes. *Environment International, 94*, 489–494.

Li, T., Horton, R. M., & Kinney, P. (2013). Future projections of seasonal patterns in temperature-related deaths in Manhattan. *Nature Climate Change, 3*, 717–721.

Martens, P., Kovats, R. S., Nijhof, S., de Vries, P., Livermore, M. T. J., & Bradley, D. J. (1999). Climate change and future populations at risk of malaria. *Global Environmental Change, 9* (Supplement 1), S89–S107.

McMichael, A. J., Campbell-Lendrum, D., Kovats, S., Edwards, S., Wilkinson, P., Wilson, T., … Andronova, N. (2004). Global climate change. In M. Ezzati, A. D. Lopez, A. Rodgers, & C. J. L. Murray (Eds.), *Comparative quantification of health risks: Global and regional burden of disease due to selected major risk factors* (Vol. 1, pp. 1543–1650). Geneva, Switzerland: World Health Organization. Retrieved from www.who.int/publications/cra/chapters/volume2/1543-1650.pdf.

McMichael, A. J., Wilkinson, P., Kovats, R. S., Pattenden, S., Hajat, S., Armstrong, B., … Nikiforov, B. (2008). International study of temperature, heat and urban mortality: The "ISOTHURM" project. *International Journal of Epidemiology, 37*(5), 1121–1131. doi: 10.1093/ije/dyn086.

Parham, P. E., & Michael, E. (2010). Modeling the effects of weather and climate change on malaria transmission. *Environmental Health Perspectives, 118*(5), 620–626. doi:10. 1289/ehp. 0901256.

Sanderson, M., Arbuthnott, K., Kovats, S., Hajat, S., & Falloon, P. (2017). The use of climate information to estimate future mortality from high ambient temperature: A systematic literature review. *PLOS One, 12*(7). doi:ARTN e018036910.1371/journal. pone.0180369.

Schwartz, J. (2000). The distributed lag between air pollution and daily deaths. *Epidemiology, 11*(3), 320–326. doi:10.1097/00001648-200005000-00016.

Wood, S. N. (2006). *Generalized additive models: An introduction with R.* Boca Raton, FL: Chapman & Hall/CRC.

Yu, W. W., Hu, W. B., Mengersen, K., Guo, Y. M., Pan, X. C., Connell, D., & Tong, S. L. (2011). Time course of temperature effects on cardiovascular mortality in Brisbane, Australia. *Heart, 97*(13), 1089–1093. doi:10.1136/hrt.2010.217166.

6 Research Methodology II
Climate and human behavioural model

The previous chapter describes research methodologies that model patterns of weather (e.g. temperature) and health outcomes. This chapter discusses how retrospective cohort data study, cross-sectional telephone survey, case study, focus group, stakeholder interview, and a number of quantitative study designs (e.g. cross-sectional, serial cross-sectional, and cohort follow-up study, and behavioural interventional design) are used in examining individual or community knowledge, attitude, and behaviour.

Cohort study: retrospective data studies

In addition to using mortality (Chan, Goggins, Kim, & Griffiths, 2012) and morbidity (e.g. hospitalisation and clinic attendance; Chan, Goggins, Yue, & Lee, 2013; Goggins & Chan, 2017) as health outcome variables, retrospective time-series Poisson generalised additive model analysis might also be constructed for behavioural outcomes and patterns (Chan, Goggins, Kim, Griffiths, & Mak, 2011) (see Case Box 6.1). Using meteorological data of the Hong Kong Observatory (HKO) and routine emergency help call data from the Hong Kong Senior Citizen Home Safety Association (SCHSA) during warm seasons (June–September) 1998–2007, analyses have been conducted.

Case Box 6.1 Temperature help-seeking model with retrospective data

Daily weather variables including mean, maximum, and minimum temperatures, dew point temperatures, and mean humidity were obtained from the HKO. Pollution data were obtained from the 11 general environmental collection stations of the Hong Kong Environmental Protection Department. Daily means of pollutants were calculated from hourly concentrations of nitrogen dioxide (NO_2), sulphur dioxide (SO_2), ozone (O_3), and PM_{10} (which is also known as respirable suspended particulates (RSP) in Hong Kong (Environmental Protection Department of the Government of the Hong Kong Special Administrative Region, n.d.)). Average weekly consultation rates of influenza-like illnesses reported by general outpatient clinics and practitioners were obtained from the Centre for Health Promotion of the Department of Health of Hong Kong, which were used as a proxy indicator to control for the influence of influenza epidemics on mortality.

Emergency call data were obtained from SCHSA of Hong Kong. SCHSA, a non-profit charitable organisation, provides the "Personal Emergency Link" ("PE Link") Service to older citizens living alone and people in need. Despite being mostly for the older population, the PE Link Service is open to applicants of all ages, home districts, and living environments with residential telephone lines. The 24-hour emergency hotline offers support to the emergency needs of callers and provides the necessary support services through referrals. In the event of an emergency, operators might: (i) call the police or ambulance centre for medical assistance; (ii) call the emergency contact person to report the latest status of the user, including hospitalisation details; or (iii) fax the medical history to the Accident & Emergency Department to facilitate rescue and medical care. If there is no response from the caller within 2 minutes of pressing the button for the PE Link Service, the centre will treat the case as an emergency and send for the Fire Services Department to undertake rescues accordingly. Within the study period, 48,261 members were enrolled in SCHSA. Over two-thirds of callers became SCHSA members with financial assistance from organisations such as the Social Welfare Department, the Housing Department, or the SCHSA Personal Emergency Link Charitable Programme, while the remaining paid on their own.

Poisson generalised additive models were used to model the association between the number of daily calls and daily temperature. Emergency calls (based on daily first-time call) were used as a proxy measurement for help-seeking behaviour. Effect modification of the temperature–call frequency association was assessed by subgroup analysis by several demographic variables.

Areas of residence were grouped into three and used as a proxy indicator to examine the impact of living area characteristics: (i) Kowloon—old district, densely populated and low-income; (ii) Hong Kong—newer district, less densely populated and middle-to-high-income; and (iii) New Territories—newest district, with urban planning, younger population, migrants, and young families. Binary variables were created from socio-economic status (whether or not a recipient of the Comprehensive Social Security Assistance (CSSA) scheme), dependency status (living alone versus not living alone), and access to a social network (member of SCHSA versus member of another organisation). Specifically, with regard to socio-economic status, the Hong Kong government's CSSA scheme provides supplemental income to people who live below the poverty line in Hong Kong and thus CSSA status represents poverty or low socio-economic status. Access to social support was defined in this study as access to a community network or services (e.g. whether SCHSA membership was obtained through government referral or through a charitable organisation). Statistical analyses were stratified into subgroups based on age, gender, area of residence, reason for calling, socio-economic status, dependency status, and access to social network.

Models were developed with smooth terms with four degrees of freedom each for weather variables including temperature, precipitation (rainfall), and relative humidity (RH). Daily maximum, mean, and minimum temperature variables were tried in the models separately to determine which of the three was most strongly associated with daily health-related calls. Daily variation in temperature (= maximum temperature – minimum temperature), change in temperature from the previous day's daily mean RH, rainfall, and lag terms for temperature up to 7 days were also considered. The models also controlled for seasonality and long-term trends using a smooth function of time, SO_2 levels, duration of heat-waves, and indicator variables for day of week and public holidays. A "heatwave duration" variable was created based on the number of consecutive days in which the daily mean, maximum, and minimum temperatures exceeded the thresholds: (i) mean temperature > 28.2°C; (ii) minimum temperature > 25.5°C; and (iii) maximum temperature > 31.5°C. The smooth terms allowed for the modelling of non-linear associations between temperature and number of calls as well as for other non-linear associations and the characteristic of seasonality that may some-times be present in long-term time trends. Temperature thresholds above and below which call frequency began to increase were estimated graphically through visual inspection of plots of the adjusted associations between call frequency and maximum temperature from the generalised additive models (Chan et al., 2011).

Methodological limitations of using data of a retrospective nature might be the limitation of the availability of variables of interest. In addition, only first-time calls made by members were used. Results may be biased toward the SCHSA population who are generally older and female. The lack of informa-tion regarding the air-conditioner ownership within the study population might also lead to potential biased findings towards expressed help needs during extreme temperature. Another potential limitation to this study is that the most vulnerable subgroups may have been excluded because the PE Link emergency service requires the possession of a landline telephone.

Cross-sectional study: telephone survey studies

In a developed urban context where the general population has stable access to a telephone communication network, telephone survey study design might be a research methodology of choice to obtain an overview of knowledge, attitude, and behavioural intents in community response behaviour patterns. Data of individual or household might effectively be collected before, during, and after the incident/event of interests. For a community with a high level of landline telephone infiltration, telephone survey may be stratified by age, gender, and district. The collected data might then be matched by age, gender, and district of the general population profile for potential generalisability of the findings for the studied community. This study method can also collect follow-up data of a study cohort, with data collection conducted during specific pre-set time intervals (see Case Box 6.2).

The *random digit dialling (RDD)* method (where samples may be gathered by computerised selection or by manual selection through random number genera-tion for dialling sequence) may ensure randomisation in data collection. Based on the landline-based telephone number list in the study community, house-holds are randomly "called" (or "picked") to be invited to participate in the study. It is important to pre-set criteria of both inclusion and exclusion of the target study participants (e.g. age, gender, and specific socio-economic demographics) before the sampling. Quota sampling may be used to ensure the demographic representation of the general population, with quotas based on age, sex, and residential district in the local context (Rubin, Amlot, Page, & Wessely, 2009). In addition, to minimise potential bias from responders at the household level (e.g. the same individual might usually respond to phone calls within the household), the *"last-birthday method"* (i.e., requesting to interview the individual in the household who has passed his/her last birthday most recently) might be used to ensure randomisation of responders (by age, gender, etc.) at the household level.

Case Box 6.2 Telephone survey methodology for cold spells in Hong Kong as a subtropical city

A population-based, stratified, and cross-sectional random digit dialling telephone survey was conducted between 28 January and 4 February 2016. Over 95% of Hong Kong households have a landline telephone, which enhances the validity of using the telephone survey methodology to conduct a representative study of the general population. Since 95.8% of the Hong Kong population are Cantonese speakers or able to use the language, the survey was conducted in the Cantonese language. The study targeted the non-institutionalised population aged 15 years old or above residing in Hong Kong, including residents holding valid work or study visas. Exclusion criteria included (i) non-Cantonese-speaking respondents; (ii) children under the age of 15; (iii) overseas visitors holding tourist visas to Hong Kong or two-way permit holders from mainland China; and (iv) those unable to be interviewed due to medical reasons.

For the sample size calculation, based on a conservative hypothesis, the prevalence of studied behaviour was assumed to be 50%. A required sample size of 784 participants was calculated, with a 3.5% margin of error and 95% confidence interval. In addition, quota sampling was used to ensure the demographic representation of the general population in Hong Kong in terms of age, gender, and district of residence. Respondents were required to be 15 years old or above and able to speak the local dialect. Up to five calls were made before the telephone number was considered invalid and all calls were made during the same time of the day (e.g. evening on weekdays and whole day on weekends) to prevent overpresentation of the unemployed segment of the population. Last-birthday method was used to ensure the interviewees might not be limited to the usual call responder of a household. To account for potential missing data and increase the modelling flexibility, 1,017 participants were recruited as the final sample (Chan, Huang, Mark, & Guo, 2017; Chan, Wang, Ho, Huang, Liu, & Guo, 2017).

Although there are many practical and feasibility advantages of using the telephone survey methodology in studying community behaviour, a number of methodological limitations exist for this kind of survey study. First, the study methodology assumes all individuals or households (or units of analysis) are represented or included in the study sampling frame (e.g. telephone number list) for potential randomisation. However, if the study design is implemented in communities of less developed information network and communication technology, the sampling frame of using "listed telephone numbers" may suffer from potential selection bias. Households that do not possess a landline telephone service might be missing. In particular, it might exclude unintentionally households/individuals who have difficulties in accessing landline telephones due to financial constraint, geographic distance, or simply personal choice to opt out of telephone access. In addition, many newly developed communities might prefer mobile phone networks rather than relying on landline telephone networks. Alternative survey methods may thus be used, e.g. postal survey, online survey, or mobile phone survey.

Moreover, whilst residing in the geographic locations of interest to the study, certain population subgroups might have phone numbers that are linked to other geographic areas (e.g. people who are residing in the study context as working migrants and transient visitors). In addition, with the increasing prevalence of low-cost mobile technology, individuals and households might have more than one telephone number in active use, which might violate the randomisation assumption that each individual/household is only represented by one telephone number. Nevertheless, as of November 2013, the penetration rate of the residential landline service in Hong Kong was 102.6% (Tam, Huang, & Chan, 2018), which implies that almost all households had at least one home-based telephone service in Hong Kong.

To ensure standardisation and a research acceptable response rate, procedures of how to manage non-contact and non-response bias should be carefully described and accounted for in research design. Repeated calling of the same number to identify the appropriate respondents (if last-birthday method or another specific pre-set selection criterion is used) might be warranted. A typical study might require up to five repeated callings to solicit response from identified respondents or simply to complete the telephone survey. The response rate calculation should at least take into account non-functional telephone lines, fax lines, or phone lines that might not be of residential use.

Another important consideration for telephone survey-based studies is the potential finding implications of a cross-sectional study design. Single, one-off cross-sectional design study can at best demonstrate associations between patterns and social-demographic predictors. Causation cannot be attributed to the findings. In addition, data collection through telephone survey is typically based on self-reported information and these data might subject to reporting bias. Missing data from non-respondents is another potential source of reporting bias. Imprecision of measurements and the absence of validation of reported answers also lead to inaccuracies. Moreover, with the finite amount of time in each telephone interview, the survey study could only collect data based on a limited number of questions, which restricted exploring and explaining reported behavioural patterns in detail. Besides, results may not be generalisable, as other countries or cities have not experienced the same epidemiology of disasters. Finally, the consistency of the responses over a long survey period may be influenced by external factors during the survey period. For example, if an outbreak of disease/ typhoon occurs in the middle of a survey period, the respondents may change their perceptions (e.g. risk perceptions) due to changes in circumstances. To reduce this potential problem, the field data collection should be completed within a short period (e.g. 2 weeks).

Other methods

Stakeholder interviews can facilitate topic exploration, obtaining insights to identify explanations for patterns and phenomena, and collection of information from particular subgroups. Stakeholders involved in these studies are usually nominated, identified, and their role in the topic of interest should be mapped out before the study. Some other common research methods of collecting stakeholders' perspectives may include Delphi study, anecdotal reports, structured surveys (written or spoken), postal mail, telephone, electronic or in-person in-depth interviews, focus groups, or group interviews, as well as direct observation (McKenna, 2004). While each method has its merits, reliability and consistency of study results might be enhanced if triangulation is achieved through multiple data sources and analyses. **Anecdotal reports** by their very nature lack any formal method but provide an opportunity for people to speak their minds. Surveys provide a way of measuring the knowledge, attitudes, beliefs, and behaviours of the target population. **Structured surveys** provide useful ways of listening to some stakeholders, but may not prove very useful in listening to others. A **focus group study** might serve to explore a largely unknown topic or to seek explanation for patterns and behaviours identified. It might be typically carried out by grouping together people with similar characteristics (e.g. gender and demographic profile) and the interview might be conducted with pre-sent templates or questionnaires (with structured or semi-structured questions/surveys). **Direct observation** records what actually happened during the frame of analysis. All methods of listening to stakeholders have two things in common: regardless of the methods, all of them require the objective of listening and the people to listen to (i.e. the population). Although these methods all help one listen to stakeholders, some methods better match particular stakeholders and particular circumstances.

Conclusion

This chapter aims to describe research methods that may be useful for understanding climate, health and behavioural outcomes. Although it is beyond the scope of this book to provide detail of each method, it serves to show how data might be collected effectively to improve understanding of how climate (e.g. temperature) may affect health in a population.

References

Chan, E. Y. Y., Goggins, W. B., Kim, J. J., & Griffiths, S. M. (2012). A study of intracity variation of temperature-related mortality and socioeconomic status among the Chinese population of Hong Kong. *Journal of Epidemiology and Community Health*, 66(4), 322–327.

Chan, E. Y. Y., Goggins, W. B., Kim, J. J., Griffiths, S., & Mak, T. K. (2011). Help-seeking behaviour during elevated temperature in Chinese populations. *Journal of Urban Health*, 88(4), 637–650.

Chan, E. Y. Y., Goggins, W. B., Yue, J. S. K., & Lee, P. (2013). Hospital admissions as a function of temperature, weather phenomena and pollution levels in an urban setting in China. *Bulletin of the World Health Organization*, 91(8), 576–584.

Chan, E. Y. Y., Huang, Z., Mark, C. K. M., & Guo, C. (2017). Weather information acquisition and health significance during extreme cold weather in a subtropical city: A cross-sectional survey in Hong Kong. *International Journal of Disaster Risk Science*, 8(2), 134–144. doi:10.1007/s13753-017-0127-8.

Chan, E. Y. Y., Wang, S. S., Ho, J. Y., Huang, Z., Liu, S., & Guo, C. (2017). Socio-demographic predictors of health and environmental co-benefit behaviours for climate change mitigation in urban China. *PLOS One*, 12(11), e0188661. doi:10.1371/journal.pone.0188661.

Environmental Protection Department of the Government of the Hong Kong Special Administrative Region (n.d.). Hong Kong air pollutant emission inventory—Definition for respirable suspended particles. Retrieved from www.epd.gov.hk/epd/english/environmentinhk/air/data/emission_inve_rsp.html.

Goggins, W. B., & Chan, E. Y. Y. (2017). A study of the short-term associations between hospital admissions and mortality from heart failure and meteorological variables in Hong Kong: Weather and heart failure in Hong Kong. *International Journal of Cardiology*, 228, 537–542.

McKenna, C. K. (2004). Listening to stakeholders: Interviews, focus groups, surveys, and direct observation. In J. T. Ziegenfuss & J. W. Sassani (Eds.), *Portable health administration* (pp. 173–184). London: Elsevier.

Rubin, G. J., Amlot, R., Page, L., & Wessely, S. (2009). Public perceptions, anxiety, and behaviour change in relation to the swine flu outbreak: Cross sectional telephone survey. *British Medical Journal*, 339, b2651. doi:10.1136/bmj.b2651.

Tam, G., Huang, Z., & Chan, E. Y. Y. (2018). Household preparedness and preferred communication channels in public health emergencies: A cross-sectional survey of residents in an Asian developed urban city. *Environmental Research and Public Health*, 15, 1598. doi:10.3390/ijerph15081598.

7 The case of Hong Kong

This chapter describes Hong Kong, a subtropical metropolis in southern China, which is the key study site of the research studies reported in this book.

Subtropical city in Southern China

Hong Kong, a subtropical metropolis, is a Special Administrative Region (SAR) of the People's Republic of China (see Table 7.1). It is situated in the southeastern tip of China and has a total geographic area of 1,106 km². Its estimated population was about 7.48 million at the end of 2018 (Hong Kong SAR Government Census and Statistics Department, 2019, 21 February). With 66.2% of its landmass protected by policy to remain as green zone, country park zone, special areas, sites of special scientific interest, conservation and protection areas (65% of which is under statutory protection), its population mainly resides in a few small developed areas. Due to its British colonial history, the city consists of three geographical areas, including the densely populated central urban area of Hong Kong Island and Kowloon Peninsula (occupying around 11.5% of the land area), and the rural New Territories (encompassing the largest Lantau Island and more than 200 outlying islands) with suburban "New Towns", some of which are also quite densely populated. The overall average population density is 6,700 per km², among the highest in the world. There are 18 administrative districts in Hong Kong, as shown in Figure 7.1. The most densely populated district, Kwun Tong, has a population density of 59,400 per km² (Hong Kong Special Administrative Region Government, 2018). The metropolis has a high-rise vertical development. With 350 completed buildings taller than 150 m, Hong Kong has the world's largest number of skyscrapers (The Skyscraper Center, 2018). Its dense-vertical urban development has resulted in significant long-term decrease in local wind speed in the past few decades. Hong Kong's relatively robust and linked-up population-based electronic hospital in-patient record system allows a systematic study of the health impact of climate change.

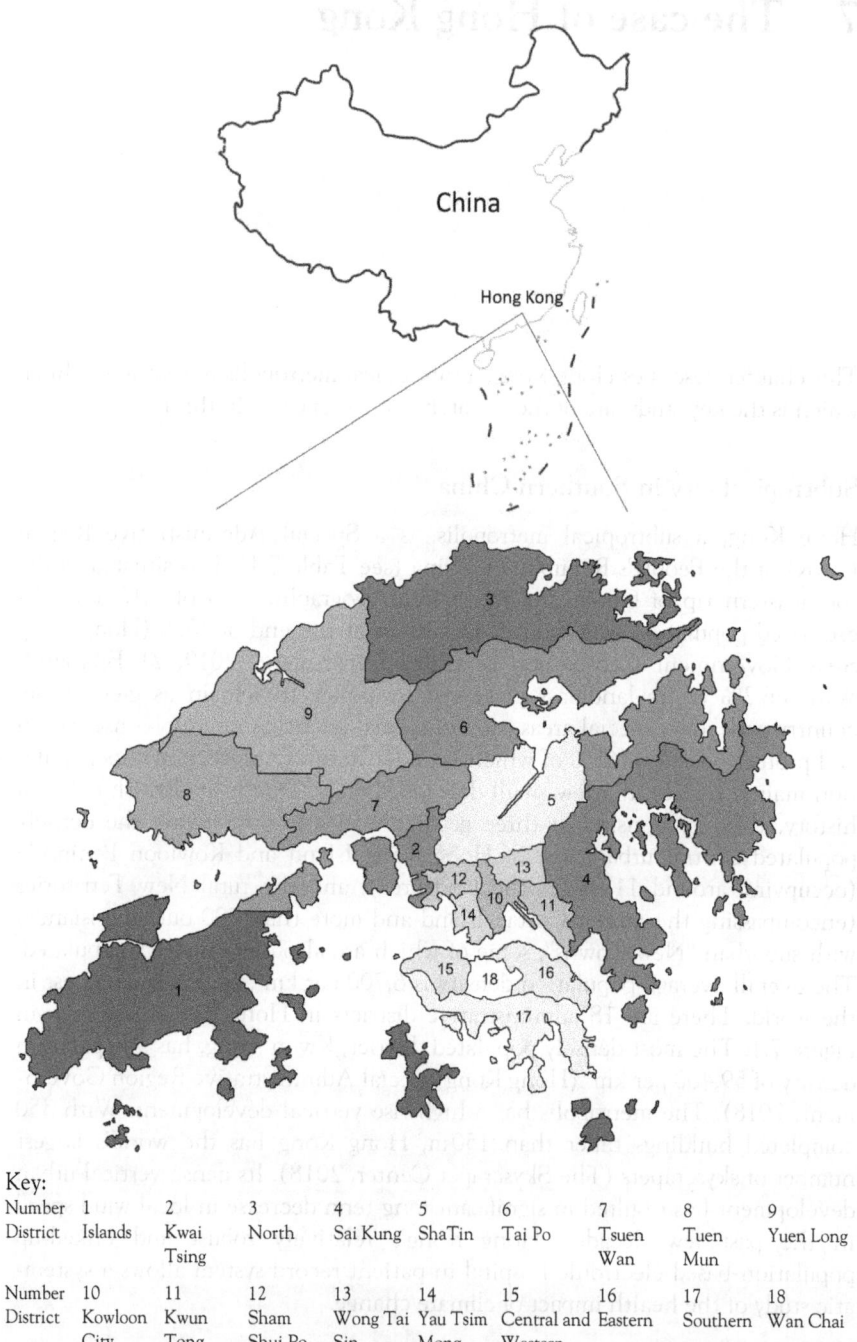

Key:

Number	1	2	3	4	5	6	7	8	9
District	Islands	Kwai Tsing	North	Sai Kung	Sha Tin	Tai Po	Tsuen Wan	Tuen Mun	Yuen Long

Number	10	11	12	13	14	15	16	17	18
District	Kowloon City	Kwun Tong	Sham Shui Po	Wong Tai Sin	Yau Tsim Mong	Central and Western	Eastern	Southern	Wan Chai

Figure 7.1 Hong Kong Special Administrative Region in China.

Table 7.1 Characteristics of Hong Kong as an urban metropolis

Issues	Situation (compared with the world)
Globalisation	Annually, almost **eight** times as many transients (58.47 million visitors in 2017) as its local population
Income inequality	**Highest income inequality** in developed regions; 9th globally
Environmental stress	One of the **highest population densities** (the fourth most densely populated country/dependency in 2018)
Urbanisation	**100%** urbanised
Emergency risk	Experiences of **global public health** crisis such as SARS outbreak (in 2003) and H7N9 outbreak (in 2012)
Impact of climate change	One of the **highest increases** in mean urban temperature in the past century

Sources: Central Intelligence Agency (n.d.); Hong Kong Special Administrative Region Government (2018); World Bank (n.d.).

Weather and climate

Hong Kong has a subtropical climate. The daily temperatures recorded in the past 50 years have been within the range of around 7–34°C. Its summer afternoon temperature often exceeds 31°C but can drop below 10°C during winter (Hong Kong Observatory, 2017, February). The summer average temperature is around 28°C (with a median of 27.8°C) and the average relative humidity is around 75%. On average, the city records about 10 very hot days annually (maximum temperature reaching over 33°C). Hong Kong recorded its hottest temperature in 50 years (36.6°C) on 22 August 2017. In winter months, the city has an average temperature of around 16°C and a medium of around 19.3°C (Hong Kong Observatory, n.d.b). Table 7.2 summarises the temperature pattern. The rainy season usually falls between April and September and especially heavy rainstorms are common between May and June (Hong Kong Observatory, 2018, 10 April). In addition, as a city in southeastern China, summer months (from July to September) are prone to the impact of tropical cyclones and heavy precipitations annually.

Studies in Hong Kong have identified 21°C as the ambient temperature with the highest self-reported thermal comfort (see Figure 7.2).

Extreme weather events

Extreme temperature

Heatwaves in Hong Kong

Heatwave is a prolonged period of excessively hot weather and it may threaten the health of human beings, animals, and plants. The Hong Kong Observatory would take different climatic elements (e.g. humidity and wind speed) into

Table 7.2 Temperature pattern of Hong Kong

Meteorological variables	Percentile									
	1st	3rd	10th	25th	Median	75th	90th	97th	99th
Cold season (November–April)									
Mean temperature (°C)	10.31	11.70	14.20	16.70	19.30	21.80	24.20	25.85	26.50
Maximum temperature (°C)	11.91	13.93	16.50	18.90	21.70	24.52	27.00	28.67	29.50
Minimum temperature (°C)	8.21	9.50	12.00	14.90	17.70	20.10	22.49	24.40	25.09
Hot season (May–October)									
Mean temperature (°C)	22.44	23.60	24.80	26.10	27.80	29.10	29.80	30.40	30.80
Maximum temperature (°C)	24.24	25.30	26.80	28.40	30.20	31.90	32.80	33.70	34.30
Minimum temperature (°C)	20.64	21.90	23.09	24.50	25.80	27.20	28.00	28.58	28.90

Temperature (°C)	<10	10–14	15–19	20–24	25–26	27–29	>29	Total
Frequency	1	43	388	484	79	14	2	1,011
Valid percentage	0.10%	4.25%	38.38%	47.87%	7.81%	1.38%	0.20%	100.00%

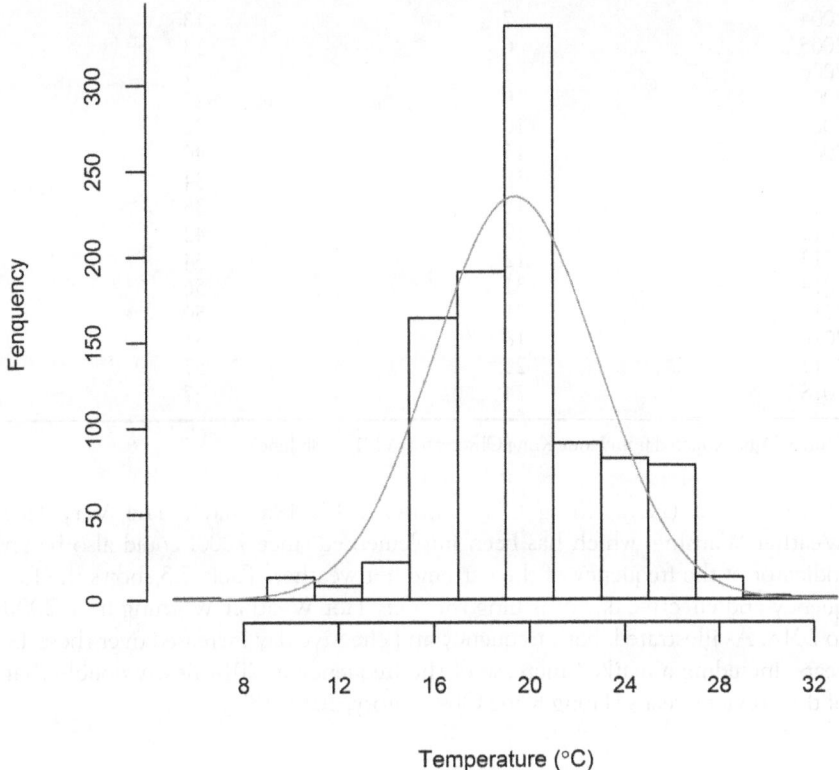

Figure 7.2 The most comfortable reported temperatures.

Source: CCOUC.

consideration when issuing the Very Hot Weather Warning, which warns its population against heatwave.

The total number of hot days (daily maximum temperature ≥33.0°C) recorded in Hong Kong has been increasing over the past few decades. From 2014 to 2017, the average number of hot days reached around 30 days a year, with the highest number of 38 days in 2016 (Hong Kong Observatory, 2018, 3b October).

The Hong Kong Observatory issues its temperature warning to alert the general public although there is no rigid temperature threshold for issuing the warning since other climatic factors such as humidity could affect the heat felt

Table 7.3 Frequency and length of very hot weather warning in Hong Kong (2000–2018)

Year	Frequency	Effective day
2000	12	30
2001	13	22
2002	7	18
2003	8	19
2004	7	13
2005	6	13
2006	3	7
2007	9	25
2008	10	22
2009	15	40
2010	18	34
2011	12	38
2012	19	42
2013	12	34
2014	31	56
2015	21	50
2016	16	51
2017	25	57
2018	24	57

Source: Data extracted from Hong Kong Observatory (2013, 18b June).

by the public (Hong Kong Observatory, 2017, 19a May). The Very Hot Weather Warning, which has been implemented since 2000, could also be an indicator of the frequency of the extreme hot weather. Table 7.3 shows the frequency and effective day of issuing the Very Hot Weather Warning from 2000 to 2018. As illustrated, both frequency and effective day increased over these 19 years, including a marked increase of the frequency in 2014 nearly double that of the previous year's (Hong Kong Observatory, 2013, 18b June).

Cold spell in subtropical city: Hong Kong

The coldest months in Hong Kong, a subtropical metropolis, typically fall in January or February and the mean minimum temperature is around 14.5°C (January) and 15°C (February) (see Figure 7.3). A cold day, in the definition of the Hong Kong Observatory, refers to one with daily minimum temperature equal to or below 12°C. In general, the number of cold days has been decreasing (Hong Kong Observatory, 2018, 3a October).

Cold Weather Warning can also be one of the indicators for extreme temperature in Hong Kong. In parallel with Very Hot Weather Warning, there is no rigid temperature threshold for issuing the cold spell warning. However, when Hong Kong is threatened by cold weather and other climatic factors such as humidity also intensify the situation, the Hong Kong Observatory issues the Cold Weather Warning, implemented since 1999 (Hong Kong Observatory, 2017, 19a May). Table 7.4 shows the frequency and effective day of issuing Cold Weather

	Data period	Jan	Feb	Mar	Apr	May	Jun	Jul	Aug	Sep	Oct	Nov	Dec
Mean maximum temperature (°C)	1981–2010	18.6	18.9	21.4	25	28.4	30.2	31.4	31.1	30.1	27.8	24.1	20.2
Mean minimum temperature (°C)	1981–2010	14.5	15	17.2	20.8	24.1	26.2	26.8	26.6	25.8	23.7	19.8	15.9
Rainfall amount (mm)	1981–2010	24.7	54.4	82.2	174.7	304.7	456.1	376.5	432.2	327.6	100.9	37.6	26.8
Days with rain	1981–2010	5.4	9.1	10.9	12	14.7	19.1	17.6	16.9	14.7	7.4	5.5	4.5

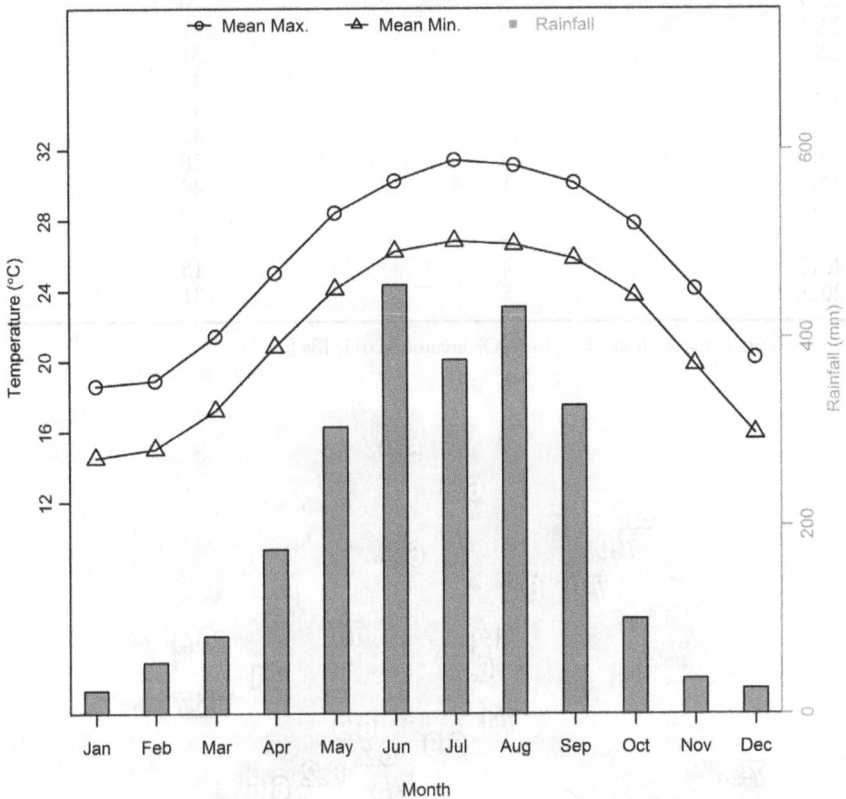

Figure 7.3 Monthly average temperature and rainfall (1981–2010).

Source: Hong Kong Observatory (n.d.a).

Warning from 2000 to 2018. Although the frequency of issuing Cold Weather Warning was fluctuating downward among these 5 years, some years experienced a markedly high frequency of Cold Weather Warning, including 11 times in 2005, 10 times in 2012, and 11 times in 2014.

In 2016, Hong Kong experienced the most severe cold spell since 1957 (see Figures 7.4 and 7.5). The coldest record was found on 24 January 2016, with

Table 7.4 Frequency and length of cold weather warning in Hong Kong (2000–2018)

Year	Frequency	Effective day
2000	7	29
2001	7	22
2002	5	18
2003	7	20
2004	6	31
2005	11	45
2006	5	20
2007	5	20
2008	8	47
2009	6	31
2010	8	32
2011	9	51
2012	10	42
2013	6	28
2014	11	40
2015	3	13
2016	8	37
2017	4	18
2018	5	31

Source: Data extracted from Hong Kong Observatory (2013, 18a June).

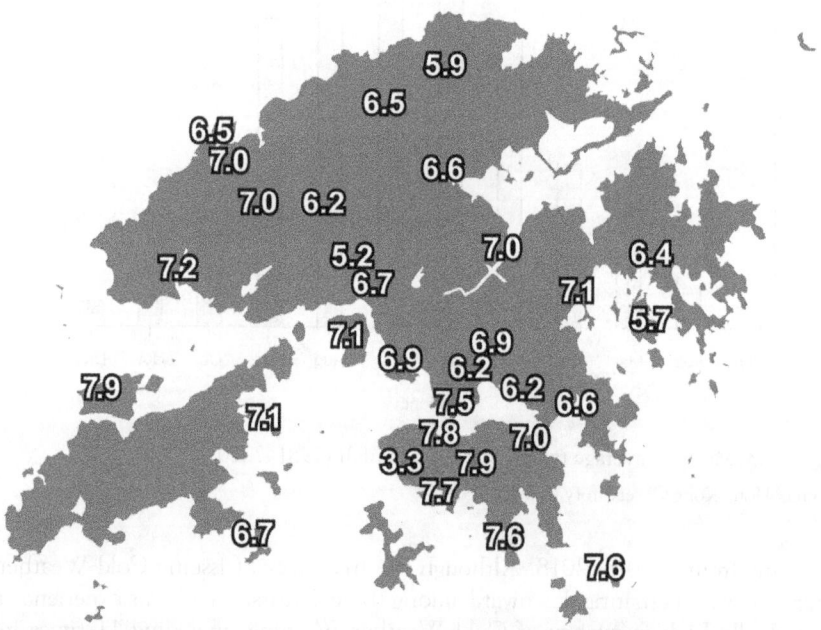

Figure 7.4 Air temperature in various locations in Hong Kong at 21:30 on 23 January 2016 (°C).

Source: Hong Kong Observatory (2016).

the daily minimum dropping to 3.1°C. Moreover, without central heating systems in most facilities of this subtropical city, widespread frost, rime, and other cold climate-related phenomena were found in some parts of New Territories (Hong Kong Observatory, 2017, 19c May). Due to the intense cold surge, more than 120 people were stranded on Tai Mo Shan, the highest hill in the territory, and nearby peaks on that day. More than 60 of them were taken to hospitals.

Rainfall

Hong Kong is among the cities with the highest rainfall in the Pacific Rim region. About 80% of its rainfall volume is recorded from May to September. The months with the most rainfall extend from June to August, while January and December are the driest months. Between 1981 and 2010, the average annual rainfall was 2,400 mm with an average of 138 rainy days, though the annual average rainfall varies greatly across Hong Kong (Hong Kong Observatory, 2015). The rainfall of Hong Kong is on the rise generally. Both the frequency of occurrence of heavy rain events and the annual number of heavy rain days are increasing (Hong Kong Observatory, 2018, 7 February). As the distribution of vector-borne disease is associated with rainfall and temperature, vectors could proliferate more quickly since heavy rain and hot weather become more frequent. For example, dengue fever was found positively associated with rainfall (Wu, Guo, Lung, Lin, & Su, 2007).

Windstorm and typhoon

Strong wind events such as tropical cyclones are the most common natural disaster in Hong Kong. From 1956 to 2017, the Hong Kong Observatory issued 16 Tropical Cyclone Warning Signals on average per year (Hong Kong Observatory, 2018, 16 April). The peak season for tropical cyclones in Hong Kong runs from July to September, but the city can be affected by gales between April and November. Tropical cyclones may also accompany storm surges, bringing the risks of flooding and in turn affecting human health. With the development of infrastructure in Hong Kong, the annual mortality of tropical cyclone has dropped below 20 since 1977 (Hong Kong Observatory, 2017, November). In terms of intensity of the typhoon, Typhoon Wanda in 1962 brought the historical minimum record of air pressure and the highest hourly mean wind speed (Hong Kong Observatory, 2018, September). Typhoon Mangkhut in 2018 triggered a record-breaking storm surge and caused severe flooding in many low-lying areas in Hong Kong (Hong Kong Observatory, 2018, September) (see Case Box 7.1).

Date	Maximum temperature (°C)	Mean temperature (°C)	Minimum temperature (°C)
1/1/2016	19.9	18.3	16.8
2/1/2016	21.7	18.9	17.2
3/1/2016	20.3	19.3	18.0
4/1/2016	22.3	20.6	19.1
5/1/2016	21.3	20.7	20.2
6/1/2016	24.3	20.9	19.2
7/1/2016	21.4	18.8	17.0
8/1/2016	21.0	18.4	16.5
9/1/2016	18.9	18.1	17.1
10/1/2016	18.5	18.0	17.2
11/1/2016	20.4	18.1	16.5
12/1/2016	18.5	17.3	16.1
13/1/2016	18.7	16.1	14.2
14/1/2016	17.5	16.5	15.6
15/1/2016	16.1	15.1	14.5
16/1/2016	17.1	16.4	15.5
17/1/2016	20.6	17.8	14.8
18/1/2016	17.8	15.2	11.9
19/1/2016	17.6	16.4	15.3
20/1/2016	16.8	15.5	14.8
21/1/2016	17.1	16.1	15.1
22/1/2016	16.2	14.1	10.3
23/1/2016	10.4	8.5	7.0
24/1/2016	7.1	4.9	3.1
25/1/2016	10.8	7.4	4.3
26/1/2016	13.5	10.4	8.1
27/1/2016	15.3	13.0	9.8
28/1/2016	17.4	16.1	14.8
29/1/2016	17.4	16.6	15.9
30/1/2016	19.9	17.6	16.2
31/1/2016	16.2	15.7	15.3
1/2/2016	15.6	12.4	10.7
2/2/2016	11.2	10.4	9.4
3/2/2016	14.3	12.5	10.3
4/2/2016	18.8	15.2	13.3

Figure 7.5 The cold wave in Hong Kong in January 2016.

Source: Hong Kong Observatory (2016, June).

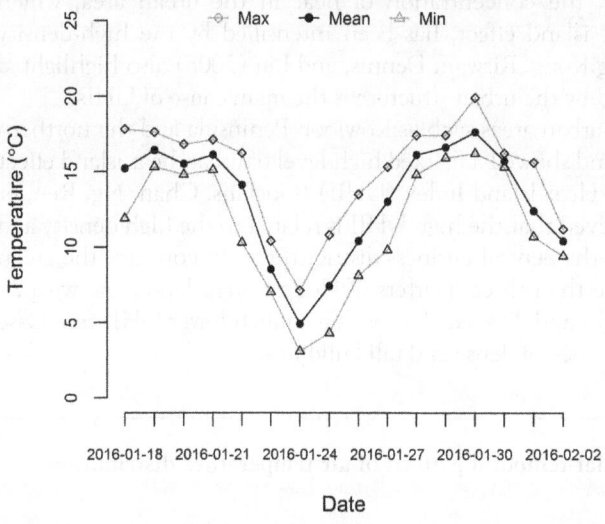

Figure 7.5 continued

Source: Hong Kong Observatory (2016, June).

Case Box 7.1 Typhoon injury study, 2018

In September 2018, Typhoon Mangkhut, the most severe typhoon affecting Hong Kong in three decades, swept across the Philippines, Hong Kong, and Macao. A population-based randomised telephone survey was conducted among Hong Kong adults soon after Typhoon Mangkhut's landing in the city in September 2018. While official report recorded 450 injuries in Hong Kong directly resulted from this typhoon, the study found an injury rate of 0.77% among its 521 respondents. Applying this event-specific injury rate to the city's 7.45 million residents during mid-2018 (Hong Kong Special Administrative Region Government Census and Statistics Department, 2019, 21 February), there might be more than 57,000 unreported injury cases of varying severity.

Source: Chan et al. (2019)

Urban environment

Heat island effect

High-rise buildings, the products of rapid urbanisation, are commonly found in Hong Kong. These high-rise structures intensify the climate change impact in Hong Kong, especially for the urban area. Urban heat islands (UHIs), a phenomenon related to the temperature of the urban area being generally higher than the surrounding rural area (Wang, Zhou, Ng, & Xu, 2016), is believed to have a close relationship with the urban setting. As Giridharan, Ganesan, and Lau (2004) explained, the concentration of heat in the urban area, which means the urban heat island effect, has been intensified by the high-density urban context in Hong Kong. Rizwan, Dennis, and Liu (2008) also highlighted that the heat generated by the urban structure is the main cause of UHIs.

In Hong Kong, the urban areas such as Kowloon Peninsula and the northern part of Hong Kong Island showed a marked high level of urban heat island effect as measured by Urban Heat Island Index (UHII) (Goggins, Chan, Ng, Ren, & Chen, 2012). It is believed that the high UHII is related to the high density and tall urban buildings in the central business district there. In contrast, the green areas constituting more than three-quarters of Hong Kong's land area, with 24 designated country parks and 22 special areas, have much lower UHII (see Case Box 7.2) due to the absence of dense and tall buildings.

Case Box 7.2 Spatial-temporal pattern of air temperature distribution in Hong Kong

By Ren Chao

Hong Kong is a high-density subtropical city. High-rise skyscrapers and a compact urban setting create its own unique built environment and complex urban morphology. How to develop a liveable high-density living environment especially under hot-humid summer time is a long-term urban development goal by local planners and government officials (Ren, 2018, August). The urban heat island (UHI) effect has been examined world-wide to indicate a temperature difference between urban and rural areas mainly caused by the impact of the built environment. However, only limited discussions in this aspect have been addressed for a spatial-temporal analysis on the intra-urban temperature variation in Hong Kong, which is important for climate-sensitive planning, as well as extremely hot weather-related heat risk management and actions (Shi et al., in press). In this study, first, hourly air temperature records from 40 Hong Kong Observatory stations from 2006 to 2015 were collected. Co-Kriging (Co-K), a geostatistical interpolation algorithm, was employed for spatial analysis of collected temperature records. Given Hong Kong's unique built environment characteristics, digital elevation model (DEM) information, sky view factor (SVF) information, and the normalised difference vegetation index (NDVI) as selected urban geometrical and environmental factors were incorporated in the Co-K interpolation to get a more comprehensive evaluation of impact of built environment on intra-urban temperature variation. The study results show that the night-time temperature of downtown area in Hong Kong cannot cool down below 28°C, which is a hot night indicator defined by the Hong Kong Observatory. It means that most of the nights in summer in Hong Kong are likely to be hot nights. This is caused by a high-density compact urban setting, which has a higher ability to trap heat in the daytime and releases less heat at night-time. Thus, the SVF among three selected urban environmental parameters is an important factor not only to intensify intra-urban temperature differences, but also to identify summer hotspot areas in Hong Kong (see Figure 7.6).

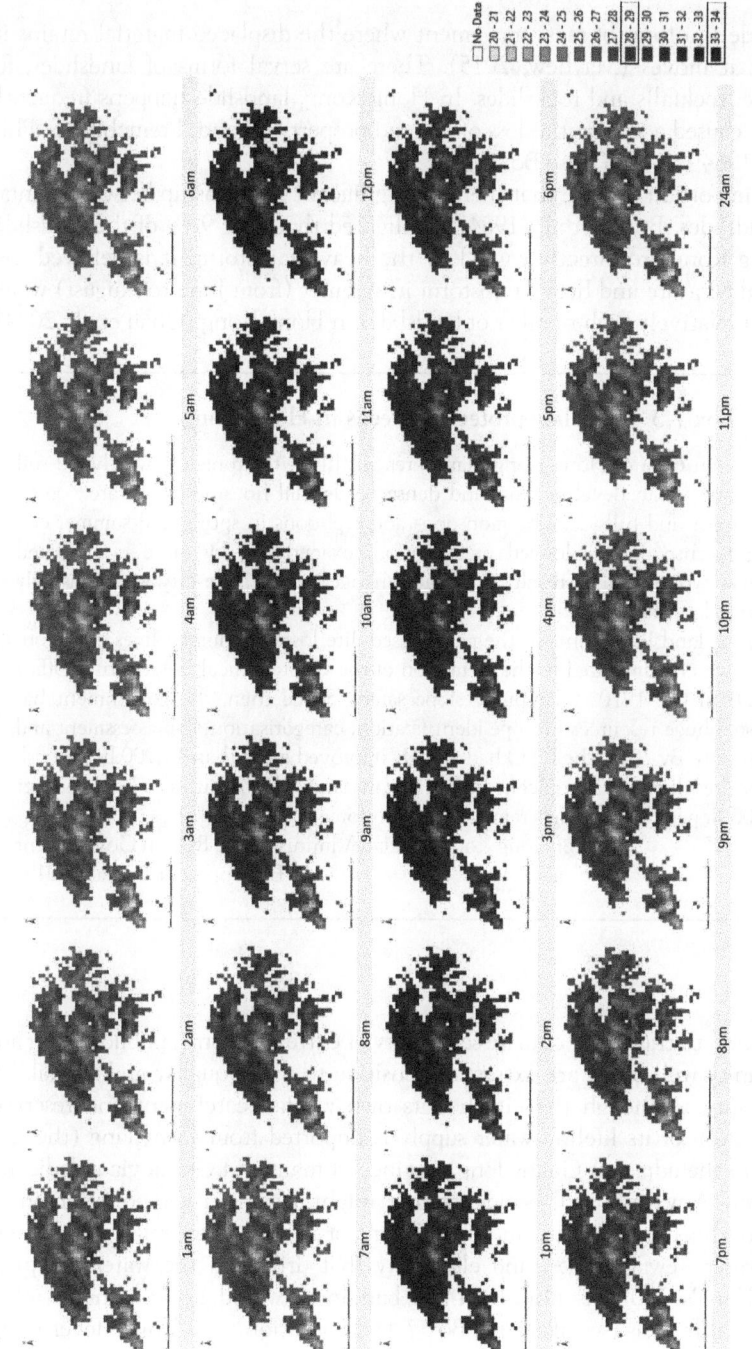

Figure 7.6 Spatial-temporal pattern of air temperature distribution in Hong Kong.

Landslides

Landslide is a form of mass movement where the displaced material retains its form as it moves (Mayhew, 2015). There are serval forms of landslides, for instance, rockfalls and rockslides. In Hong Kong, landslide happens frequently and has caused a substantial loss of life and property (Brand, Premchitt, & Phillipson, 1984 (see also Case Box 7.3).

It is important to note that there is a significant relationship between rainfall and landslides. Brand et al. (1984) highlighted that over 90% of the landslides in Hong Kong are directly caused by the heavy rainstorm. It is believed that high temperature and heavy rainstorm in summer (from June to August) would trigger a relatively high number of landslides in Hong Kong (Chau et al., 2004).

Case Box 7.3 Landslide protection needs in Hong Kong

More than 60% of Hong Kong's land area is hilly with tropically weathered soil and many urban developments and dense residential housing are located on or near slopes and hillside. The monsoons and typhoons in spring and summer can bring intense and prolonged precipitation, exacerbated by more rainfall and stronger typhoons as a result of climate change. Hence, the city is increasingly prone to landslide hazards.

Some landslide events in the past caused dire losses in human lives and properties, which cumulated in the formation of the Geotechnical Engineering Office (GEO) in the 1970s to improve slope safety. Since then, the government has invested huge resources in slope identification, categorisation, risk assessment and protection. By 2015, the GEO had already improved more than 11,000 higher risk slopes, resulting in significant reduction in landslide fatalities, while another 17,000 slopes close to roads remain to be reinforced.

Source: Hong Kong Special Administrative Region Government
Environment Bureau (2015)

Water

In addition to the urban climate sensitivity of extreme events, public health and community well-being are extremely sensitive to water quality and availability in this city. Although the city has its own rainfall catchment and reservoir system, 80% of its lifeline water supply is imported from Dongjiang (the East River) in the adjacent Guangdong province of mainland China via a dedicated aqueduct. Any industrial accidents that might lead to river pollution in its neighbourhood community and breakdowns of lifeline water-related infrastructure (water, sewage pipes, and electricity that drives all the water pumps in Hong Kong's 300 plus ultra-high-rise buildings) would bring a major urban public health crisis (see also Case Box 7.4). In addition, as a dengue-fever-prone coastal metropolis, stagnant water management and water quality of its beaches, marine, and rivers are all significant to human health.

Case Box 7.4 Lifeline infrastructure: water and sewage in Hong Kong

A safe, reliable, affordable, and easily accessible water supply is essential for good health. In cities, community well-being and public health protection rely heavily on the integrity and reliability of lifeline infrastructure that supports water supply and sewage systems.

Hong Kong is one of the most densely populated vertical cities globally with the highest number of high-rise buildings that exceed 150 metres. Public health and community well-being in this city are extremely sensitive to water availability. Although the city has its own rainfall catchment and reservoir system, 80% of its water supply relies on Dongjiang (the East River) of Guangdong Province of mainland China via a dedicated aqueduct. Any industrial accidents that might lead to the pollution of Dongjiang and breakdowns of lifeline water-related infrastructure (e.g. water, sewage pipes, and electricity which drives all the water-related pumps within Hong Kong's 300-plus ultra-high-rise buildings) would bring a major urban public health crisis to the city. In addition, as a dengue fever-prone, sea-side metropolis, stagnant water management and water quality of its beaches, marine, rivers, and sewage are all significant for human health. The potential impact of climate change on rainfall and on vector-borne disease highlights the vulnerability and urban resilience towards water and sewage issues in this urban context.

Source: Chan and Ho (2019)

Case Box 7.5 Lifeline infrastructure: electricity supply in Hong Kong

Losing electricity power even on a modest scale can have disastrous consequences in a metropolis like Hong Kong, and a large-scale power loss due to an extreme weather event could lead to multiple failures. In Hong Kong, the two power companies conduct regular weather-related assessments and drills, particularly ahead of each year's typhoon season.

CLP Power Hong Kong (CLP) supplies electricity to 80% of the city's residents in Kowloon and the New Territories. The Hongkong Electric Company (HEC) provides electricity to the rest of the residents on Hong Kong Island and Lamma Island. For the former, more than 30% of its network is carried through overhead lines, with more than 700 transmission pylons. While these overhead lines and transmission pylons are vulnerable to extreme weather events, the power supply system was designed to allow for an alternative pylon or supply circuit to maintain electricity supplies in the event of the failure of a pylon or a circuit due to strong winds or landslips. For HEC, overhead lines have been gradually phased out since 2012. Its power transmission and distribution network now consists mainly of cable tunnels and underground power cables, which are more resilient against adverse weather conditions. Both companies have also deployed advanced cable diagnostic techniques to identify and replace weak components to reduce risk of failure.

Source: Hong Kong Special Administrative Region Government
Environment Bureau (2015)

Socio-economic demographic patterns

Hong Kong, a highly developed city in China, has one of the world's highest intra-city income inequalities and one of the world's highest average increase of urban ambient temperatures during the past century. It also has one of the lowest birth rates (53.7 per 1,000 at the end of 2018) and fertility rates (1,125 per 1,000 female population in 2017) in the world. At the end of 2018, the death rate was 47.0 per 1,000; children below the age of 10 and teens each constituted 7.7% of the population, while those above the age of 59 accounted for 24.9% (Hong Kong Special Administrative Region Government Census and Statistics Department [CSD], 2019, 19, 21 February). In 2017, the life expectancies at birth for males and females were 81.9 and 87.6 years respectively, and the proportion of educational attainment at degree level for population aged 15 and over was 24.4% (Hong Kong Special Administrative Region Government Centre for Health Protection [CHP], n.d.b; Hong Kong Special Administrative Region Government Education Bureau, 2018, April).

The public and private health expenditures were estimated to be 3.7% and 2.8% of the GDP respectively in 2015 (Hong Kong Special Administrative Region Government Food and Health Bureau [FHB], 2008). The top 10 killers in 2017 in descending order were malignant neoplasms, pneumonia, diseases of heart, cerebrovascular diseases, external causes of morbidity and mortality, nephritis, nephrotic syndrome, and nephrosis, chronic lower respiratory diseases, dementia, septicaemia, and diabetes (CHP, n.d.a.).

In 2016, migrants residing in Hong Kong for fewer than 10 years from mainland China, Macao, and Taiwan constituted 5.4% of the population, while those from other places accounted for 5.3% (CSD, 2017, February), and there were more than 700,000 migrants from mainland China from 2002 to 2016, who had lower education attainment than the overall population, median monthly employment earnings, and median monthly household income (Hong Kong Special Administrative Region Legislative Council Secretariat Research Office, 2018, March). They may also have a lower vaccination rate.

As to the city's economic base, service industries constituted 92.4% of the GDP in 2017, while agriculture, fishing, mining, and quarrying was 0.1%, manufacturing 1.1%, electricity, gas and water supply, and waste management 1.4%, and construction 5.1% (CSD, 2019, 27 February).

It is notable that socio-economic characteristics of Hong Kong people were found to be associated with various disparities in health outcomes. If there is a 1°C increase in the daily mean temperature above 28.2°C, it is estimated that the mortality rate will increase by 1.8%. Some vulnerable groups were found to have higher heat-mortality rate, including those of lower socio-economic status and unknown residence, and married people (Chan et al., 2010). Chen, Ding, Yang, Hu, and Qi (2018) also indicated that with a high social vulnerability, the heat health risks in some less urbanised cities and suburban areas in China would also be increased.

Potential impact of climate change on health

In addition to the common meteorological impact of temperature, rainfall, and sea-level rise on its population, extreme weather events might also affect the well-being of urban population in this city. There have been a number of observable climate-related pattern changes during the past few decades. Table 7.5 highlights some of these patterns. With all its essential service and lifeline support of water, electricity, and sewage hinging on its modern but potentially vulnerable infrastructure, ensuring the resilience of such infrastructure is essential to protect well-being and health in the city (see Cases Boxes 7.4, 7.5, and 7.6).

Case Box 7.6 Climate change policies in Hong Kong

The Hong Kong government issued an action in 2017, outlining the mitigation, adaptation, and resilience-building policies to reduce carbon emissions and the potential impact of climate change by the year 2030. The mitigation policies include phasing down coal in local electricity production, the use of renewable energy, making buildings and infrastructure of the city more energy efficient, improving public transport, controlling private car growth, promoting walking and cycling, reducing urban heat island effect through landscaping, and promoting low carbon footprint lifestyle choices in clothing, food, and overseas travel, The aim is to reduce Hong Kong's carbon intensity by 65–70% from the 2005 level and per capita carbon emission to 3.3–3.8 tonnes by 2030. This involves the reduction of energy intensity by 40% by 2050. The adaptation policies cover infrastructure improvement such as slope safety, integrating drainage and flood management, sea-level rise and coastal protection, and green roofs; city planning like a new code of practice on wind effects, urban climatic planning, and urban regeneration; water security in terms of multi-source water supply structure and water conservation campaign; and promoting conservation and biodiversity. Resilience-building policies include preparing for emergencies, dealing with extreme heat, and raising community awareness.

Source: Hong Kong Special Administrative Region Government
Environment Bureau (2015)

Conclusion

The following chapters will use climate and health studies conducted in Hong Kong as examples to discuss the patterns and impacts of implications of climate change in this urban city.

Table 7.5 Some examples of changes in climate-related patterns in Hong Kong observed within the past few decades

Temperature	Rainfall	Sea-level rise	Disasters and extreme weather events
Increased by 1°C, extreme high temperature days (above 33°C) increased by 10 times (Hong Kong Observatory, 2017, 20b July; 2018, 3b October)	Number of very wet years (annual rainfall > 3,168 mm): increased by 4 times from last century to this century (Hong Kong Observatory, 2017, 20a July) Annual total rainfall rose 40 mm per decade (Hong Kong Observatory, 2018, 7 February) Annual number of heavy rain days (hourly rainfall > 30mm) increased 0.3 days per decade (Hong Kong Observatory, 2018, 7 February)	Sea-level rise: 31 mm per decade (Hong Kong Observatory, 2018, 9 January) Maximum sea level during storm surge: 3.53 m for Typhoon Hagupit (2008); 3.88 m for Typhoon Mangkhut (2018); 3.96 m for Typhoon Wanda (1962); 4.05 m for an unnamed typhoon (1937) (Hong Kong Observatory, 2017, 19b May; 2018, 3c October)	More extreme events: Typhoon Hagupit (2008): • 16 major urban floods with island population evacuated; • 58 injuries; • 4,500 trees collapsed Typhoon Mangkhut (2018): • 46 reported floods • more than 450 injured • 46,000 trees collapsed • 600 roads blocked • a sewage plant damaged • railway system and transport system paralysed

Source: Hong Kong Observatory (2016, June).

References

Brand, E. W., Premchitt, J., & Phillipson, H. B. (1984). Relationship between rainfall and landslides in Hong Kong. *Proceedings of the 4th International Symposium on Landslides* (pp. 276–284). Toronto.

Central Intelligence Agency. (n.d.). *The world factbook* [online]. Retrieved from www.cia.gov/library/publications/the-world-factbook/rankorder/2172rank.html.

Chan, E., Goggins, W., Kim, J., & Griffiths, S. (2010). A study of intracity variation of temperature-related mortality and socioeconomic status among the Chinese population in Hong Kong. *Journal of Epidemiology and Community Health, 66*(4), 322–327.

Chan E. Y. Y., & Ho, J. Y. (2019). Urban water and health issues in Hong Kong. In B. Ray & R. Shaw (Eds.), *Urban drought: Emerging water challenges in Asia* (pp. 241–262). Singapore: Springer.

Chan, E. Y. Y., Man, A. Y. T., Lam, H. C. Y., Chan, G. K. W., Hall, B. J., & Hung, K. K. C. (2019). Is urban household emergency preparedness associated with short-term impact reduction after a super typhoon in subtropical city? *International Journal of Environmental Research and Public Health, 16*(3), 596.

Chau, K., Sze, Y., Fung, M., Wong, W., Fong, E., & Chan, L. (2004). Landslide hazard analysis for Hong Kong using landslide inventory and GIS. *Computers & Geosciences, 30*(4), 429–443.

Chen, Q., Ding, M., Yang, X., Hu, K., & Qi, J. (2018). Spatially explicit assessment of heat health risk by using multi-sensor remote sensing images and socioeconomic data in Yangtze River Delta, China. *International Journal of Health Geographics, 17*(1).

Giridharan, R., Ganesan, S., & Lau, S. (2004). Daytime urban heat island effect in high-rise and high-density residential developments in Hong Kong. *Energy and Buildings, 36*(6), 525–534.

Goggins, W., Chan, E., Ng, E., Ren, C., & Chen, L. (2012). Effect modification of the association between short-term meteorological factors and mortality by urban heat islands in Hong Kong. *PLOS One, 7*(6), e38551.

Hong Kong Observatory. (n.d.a). Local climate highlight [online]. Retrieved from www.hko.gov.hk/m/hkclimate.htm.

Hong Kong Observatory. (n.d.b). Temperature categories for Hong Kong in various seasons [online]. Retrieved from www.hko.gov.hk/wxinfo/season/catTT_81-10_e.htm.

Hong Kong Observatory. (2013, 18a June). HKO Warnings and signals database: Cold Weather Warning [online]. Retrieved from www.hko.gov.hk/cgi-bin/hko/warndb_e1.pl?opt=12&start_ym=200001&end_ym=201812&submit=Submit+Query.

Hong Kong Observatory. (2013, 18b June). HKO Warnings and signals database: Very Hot Weather Warning [online]. Retrieved from www.hko.gov.hk/cgi-bin/hko/warndb_e1.pl?opt=13&start_ym=200001&end_ym=201810&submit=%E6%90%9C%E5%B0%8B.

Hong Kong Observatory. (2015). Climate of Hong Kong [online]. Retrieved from www.hko.gov.hk/cis/climahk_e.htm.

Hong Kong Observatory. (2016). Automatic regional weather forecast [online]. Retrieved from www.hko.gov.hk/contente.htm.

Hong Kong Observatory. (2016, June). Daily extract of meteorological observations, January 2016 [online]. Retrieved from www.hko.gov.hk/cis/dailyExtract_e.htm?y=2016&m=1.

Hong Kong Observatory. (2017, February). Climatological information services: Extract of annual data [online]. Retrieved from www.hko.gov.hk/cis/yearlyExtract_e.htm#table2.

Hong Kong Observatory. (2017, 19a May). Cold and Very Hot Weather Warnings [online]. Retrieved from www.hko.gov.hk/wservice/warning/coldhot.htm.

Hong Kong Observatory. (2017, 19b May). Significant storm surge events in Hong Kong before 1954 [online]. Retrieved from www.hko.gov.hk/wservice/tsheet/pms/storm surgedb_notes_e.htm.

Hong Kong Observatory. (2017, 19c May). The year's weather—2016 [online]. Retrieved from www.hko.gov.hk/wxinfo/pastwx/2016/ywx2016.htm.

Hong Kong Observatory. (2017, 20a July). Climate projections for Hong Kong: Rainfall [online]. Retrieved from www.hko.gov.hk/climate_change/proj_hk_rainfall_e.htm.

Hong Kong Observatory. (2017, 20b July). Climate projections for Hong Kong: Temperature [online]. Retrieved from www.hko.gov.hk/climate_change/proj_hk_temp_e.htm.

Hong Kong Observatory. (2017, November). Casualties and damage caused by tropical cyclones in Hong Kong since 1960 [online]. Retrieved from www.weather.gov.hk/informtc/historical_tc/cdtc.htm.

Hong Kong Observatory. (2018, 9 January). Climate change in Hong Kong: Mean sea level [online]. Retrieved from www.hko.gov.hk/climate_change/obs_hk_sea_level_e.htm.

Hong Kong Observatory. (2018, 7 February). Climate change in Hong Kong: Rainfall [online]. Retrieved from www.hko.gov.hk/climate_change/obs_hk_rainfall_e.htm.

Hong Kong Observatory. (2018, 10 April). Rainstorm warning system [online]. Retrieved from www.hko.gov.hk/wservice/warning/rainstor.htm.

Hong Kong Observatory. (2018, 16 April). Frequency and total duration of display of tropical cyclone warning signals: 1956–2017 [online]. Retrieved from www.hko.gov.hk/informtc/historical_tc/fttcw.htm.

Hong Kong Observatory. (2018, September). Typhoons necessitating the issuing of the Hurricane Signal No. 10 [online]. Retrieved from www.hko.gov.hk/informtc/historical_tc/histtype.htm.

Hong Kong Observatory. (2018, 3a October). Climatological information services: Number of cold days observed at the Hong Kong Observatory since 1884, exclude 1940–1946 [online]. Retrieved from www.weather.gov.hk/cis/statistic/coldday_statistic_e.htm.

Hong Kong Observatory. (2018, 3b October). Climatological information services: Number of very hot days observed at the Hong Kong Observatory since 1884, exclude 1940–1946 [online]. Retrieved from www.hko.gov.hk/cis/statistic/vhotday_statistic_e.htm.

Hong Kong Observatory. (2018, 3c October). Storm surge records in Hong Kong during the passage of tropical cyclones: Database record since 1954 [online]. Retrieved from www.hko.gov.hk/wservice/tsheet/pms/stormsurgedb_e.htm.

Hong Kong Special Administrative Region Government. (2018). *Hong Kong 2017*. Hong Kong: Author. Retrieved from www.yearbook.gov.hk/2017/en/index.html.

Hong Kong Special Administrative Region Government Census and Statistics Department [CSD]. (2017, February). 2016 population by-census: Main tables [online]. Retrieved from www.bycensus2016.gov.hk/en/bc-mt.html.

Hong Kong Special Administrative Region Government Census and Statistics Department. (2019, 19 February). Population estimates: Publications and tables [online]. Retrieved from www.censtatd.gov.hk/hkstat/sub/sp150.jsp?tableID=004&ID=0&productType=8.

Hong Kong Special Administrative Region Government Census and Statistics Department. (2019, 21 February). Population: Overview: Latest statistics [online]. Retrieved from www.censtatd.gov.hk/hkstat/sub/so20.jsp.

Hong Kong Special Administrative Region Government Census and Statistics Department. (2019, 27 February). National income: Publications and tables [online].

Retrieved from www.censtatd.gov.hk/hkstat/sub/sp250.jsp?tableID=036&ID=0&product Type=8.

Hong Kong Special Administrative Region Government Centre for Health Protection [CHP]. (n.d.a). Death rates by leading causes of death, 2001–2017 [online]. Retrieved from www.chp.gov.hk/en/statistics/data/10/27/117.html.

Hong Kong Special Administrative Region Government Centre for Health Protection. (n.d.b). Life expectancy at birth (male and female), 1971–2017 [online]. Retrieved from www.chp.gov.hk/en/statistics/data/10/27/111.html.

Hong Kong Special Administrative Region Government Education Bureau. (2018, April). Distribution of educational attainment of population aged 15 and over [online]. Retrieved from www.edb.gov.hk/en/about-edb/publications-stat/figures/educational-attainment.html.

Hong Kong Special Administrative Region Government Environment Bureau. (2015). *Hong Kong climate change report 2015*. Retrieved from www.enb.gov.hk/sites/default/files/pdf/ClimateChangeEng.pdf.

Hong Kong Special Administrative Region Government Environment Bureau. (2017). *Hong Kong's climate action plan 2030+*. Retrieved from www.enb.gov.hk/sites/default/files/pdf/ClimateActionPlanEng.pdf.

Hong Kong Special Administrative Region Government Food and Health Bureau [FHB]. (2008). *Projection of Hong Kong's healthcare expenditure*. Retrieved from www.fhb.gov.hk/beStrong/files/consultation/projecthealthexp_eng.pdf.

Hong Kong Special Administrative Region Legislative Council Secretariat Research Office. (2018, March). *Livelihood of new arrivals from the Mainland*. Retrieved from www.legco.gov.hk/research-publications/english/1718issh18-livelihood-of-new-arrivals-from-the-mainland-20180323-e.pdf.

Mayhew, S. (2015). Landslide. In *A Dictionary of Geography*, 5th ed. Oxford, United Kingdom: Oxford University Press. Retrieved from www.oxfordreference.com/view/10.1093/acref/9780199680856.001.0001/acref-9780199680856-e-1804?rskey=3d1Yxa&result=1.

Ren, C., (2018, August). Urban climate science for planning healthy cities in Asia. Paper presented at the 10th International Conference on Urban Climate, New York, NY.

Rizwan, A., Dennis, L., & Liu, C. (2008). A review on the generation, determination and mitigation of urban heat island. *Journal of Environmental Sciences*, 20(1), 120–128.

Shi, Y., Ren, C., Meng, C., Lau, K. K.-L., Lee, T. C., Choy, C.-W., Ng, E. (in press). Assessing spatial variability of extreme hot weather conditions in Hong Kong: A land use regression approach. *Environmental Research*.

The Skyscraper Center. (2018). Cities ranked by number of 150m+ completed buildings [online]. Retrieved from www.skyscrapercenter.com/cities.

Wang, W., Zhou, W., Ng, E., & Xu, Y. (2016). Urban heat islands in Hong Kong: Statistical modeling and trend detection. *Natural Hazards*, 83(2), 885–907.

World Bank. (n.d.). *Indicators* [online]. Retrieved from https://data.worldbank.org/indicator.

Wu, P. C., Guo, H. R., Lung, S. C., Lin, C. Y., & Su, H. J. (2007). Weather as an effective predictor for occurrence of dengue fever in Taiwan. *Acta Trop, 103*, 50–57.

8 Health impact of extreme temperature and heat island effect on mortality

Published literature has shown human mortality varies with acclimatisation, demographics, and socio-economic characteristics. The International Panel on Climate Change (IPCC) projects that changing weather patterns will increase temperature-related mortality risks around the world (IPCC, 2007). A number of articles have demonstrated the heat-related health impact in urban context (Braga, Zanobetti, & Schwartz, 2001; McMichael et al., 2008) and a multi-country comparative study found that the pattern of heat-related mortality varied with average city income in urban settings (Hajat, Armstrong, Gouveia, & Wilkinson, 2005). In high-income cities, older people were more vulnerable to heat-related mortality, while in low-income cities mortality tended to accumulate for young population. Extreme temperature events and periods of elevated temperature, in particular, are expected to contribute to a greater burden of mortality and morbidity in both high- and low-income settings (McMichael et al., 2008; Pirard et al., 2005).

Asia is the region with the fastest growing metropolis around the world. Hong Kong, a major city in southern China, has one of the world's highest income inequalities and one of the world's highest average increases in urban ambient temperatures (see also Chapter 7). This chapter describes a number of studies that investigated the temperature impact on mortality in this city. Both hot and cold temperature impacts on this subtropical city and intra-city variation of mortality patterns in this vertical-based urban community and socio-demographic predictors of intra-city impacts will be discussed. Findings of how the "heat island effect" associated with unintended urban design may have impacts on health outcomes for certain segments of the community will also be explored.

The temperature–morbidity model in Hong Kong

Hong Kong has one of the world's highest average increase of urban ambient temperature during the past century. For the 21st century, the Hong Kong Observatory (HKO) predicts that annual mean temperature will rise by 3–6°C (Hong Kong Observatory, 2015). To understand the temperature mortality relationship in urban context, a number of retrospective ecological studies based on routine mortality, temperature, and pollution data were conducted (Chan, Goggins, Kim, & Griffiths, 2012). In the models used in these studies, mortality data (including age, gender, marital status, reported previous country of residence, area of residence, and cause of death) between 1998 and 2006 were obtained from the Hong Kong Census and Statistics Department. Mean daily temperatures, dew point temperatures, and mean humidity were obtained from the HKO. Pollution levels in daily means were calculated from hourly concentrations of nitrogen dioxide (NO_2), sulphur dioxide (SO_2), ozone (O_3), and PM_{10} (also known as respirable suspended particulates (RSP)) from 11 general environmental collection stations of the Hong Kong Environmental Protection Department (EPD). Average weekly consultation rates for influenza-like illnesses reported by general outpatient clinics (GOPCs) and general practitioners (GPs) were obtained from the Centre for Health Promotion to use as a proxy indicator to control for the influence of influenza epidemics on mortality. Median monthly domestic household incomes according to government tertiary planning units (TPUs), the smallest geographic unit for which data may be available for analysis, were obtained as a measure of neighbourhood socioeconomic status.

Socio-demographic variables were classified as ≥85, 75–84, and 0–74 and marital status as married or non-married. Neighbourhood socio-economic status (SES) was obtained from the median monthly domestic household income in the TPU of area of residence, which was categorised as "SES Low" (≤HK$15,000 per month/US$23,077 per year), "SES Medium" (HK$15,001–25,000 per month/US$23,077–38,462 per year) and "SES High" (>HK$25,000 per month/US$28,462 per year). Migration status was derived from "reported previous country of residence" as "locals", "migrants from China", and "other countries". A measure of urban design was created by grouping "areas of residence" into: (i) Hong Kong Island (less densely populated coastal residence with good ambient air ventilation, younger population); (ii) Kowloon (most densely populated area, with urban planning characterised by rows of 80+ storey buildings that block district ambient air ventilation); (iii) New Territories (less densely populated new towns, younger population); and (iv) Unknown (including population who were homeless, street sleepers, with transient status, living in area with no official residence district or with unknown residence status). Cause of death was considered as cancer and non-cancer, and further divided into 10 subtypes (cardiovascular, respiratory, nephritis, diabetes, septicaemia, aortic aneurism, cirrhosis, respiratory infections, stroke, and others).

Poisson generalised additive models (GAMs) were constructed to examine the association between daily mean temperature and daily deaths from natural causes during the warm season (May through October). Confounders considered were air pollution, day of the week, and influenza circulation. In several Asian cities, using an average lag of 0–1 days for pollutants had the strongest effect on mortality. NO_2, SO_2, RSP, and O_3 were controlled for by using linear terms for the average of the same day and a lag of 1 day for each pollutant. Day of the week and holidays were controlled for by using indicator variables. Influenza was controlled for using a linear function of the average weekly cases reported to GPs and GOPCs.

Cubic smoothing spline functions with 40 degrees of freedom (df) were used to control for seasonality and long-term time trends. For annual data, 7 df per year is often used; but since the study model only considered 6 months, we used 3.5 df per year plus 8 df for bridging the gap between adjacent years. The assumptions of the quasipoisson distribution family were used to account for possible data overdispersion. Model residuals were checked for autocorrelation. Sensitivity analysis was performed by varying the degree of freedom for smooth functions of time and temperature for the models (Chan et al., 2012). In the final models, two linear terms were adopted to model the temperature effect on mortality. To account for the heat effect, "same day mean daily temperature − 28.2 for days > 28.2°C and 0 for days ≤ 28.2°C" was used. For modelling the cool effect, a linear term, "28.2 − average of mean temperature for lags 0–7 for days with average of mean lag 0–7 temperature < 28.2°C, 0 for days for which this average ≥ 28°C" was used. The threshold temperature was estimated graphically. For more details, refer to Chan et al. (2012).

Results of the Chan et al. (2012) study found 28.2°C to be a critical threshold for elevated non-accidental mortality during the warm season in Hong Kong—a city that has had one of the highest income inequalities globally and the fastest increase of ambient urban temperature within the past century (United Nations Development Programme, 2006). The overall temperature–mortality threshold was found to be slightly higher than that found for stroke death using maximum temperature in Hong Kong (Leung, Yip, & Yeung, 2008) and higher than the threshold found for European cities (Hajat et al., 2006). Nevertheless, the Hong Kong model findings are consistent with other Asia-specific studies (Kan, Jia, & Chen, 2003; Kim, Ha, & Park, 2006; McMichael et al., 2008; Simon, 2006; Tan et al., 2007) that found mortality thresholds for Bangkok (29°C) and Chiang Mai (28°C) in Thailand and Delhi in India (29°C). Perhaps due to better infrastructure development and greater access to air conditioning in Hong Kong (Electric and Mechanical Services Department [EMSD] of the Government of the Hong Kong Special Administrative Region, 2007), the percentage increase in daily mortality for 1°C increase above these thresholds was higher in these Asian cities (range from 2.4% to 5.8%) than in Hong Kong (1.8%). A study in Shanghai, China also hypothesised that the increased use of air conditioning might have contributed to the lower heatwave-related mortality rate in 2003 when compared with 1998 (Kan et al., 2007). Meanwhile, in the Chan et al. (2012) study, the mortality in Hong Kong was found to increase as temperature increased between 22.0°C and 28.2°C, but the mortality increase appeared higher on the same day when compared with the mortality increase in later days (i.e. days 2–7). This mortality displacement could be due to "harvesting" (Braga et al., 2001), where mortality is concentrated on the day of elevated temperature but subsequently decline because very vulnerable individuals have been removed from the population. Another possible explanation for the temperature–mortality association difference above and below 28.2°C may be related to the potential longer-term cool effects that may have offset the short-term heat effects at temperatures lower than 28.2°C.

Table 8.1 shows the relative risks of temperature-related mortality per 3°C increase and decrease in a single day's average daily temperature above 28.2°C for Hong Kong during 1998–2006. On average, a 1.0°C increase in mean temperature above 28.2°C for a particular day was associated with an estimated 1.8% increase in mortality. Deaths among women (RR = 1.068, 95% CI: 1.017–1.121, $p = 0.008$) were more sensitive to higher temperatures than among men (RR = 1.045, 95% CI: 1.001–1.092, $p = 0.046$). Age was collapsed into two groups (0–74 and ≥75) because estimates for the 75–84 and >85 age groups were almost identical.

After stratification, minor differences were found between males and females of those less than 75 years old in terms of sensitivity of daily mortality to higher temperature (RR (male) = 1.067 versus RR (female) = 1.061) but a much larger gender difference in sensitivity for those ≥75 (RR (male) = 1.014 versus RR (female) = 1.076). Temperature-related mortality was negatively associated with socio-economic status (SES) with the strongest effects for those living in low SES areas, a weaker effect for those in medium SES areas, and no apparent effect for those in high SES areas. Urban design had little effect on the temperature–mortality relationship but those with unknown residence (RR = 1.278, 95% CI: 1.058–1.545, $p = 0.011$) were more vulnerable to heat effects, as were married people. Some groups were found to be more vulnerable to heat-related mortality within the urban community, specifically those with lower socio-economic status, perhaps due to chronic health problems, their inability to afford air conditioners or their greater reluctance to use air conditioners owing to the electricity costs. As such, specific health protection strategies may be necessary to protect vulnerable groups from the adverse health impact of elevated temperature.

In addition, similar to other studies, cardiovascular and respiratory deaths were found to be more sensitive to daily temperature fluctuations (Braga, Zanobetti, & Schwartz, 2002; Hajat, Kovats, & Lachowycz, 2007; Saez, Sunyer, Castellsagué, Murillo, & Antó, 1995). Findings indicated that heat might affect several other non-cancer causes of death. Stratification by cause of death showed that cancer deaths were insensitive to temperature changes while non-cancer deaths (RR = 1.086, 95% CI: 1.041–1.132, $p < 0.001$) were associated with elevated temperature. Table 4.3 shows relative risks of cause-specific mortality corresponding to 3°C increases and decrease in a single day's average daily temperature above 28.2°C for Hong Kong, 1998–2006. Deaths from cardiovascular diseases (RR = 1.085, 95% CI: 1.014–1.162) and respiratory infections (RR = 1.102, 95% CI: 0.997–1.217, $p = 0.053$) were sensitive to elevated temperature above 28.2°C. However, there was a different pattern of temperature mortality for decreasing mean temperature below 28.2°C during the warm season. Whilst migrant status and SES status were not significant effect modifiers, deaths among men (RR = 1.039, 95% CI: 0.995–1.085, $p = 0.021$), those aged ≥75 (RR = 1.040, 95% CI: 1.007–1.075, $p = 0.019$), those with unknown

Table 8.1 Relative risks of mortality corresponding to 3°C increase and decrease in a single day's average daily temperature above 28.2°C for Hong Kong during 1998–2006

Variables	3.0°C increase above 28.2°C		3.0°C decrease below 28.2°C		$N^\dagger$
	Relative risk (95% CI)	p-value	Relative risk (95% CI)	p-value	
All	1.055 (1.022,1.090)	0.001	1.021 (0.997,1.046)	0.022	129,688
Previous residence‡ (proxy for migration status)					
Hong Kong	1.057 (0.981, 1.140)	0.146	1.024 (0.968, 1.083)	0.406	24,393
China	1.050 (1.012,1.090)	0.010	1.022 (0.994,1.051)	0.127	99,195
Gender					
Male	1.045 (1.001,1.092)	0.046	1.039 (0.995,1.085)	0.021	72,148
Female	1.068 (1.017,1.121)	0.008	1.000 (0.964,1.037)	0.990	57,538
Age					
≥75 yrs.	1.047 (1.002,1.094)	0.043	1.040 (1.007,1.075)	0.019	70,466
<75 yrs.	1.065 (1.015,1.118)	0.011	0.998 (0.963,1.035)	0.928	52,793
Gender and age					
Male ≥75 yrs.	1.014 (0.951,1.082)	0.666	1.058 (1.008,1.110)	0.023	33,254
Male <75 yrs.	1.067 (1.005,1.133)	0.034	1.023 (0.979,1.070)	0.308	38,546
Female ≥75 yrs.	1.076 (1.012,1.143)	0.019	1.025 (0.979,1.072)	0.297	37,212
Female <75 yrs.	1.061 (0.976,1.153)	0.117	0.952 (0.895,1.013)	0.117	20,070

	Model A HR (95% CI)	p	Model B HR (95% CI)	p	N
SES of residential area*					
Low	1.065 (0.998,1.909)	0.056	0.981 (0.934,1.032)	0.461	38,249
Medium	1.038 (0.989,1.089)	0.129	1.029 (0.991,1.067)	0.135	68,952
High	1.003 (0.904,1.112)	0.961	1.015 (0.938,1.099)	0.708	15,080
Area of residence (proxy for urban design)					
Hong Kong	1.043 (0.964,1.129)	0.296	1.022 (0.962,1.085)	0.489	25,954
Kowloon	1.041 (0.981,1.104)	0.183	1.004 (0.960,1.051)	0.852	46,974
New Territories	1.042 (0.984,1.103)	0.158	1.015 (0.972,1.061)	0.496	49,172
Unknown	1.278 (1.058,1.545)	0.011	1.313 (1.129,1.528)	0.000	7,261
Marital status					
Married	1.055 (1.007,1.105)	0.023	1.036 (1.001,1.072)	0.043	64,816
Unmarried	1.042 (0.989,1.099)	0.121	1.020 (0.981,1.061)	0.319	50,185
Cause of death					
Cancer	1.010 (0.959,1.064)	0.715	1.002 (0.964,1.041)	0.938	50,619
Non-cancer	1.086 (1.041,1.132)	<0.001	1.034 (1.104,0.968)	0.035	79,069

Source: Adapted from Chan et al. (2012).

Notes

† N = 129,688 non-accidental deaths were included in the analysis. Subgroups totals may not add up due to other or unknown cases.

‡ Not shown in this table: reported previous residence from other countries. Information available upon request.

* The proxy socio-economic status (SES) variable was created first by matching individual "area of residence" within the mortality data to the median monthly domestic household income within that area of residence as reported by government tertiary planning units (TPUs, the smallest geographic unit for which data are available). Resulted proxy SES was then categorised into SES Low (≤HK$15,000 per month/US$23,077 per year), SES Medium (HK$15,001–25,000 per month/US$23,077–38,462 per year) and SES High (>HK$25,000 per month/US$28,462 per year).

residence (RR = 1.313, 95% CI: 1.129–1.528, $p = 0.000$), marital status (RR = 1.036, 95% CI: 1.001–1.072, $p = 0.043$), and non-cancer-related causes (RR = 1.034, 95% CI: 1.104–0.968, $p = 0.024$) were more sensitive to drops in temperature. Overall, the temperature–mortality threshold in Hong Kong was 28.2°C and the average per 1°C temperature increase was associated with 1.8% increase in mortality above this threshold.

Subgroup analyses showed that mortality among women, those with unknown residence, and married individuals were more sensitive to high temperature effects. An inverse gradient relationship was observed between area-level SES and heat-related mortality. Non-cancer-related causes such as cardiovascular- and respiratory infection-related death were significantly associated with temperature-related morality in urban Hong Kong, China. Whilst area of residence (a proxy for urban design) was not found to be significantly associated with heat-related mortality, further study might be necessary as the current model cannot ascertain its true impact due to design limitations.

Epidemiological patterns of mortality in elevated temperature highlight vulnerable population subgroups in urban settings who may need targeted health protection strategies to protect their well-being. Strategies such as the establishment of heat health warning systems, public service announcements (e.g. mass media messages, distribution of educational materials, automated notification systems), cooling centres, information phone lines, hospital alerts (for emergency preparedness), outreach services to vulnerable groups (e.g. homeless), distribution of cooling methods (e.g. fans or air-conditioner donations), and environmental projects (e.g. urban planning) might be helpful to protect the general public from the adverse impact of elevated temperature. However, the cost-effectiveness of these strategies and the receptiveness of different population subgroups towards these strategies would need to be evaluated.

Disease-specific temperature mortality: heart failure

Heart failure (HF) is a syndrome in which the heart is not able to pump blood sufficiently to meet the patient's needs and is an end-stage disease and is responsible for considerable morbidity and mortality worldwide (McMurray & Pfeffer, 2005). The condition reduces quality of life and causes high risk for death. Common causes of HF include myocardial infarction and hypertension. It accounts for about 2% of healthcare spending in developed countries such as the United States. In the developing context, the incidence of HF has been increasing, particularly in Asia, largely due to an ageing population (Qiu, Yu, Tse, Tian, Wang, & Wong, 2013). Numerous studies have examined short-term and seasonal associations between ambient temperatures and HF-related morbidity and/or mortality, and most have found that mortality and hospitalisations increase during periods of both hot and cold weather. Results showed the nature of the associations and the minimum mortality/morbidity temperatures vary between study locations. A study from Scotland (Stewart, McIntyre, Capewell, & McMurray, 2002) found that HF hospitalisations and mortality peaked in winter and reached a nadir in summer, with stronger seasonal effects noted for women and those over 75 years of age. A French study (Boulay, Berthier, Sisteron, Gendreike, & Gibelin, 1999) also found a winter peak in mortality and hospitalisation with slightly stronger seasonal differences evident for women and those over 85 years of age. A study from a hot climate area in South Australia found stronger seasonal patterns than those observed in Europe, with the winter peak months hospitalisation and mortality rates nearly double those of the nadir summer months (Inglis et al., 2008).

Association between meteorological variables and HF mortality or morbidity were also examined in a number of studies. A study using data from three cities in Bavaria, Germany found that HF mortality increased during both extreme hot and cold weather, with the increase being significant in Munich and non-significant in the other two cities (Breitner, Wolf, Peters, & Schneider, 2014). A study of emergency room visits during the hot season in California (Basu, Pearson, Malig, Broadwin, & Green, 2012) and a study of hospital admissions in New York City (Lin et al., 2009) both found non-significant decreases in HF admissions with increases in temperatures. A study using city-wide hospitalisation data from Hong Kong found that HF admissions peaked in the winter and that greater diurnal temperature variation (DTR) was associated with more admissions, with stronger associations evident in the cold season, and for females and older people (Qiu et al., 2013). A study from Israel using data from a single urban hospital found that HF admissions were significantly higher on days with a lower night-time minimum temperature (Milo-Cotter et al., 2006). A study using clinical trials data from 30 European, Asian, and American countries (Das et al., 2014) found that temperature fluctuations were associated with acute HF with more admissions being associated with warmer temperatures at lags 1–3 but colder temperatures at lags 6–7. Meanwhile, a large study examining hospital admissions among older Medicare enrollees in the United States found that chronic HF admissions were significantly lower during heatwave periods (Bobb, Obermeyer, Wang, & Dominici, 2014). These studies seem to highlight that morbidity associated with HF has a tendency to affect older people, patterns change with daily temperature variation, and it is more significant on colder days.

Previous research has shown winter peaks for both hospitalisations and mortality from HF, but few studies have examined the association between multiple meteorological parameters and HF. A study by Goggins and Chan (2017) examined daily HF admissions to Hong Kong public hospitals, which covered about 83% of total admissions, and daily HF deaths, which were obtained for 2002–2011. Poisson generalised additive regression models were used with daily HF admissions/mortality as outcomes and daily mean temperature, humidity, and wind speed as predictors, while controlling for pollutant levels, time trend, season, day of the week, and holiday. Non-linear distributed lag functions were used for predictors to allow for non-linear and delayed associations. Lower mean daily temperatures were found to be strongly associated with increased HF admissions and mortality with a cumulative (to 23 days) relative risk (RR) (95%

confidence interval (CI)) for HF admissions of 2.63 (2.43, 2.84) for an 11°C versus a 25°C day, and cumulative (42 days) RR (95% CI) = 3.13 (1.90, 5.16) for HF mortality. The association with cold weather was stronger among older age groups and for new hospitalisations when compared with recurrent ones, while presence of co-morbidities did not modify the association. Both high and low relative humidity were modestly associated with more admissions. Study findings indicated both HF admissions and mortality in Hong Kong were very strongly associated with cold temperatures. Reducing exposure to cold temperatures among those at risk for HF has the potential to reduce hospitalisations and mortality.

Heat island effect in Hong Kong

Studies on the short-term association between weather conditions and mortality have generally found that human mortality tends to increase during periods of cold or hot weather with a U-, J-, or reversed J-shaped association being evident (Anderson & Bell, 2009; Braga et al., 2001; Chan et al., 2012; Chan et al., 2013; Curriero et al., 2002; Goggins, Chan, Yang, & Chong, 2013). While it has been well established that mortality tends to rise in urban areas when the temperature exceeds a certain threshold, which varies from city to city, few studies have looked at variation in this effect within cities. An important potential modifier of these heat effects is the presence of the urban heat island (UHI) effect due to the thermal capacity of buildings and sealing surfaces with artificial materials. This effect can cause temperatures in parts of cities characterised by large areas covered by buildings, roadways, parking areas, narrow streets, and lack of green space to exceed substantially those of greener and less dense rural and suburban areas. A study by Smargiassi et al. (2009) conducted in Montreal looked at the association between mortality and high temperatures in the summertime and conducted stratified analyses where the strata were defined according to surface temperatures recorded from two thermal surface images. This study found that the elevated risk of death on hot days was significantly greater in heat island areas, defined as areas of the city with higher thermal surface temperatures. A study of heatwave-related mortality in Berlin, Germany found that mortality increases during heatwaves were greater in districts with a higher proportion of land area covered by sealed surfaces (Gabriel & Endlicher, 2011), while a case-control study found that higher surface temperatures around residences estimated from satellite images were a significant risk factor for mortality during the 2003 heatwave in France (Vandentorren et al., 2006). Prior studies from around the world have indicated that very high temperatures tend to increase summertime mortality. However, possible effect modification by urban micro heat islands has only been examined by a few studies in North America and Europe.

As highlighted in Chapter 7, Hong Kong is a Special Administrative Region (SAR) of China with a total land area of 1,106 km^2 and a 2018 population of 7.48 million. The SAR consists of a densely populated central urban area (occupying around 25% of the land area), suburban "new towns" (occupying around 30% of the land area), which are also sometimes quite densely populated, and villages and rural areas (occupying around 45% of the land area). Hong Kong has a subtropical climate with hot and humid summers. The summer average temperature is around 28°C and the average relative humidity is around 75% and had one of the world's highest average increases in urban ambient temperature during the past century. As previous studies of micro heat island effects on mortality increases during hot weather have all been conducted in Europe or North America, in cities with cooler climates and lower population densities, little is known about this effect in the generally more densely populated and hotter cities in Asia. In the following study, the Hong Kong team examined the way in which the association between hot weather and mortality varied between areas of Hong Kong with different degrees of Urban Heat Island Index (UHII) for the period 2001–2009.

The temperature heat island and mortality model

Microdata sets containing data on all deaths in Hong Kong from 2001 to 2009 were obtained from the Hong Kong Census and Statistics Department. Variables available in the data include date of death, cause of death (ICD-10), gender, age and tertiary planning unit (TPU) of residence for each decedent. Data on meteorological variables including mean daily temperature, mean relative humidity (RH), total daily global solar radiation (GSR), and mean daily wind speed were obtained from the Hong Kong Observatory. Mean temperature and relative humidity were measured at the centrally located Hong Kong Observatory headquarters. Total GSR was measured at King's Park, which is also centrally located, while mean wind speed was measured at Waglan Island, which is away from the city. Data on average daily pollutants including particulate matter < 10 μm (PM_{10}), nitrogen dioxide (NO_2), sulphur dioxide (SO_2), and ozone (O_3) for 14 monitoring stations were obtained from the Hong Kong Environmental Protection Department. The levels for each day were then computed as the average across the 14 stations. Data on influenza consultation rates per 1,000 consultations for general practitioners in Hong Kong were obtained from the Hong Kong Department of Health website.

Physiological Equivalent Temperature (PET) has been used to assess urban human thermal comfort (Höppe, 1999). The model takes into account environmental factors like air temperature, air humidity, wind velocity, and mean radiant temperature to assess the thermal comfort levels of an individual. Based on user surveys, it is possible to establish the neutral PET value of inhabitants of the city. For example, in hot and humid summer months of Hong Kong, the neutral PET is around 27–29°C (Cheng, Ng, Chan, & Givoni, 2011). For this study, the UHII for each of the tertiary planning units in Hong Kong was calculated using land use and building geometry data provided by the Planning Department of the Hong Kong SAR Government. By correlating urban morphological data with the sky view factor (SVF) at an area average grid cell of

100 m × 100 m, the UHIIs can be predicted (Chen et al., 2010). Greenery's contribution to lowering UHII was factored based on the area average greening coverage of the urban areas (Ng, Liang, Wang, & Yuan, 2012). The area average wind velocity was assessed based on the frontal area densities (FAD) of the urban forms. The mean radiant temperature (Tmrt) was assumed to be 2–4°C above air temperature based on the human body standing under shades provided by the surrounding buildings. By feeding the various environmental parameters into the PET model, a bioclimatic map of the urban areas can be drawn. The bioclimatic map indicates the intra-urban PET differences of the urban areas. The difference is due purely to buildings and the physical and artificial urban development. In a nutshell, class 8 areas, which are all dense urban areas, can have a PET value 8°C higher than class 1 areas, which are all rural and landscaped areas. The map gives a good indication of the thermal environment inhabitants may experience. Given the same ambient thermal environment, those living in class 8 areas would experience higher heat stress than those living in class 3 areas.

Poisson generalised additive models (GAMs) were used to model the association between meteorological variables and mortality while controlling for important confounders (Goggins, Chan, Ng, Ren, & Chen, 2012). Analyses were restricted to the hot season, June–September, and included the years from 2001 to 2009. Models were fit for all daily natural deaths and daily non-cancer natural deaths, as non-cancer mortality was found to be more sensitive to heat effects in our previous study. Natural and non-cancer deaths were stratified according to the UHII for the tertiary planning unit of residence of the decedent. Specifically, TPUs the UHII of which was greater than the median of 3.67 were classified as "hot" areas and those below the median as "cool" areas. Separate models were then fit for each of four outcomes: (1) natural deaths in "cool" TPUs, (2) natural deaths in "hot" TPUs, (3) non-cancer deaths in "cool" TPUs, and (4) non-cancer deaths in "hot" TPUs. Other than the stratification of the analysis according to the UHII of each TPU, there was no spatial element in the models. Initial models included a day of the year indicator, 1, ..., 365 (or 366 for leap years) with maximum degrees of freedom (df) = 4 to control for seasonality, a day of study variable, 1, ..., 1098, also with maximum df = 4 to control for long-term trends due to changes in population size, age structure, and medical advances, and a day of the week indicator that was treated as a categorical variable.

Meteorological variables included in the models included mean temperature, mean relative humidity, daily total solar radiation, and the natural logarithm of mean wind speed (log transformed to reduce the influence of outliers). After examination of the time course of associations using distributed lag models, it was decided to use the mean of the same day and previous 4 days (lags 0–4) for each of these variables in subsequent models. Each meteorological variable was initially allowed a maximum of 4 df. After graphical examination of the associations it was decided to use linear terms for log wind speed and solar radiation, and two hockey stick terms for mean temperature, one term $T_{HOT} = T - 29$ if mean daily temperature > 29°C and 0 otherwise, and $T_{COLD} = 28 - T$ if mean temperature < 28°C and 0 otherwise. Relative humidity was modelled using a smooth term as its relationship with mortality was inverse U-shaped and very non-significant thus it was included as a confounder only. Mean daily respirable particle (rsp) concentrations were included to control for pollutant levels. The means of same day and previous day's concentration were used as a previous study (Ng & Cheng, 2012) found this to be the strongest predictor of mortality and this variable was log10 transformed to reduce the influence of outliers. R version 2.9.2 statistical software was used for all analyses.

Overall natural cause heat island mortality

Results for models fit for natural cause mortality are shown in Table 8.2. Results of stratified analyses show that the high temperature effect is significant only for the heat island areas, with an average rise in mortality of 4.1% for a 1°C rise in lag 0–4 temperature above 29°C ($p = 0.019$). The high temperature effect in the non-heat island areas is lower; 0.7% rise for 1°C increase above 29°C, and non-significant ($p = 0.66$). However, the difference in coefficients is not statistically significant ($p = 0.16$). The cool temperature effect below 28°C was non-significant in the all-Hong Kong analysis, and in both of the stratified analyses. The biggest difference between heat island and non-heat island areas is in the association of wind speed with mortality. For heat island areas, the association is highly significant ($p = 0.0002$) with very calm recent conditions (5th percentile lag 0–4 mean wind speed) being associated with a 5.7% higher average mortality than very windy recent conditions (95th percentile lag 0–4 mean wind speed). For non-heat island areas, the association with wind speed is slight and non-significant ($p = 0.83$). Moreover, the difference in wind speed coefficients between hot and cool areas is statistically significant ($p = 0.0052$). The solar radiation effect was not significant ($p = 0.48$) overall with 1.5% (95% CI = –2.5, 5.6) higher mortality when lag 0–4 solar radiation was at the 95th percentile versus the 5th percentile. The solar radiation effect was also not significant in the stratified analyses but the magnitude of effect was stronger for cool areas. The partial autocorrelation of the residuals for both models were all < 0.1 and non-significant, indicating that adding autoregressive terms to the model was not necessary (Goggins et al., 2012).

There was a slight tendency for TPUs classified as "hot" based on UHII to have lower SES as well. Of the deaths in "hot" TPUs, 54.3% were in low SES TPUs whereas only 45.6% of deaths in "cool" TPUs were also in low SES TPUs. The results of analyses stratified by UHII and SES indicated that both high UHII and low SES appeared to exacerbate the adverse high temperature and low wind speed effects. For temperature, the estimated mortality increases per 1°C increase above 29°C were 5.6% for high UHII/low SES, 2.6% for low UHII/low SES, 3.0% for high UHII/high SES, and –1.2% for low UHII/high SES. For wind speed, the estimated mortality increases for lag 0–4 mean wind speed = 11.0 km/hr (5th percentile) versus 33.6 km/hr (95th percentile) were

Table 8.2 Results of generalised additive models for all natural causes mortality and non-cancer mortality in Hong Kong, June–September 2001–2009*

	All Hong Kong		Hot areas		Cool areas		P comparing hot and cool coefficients
	% increase (95% CI)	P	% increase (95%CI)	P	% increase (95% CI)	P	
All natural cause mortality							
Temp >29°C (per 1°C)	2.1 (−0.3, 4.6)	0.080	4.1 (0.7, 7.6)	0.0190	0.7 (−2.4, 3.9)	0.66	0.1600
Temp <28°C (per 1°C)	0.9 (−0.6, 2.5)	0.240	0.6 (−1.2, 2.8)	0.6300	0.8 (−1.1, 2.8)	0.43	0.8800
Mean wind speed (5th vs. 95th percentile)	2.3 (0.2, 4.5)	0.030	5.7 (2.7, 8.9)	0.0002	−0.3 (−3.2, 2.6)	0.83	0.0052
Natural non-cancer mortality							
Temp >29°C (per 1°C)	2.3 (−0.7, 5.3)	0.130	5.2 (0.9, 9.8)	0.018	2.3 (−1.7, 6.6)	0.26	0.350
Temp <28°C (per 1°C)	2.4 (0.5, 4.3)	0.012	1.4 (−1.3, 4.0)	0.310	0.8 (−1.7, 3.4)	0.52	0.770
Mean wind speed (5th vs. 95th percentile)	2.3 (−0.3, 5.1)	0.083	4.7 (0.9, 7.6)	0.019	−1.6 (−5.3, 2.2)	0.40	0.024

Source: Adapted from Goggins et al. (2012).

Note

* Adjusted for solar radiation, humidity, RSP, season, trend, and day of the week.

8.0% for high UHII/low SES, 3.3% for low UHII/low SES, 2.6% for high UHII/ high SES, and –3.2% for low UHII/high SES (Goggins et al., 2012).

Heat island impact on non-cancer mortality

Table 8.2 also shows the results of the models applied to daily non-cancer natural mortality. As expected, non-cancer mortality showed greater sensitivity to temperature than all natural mortality. The high temperature effect was sta- tistically significant for heat island ($p = 0.018$) but not for non-heat island ($p = 0.26$) areas and the estimated effect was stronger for heat island (5.2% higher per 1°C rise above 29°C) than for non-heat island (2.3% higher per 1°C rise above 29°C) areas. However, the difference in coefficients between the two groups was not significant ($p = 0.35$). As was the case for all natural mortality, the biggest difference between heat island and non-heat island areas for non- cancer mortality was for wind speed, with calm conditions again strongly associ- ated with higher mortality in heat island areas ($p = 0.019$) but not in non-heat island areas ($p = 0.40$). The difference between coefficients was statistically significant ($p = 0.024$). Solar radiation was not significant in any of the analyses and was slightly stronger for heat island areas, but the difference was not signi- ficant. The partial autocorrelation of the residuals for both models were all < 0.1 and non-significant indicating that adding autoregressive terms to the model was not necessary. Cool temperature effects were also stronger in heat island areas, but this difference was not significant (Goggins et al., 2012).

Although relative humidity or solar radiation was not found to be signifi- cantly associated with mortality in any of the models, overall study findings showed that by far the largest difference between heat island and non-heat island areas in effects of meteorological conditions was for wind speed. With certain wind speed contexts, significantly higher natural and non-cancer mor- tality in heat island areas may result but there is almost no change in natural and non-cancer mortality in non-heat island areas. This finding is not surprising as studies have found that the urban heat island effect is more intense when the wind speeds are lower (Armstrong, 2006; Zeileis, Kleibe, & Jackman, 2008). High temperature effects were also considerably stronger for heat island areas, particularly for all natural mortality models, although the differences in temper- ature effects between heat island and non-heat island areas were non-significant. The finding that the cool temperature effect on increasing mortality was non- significantly stronger in UHI areas is surprising, but the difference may represent a spurious finding. Analysis of the effect of colder temperatures during the cool season in Hong Kong (November–March) found that this effect was virtually identical for the UHI and non-UHI areas (data not shown). While the range of mean temperatures above 29°C in Hong Kong is quite narrow (maximum lag 0–4 average = 30.9°C) about one-third of days during June–September have mean temperatures above this threshold.

A study of the heat island effect on mortality during heatwaves in Shanghai found that estimated excess mortality due to the 1998 heatwave was 27.3 per

100,000 in urban areas but only 7.0 per 100,000 in exurban areas (Tan et al., 2010). A study from Bangladesh (Hashizume et al., 2009) estimated a 7.5% rise in all-cause mortality per 1°C increase in lags 0–6 mean temperature above the threshold of 28.8°C in urban areas versus a 1.5% rise for rural areas (with a lower threshold of 28.1°C) (Arnfield, 2003). There are limitations to studying heat island effects through examining urban versus suburban/rural difference in heat-mortality associations. Misclassification of urban/suburban areas may mask the impact of how areas may be affected. Some areas of Hong Kong's suburban "new towns", which often consist of densely populated housing estates with high-rise apartment buildings, had higher UHI than some of the urban areas. Similar conditions may also exist in other densely populated Asian cities. Another issue is that urban, suburban, and rural populations generally differ from each other in socio-economic, demographic, and other characteristics that modify the high temperature–mortality association.

The study found that the association between daily mortality and two meteorological variables: mean daily wind speed and mean daily temperature, was stronger in areas with higher UHII. This suggests that better urban planning designed to reduce the urban heat island effect may help mitigate the negative health consequences of high temperatures. While the current magnitude of excess heat-related mortality in Hong Kong is relatively small, due to the small number of days with mean temperature much higher than the threshold temperature of 29°C, the high rate of percentage increase in mortality, particularly non-cancer mortality, per 1°C rise in temperature suggests that heat-related mortality is likely to be a considerable problem with the impact of future global warming.

Cool season study

Global climate change has led to an increased interest in the effect of weather and climate on human health with the health effects of heat and heatwaves being a particular focus. However, the effects of cold weather on health are also important and should not be forgotten. A short-term association between temperature and mortality from natural causes has been noted in many previous studies with mortality increases generally being noted for both hot and cold temperatures. However, the actual thresholds and magnitude of heat and cold effects have been found to vary across locations, with heat effects being generally stronger in colder climates and cold effects stronger in warmer climates (Anderson & Bell, 2009; Carder et al. 2005; Curriero et al., 2002; McMichael et al., 2008). Specific studies of cold temperatures' effects on mortality include a recent multi-city European study that found stronger cold effects for older people and for those living in warmer climates, and cold temperature effects persisted at lags up to 23 days (Analitis et al., 2008). A multi-city study of temperature effects in cities in Thailand, India, Latin America, and Eastern Europe (McMichael et al., 2008) found that heat and cold effects on mortality were apparent in almost all of the cities considered but that the threshold at which these effects became apparent varied considerably. A recent study of associations between apparent temperature and mortality in Beijing, Taipei, Seoul, and Tokyo (Chung et al., 2009), found strong heat effects on mortality with thresholds ranging from 30 to 31°C. However, they did not examine cold effects in detail and did not consider lags beyond 2 days, a serious limitation for studies of cold effects on mortality. A study conducted using data from rural areas of Bangladesh estimated a 3.2% increase in all-cause mortality for each 1°C drop (average of lags 0–13 mean temperature) below a threshold of 21°C (Hashizume et al., 2009).

In addition, studies that examine temperature–mortality relationships measure the specific effect of cold spells, defined as sustained periods of cold temperature over a period of several days (the number of days and thresholds vary between studies). A study using data from the Netherlands (Huynen, Martens, Schram, Weijenberg, & Kunst, 2001) estimated a 12.8% increase in natural mortality during cold spells, and found greater excess for mortality due to cardiovascular causes and mortality in those >65 years of age. In contrast, a Czech study (Kysely, Pokorna, Kyncl, & Kriz, 2009) found excess mortality during cold spells of about 6.3% overall with the greatest excess for men aged 25–59. A study done in Moscow reported significant increases in mortality of 8.9% and 9.9% for those in the 75+ age group during two cold spells (Revich & Shaposhnikov, 2008). There was no significant increase for those under 75 years old observed in this study. A Chinese study examined the effects of a prolonged cold spell in 2008 on mortality in three cities in Guangdong province, a southern China province situated next to Hong Kong. The study estimated a 60% increase in mortality due to the cold spell in two of three cities examined with larger increases for females, older people, and for respiratory mortality (Xie et al., 2013).

Hong Kong and Taipei have subtropical climates and generally experience mean daily temperatures varying between 10 and 20°C during the December–March cool season. While cold temperatures usually only last for a few days, in 2008 Hong Kong experienced its longest cold spell in 40 years, with mean temperatures < 14°C for 24 consecutive days. Hong Kong and Taiwan have roughly similar distributions of causes of death with malignant neoplasms being the number one cause of death in both places and heart disease second (Department of Health of the Government of the Hong Kong Special Administrative Region, Centre for Health Protection, 2018; Wong et al., 2013). The Hong Kong Hospital Authority, a public organisation, accounts for more than 90% of hospital admissions (Wong et al., 2013) and their fees are heavily subsidised. Taiwan implemented the compulsory National Health Insurance (NHI) in 1995, which extended coverage to all residents (Hsiao & Cheng, 2013).

While an association between cold temperatures and higher mortality is well established, relatively few studies have examined the independent effect of cold waves, after controlling for the effect of individual cold days in subtropical and tropical cities, especially in Asia. In addition, few studies have examined the association between mortality and other meteorological variables such as relative humidity, solar radiation, and wind speed. In this study, we use modern statistical methods to investigate the associations between mortality and temperature, cold waves, and other meteorological and pollutant variables during the cool season in Hong Kong and Taipei. Goggins, Chan et al. (2013) examined the impact of cold temperatures, cold waves, and other meteorological and environmental variables on cool season mortality in two subtropical Asian cities. Separate analysis of daily mortality time series from Hong Kong and Taipei using Generalised Additive Models with natural mortality as the outcome, daily mean temperature as the main explanatory variable, and relative humidity, solar radiation, wind speed, pollutants (nitrogen dioxide (NO_2), sulphur dioxide (SO_2), respirable suspended particulates (PM_{10}), ozone (O_3), seasonality, and day of the week controlled as potential confounders. Lags up to 35 days were considered for temperature, and distributed lag models were used to determine the number of lags for final models. Subgroup analyses were also done by gender, age group, cause of death, and geographical area of residence.

Results indicated cold temperatures were strongly associated with higher mortality with lagged effects persisting up to 3 weeks in Hong Kong and 2 weeks in Taipei. Cold effects were much stronger for deaths among older people and non-cancer deaths. Prolonged cold spells modestly but significantly raised mortality after accounting for the effects of individual cold days. Higher daily ozone levels were also strongly associated with higher short-term mortality in Taipei and Hong Kong, while relative humidity and solar radiation were weakly and inconsistently associated with mortality. The study findings indicated cold temperatures and cold spells substantially increase short-term mortality in subtropical Asian cities particularly among older people. Greater attention needs to be paid to the adverse health effects of cold temperatures. Interventions including provisions of shelters, cold weather warnings, and education about the possible health effects of cold temperature should be carried out in subtropical areas.

Conclusion

This chapter describes some key scientific research evidence of temperature mortality in Hong Kong. Although there remain a number of research gaps in the current understanding of the temperature-morbidity association in urban context, intra-city mortality variations are found to be associated with socio-economic determinants. These results show urban planning decisions may have important implications on mortality outcomes. Evidence-based service planning and land-use decisions should consider impact associated with climate and health research.

References

Analitis, A., Katsouyanni, K., Biggeri, A., Baccini, M., Forsberg, B., Bisanti, L., … Michelozzi, P. (2008). Effects of cold weather on mortality: Results from 15 European cities within the PHEWE Project. *American Journal of Epidemiology*, 168(12), 1397–1408. doi:10.1093/aje/kwn266.

Anderson, B. G., & Bell, M. L. (2009). Weather-related mortality: How heat, cold, and heat waves affect mortality in the United States. *Epidemiology*, 20(2), 205–213. doi: 10.1097/ede.0b013e318190ee08.

Armstrong, B. (2006). Models for the relationship between ambient temperature and daily mortality. *Epidemiology*, 17(6), 624–631. doi:10.1097/01.ede.0000239732. 50999.8f.

Arnfield, A. J. (2003). Two decades of urban climate research: A review of turbulence, exchanges of energy and water, and the urban heat island. *International Journal of Climatology*, 23(1), 1–26. doi:10.1002/joc.859.

Basu, R., Pearson, D., Malig, B., Broadwin, R., & Green, R. (2012). The effect of high ambient temperature on emergency room visits. *Epidemiology*, 23(6), 813–820. doi:10.1097/ede.0b013e31826b7f97.

Bobb, J., Obermeyer, Z., Wang, Y., & Dominici, F. (2014). Cause-specific risk of hospital admission related to extreme heat in older adults. *JAMA*, 312(24), 2659–2667. doi: 10.1001/jama.2014.15715.

Boulay, F., Berthier, F., Sisteron, O., Gendreike, Y., & Gibelin, P. (1999). Seasonal variation in chronic heart failure hospitalizations and mortality in France. *Circulation*, 100(3), 280–286. doi:10.1161/01.cir.100.3.280.

Braga, A. L., Zanobetti, A., & Schwartz, J. (2001). The time course of weather-related deaths. *Epidemiology*, 12(6), 662–667. doi:10.1097/00001648-200111000-00014.

Braga, A. L., Zanobetti, A., & Schwartz, J. (2002). The effect of weather on respiratory and cardiovascular deaths in 12 U.S. cities. *Environmental Health Perspectives*, 110(9), 859–863. doi:10.1289/ehp. 02110859.

Breitner, S., Wolf, K., Peters, A., & Schneider, A. (2014). Short-term effects of air temperature on cause-specific cardiovascular mortality in Bavaria, Germany. *Heart*, 100(16), 1272–1280. doi:10.1136/heartjnl-2014-305578.

Carder, M., McNamee, R., Beverland, I., Elton, R., Cohen, G. R., Boyd, J., & Agius, R. M. (2005). The lagged effect of cold temperature and wind chill on cardiorespiratory mortality in Scotland. *Occupational and Environmental Medicine*, 62(10), 702–710. doi: 10.1136/oem.2004.016394.

Chan, E., Goggins, W., Kim, J., & Griffiths, S. (2012). A study of intracity variation of temperature-related mortality and socioeconomic status among the Chinese population in Hong Kong. *Journal of Epidemiology and Community Health*, 66(4), 322–327. doi:10.1136/jech.2008.085167.

Chan, E., Goggins, W., Yue, J., & Lee, P. (2013). Hospital admissions as a function of temperature, other weather phenomena and pollution levels in an urban setting in China. *Bulletin of the World Health Organization*, 91(8), 576–584. doi:10.2471/blt.12. 113035.

Chen, L., Ng, E., An, X., Ren, C., Lee, M., Wang, U., & He, Z. (2010). Sky view factor analysis of street canyons and its implications for daytime intra-urban air temperature differentials in high-rise, high-density urban areas of Hong Kong: A GIS-based simulation approach. *International Journal of Climatology*, 32(1). doi:10.1002/joc.2243.

Cheng, V., Ng, E., Chan, C., & Givoni, B. (2011). Outdoor thermal comfort study in a sub-tropical climate: A longitudinal study based in Hong Kong. *International Journal of Biometeorology*, 56(1), 43–56. doi:10.1007/s00484-010-0396-z.

Chung, J.-Y., Honda, Y., Hong, Y.-C., Pan, X.-C., Guo, Y.-L., & Kim, H. (2009). Ambient temperature and mortality: An international study in four capital cities of East Asia. *Science of the Total Environment*, 408(2), 390–396. doi:10.1097/01.ede. 0000362459.93891.48.

Curriero, F., Heiner, K., Samet, J., Zeger, S., Strug, L., & Patz, J. (2002). Temperature and mortality in 11 cities of the Eastern United States. *American Journal of Epidemiology*, 155(1), 80–87. doi:10.1093/aje/155.1.80.

Das, D., Bakal, J., Westerhout, C. M., Hernandez, A., O'Connor, C. M., Atar, D., … Ezekowitz, J. (2014). The association between meteorological events and acute heart failure: New insights from ASCEND-HF. *International Journal of Cardiology*, 177(3), 819–824. doi:10.1016/j.ijcard.2014.11.066.

Department of Health of the Government of the Hong Kong Special Administrative Region, Centre for Health Protection. (2018). Number of deaths by leading causes of death, 2001–2017 [online]. Retrieved from www.chp.gov.hk/en/statistics/data/10/27/380.html.

Electric and Mechanical Services Department of the Government of the Hong Kong Special Administrative Region. (2007). Hong Kong energy end-use data 2007 [online]. Retrieved from www.emsd.gov.hk/emsd/eng/pee/edata.shtml.

Gabriel, K. M. A., & Endlicher, W. R. (2011). Urban and rural mortality rates during heat waves in Berlin and Brandenburg, Germany. *Environmental Pollution*, 159(8–9), 2044–2050. doi:10.1016/j.envpol.2011.01.016.

Goggins, W., & Chan, E. (2017). A study of the short-term associations between hospital admissions and mortality from heart failure and meteorological variables in Hong Kong. *International Journal of Cardiology*, 228, 537–542. doi:10.1016/j.ijcard.2016.11.106.

Goggins, W., Chan, E., Ng, E., Ren, C., & Chen, L. (2012). Effect modification of the association between short-term meteorological factors and mortality by urban heat islands in Hong Kong. *PLOS One*, 7(6), e38551. doi:10.1371/journal.pone.0038551.

Goggins, W., Chan, E., Yang, C., & Chong, M. (2013). Associations between mortality and meteorological and pollutant variables during the cool season in two Asian cities with sub-tropical climates: Hong Kong and Taipei. *Environmental Health*, 12(1). doi:10.1186/1476-069x-12-59.

Hajat, S., Armstrong, B., Baccini, M., Biggeri, A., Bisanti, L., Russo, A., … Kosatsky, T. (2006). Impact of high temperatures on mortality: Is there an added heat wave effect? *Epidemiology*, 17(6), 632–638. doi:10.1097/01.ede.0000239688.70829.63.

Hajat, S., Armstrong, B., Gouveia, N., & Wilkinson, P. (2005). Mortality displacement of heat-related deaths. *Epidemiology*, 16(5), 613–620. doi:10.1097/01.ede.0000164559.41092.2a.

Hajat, S., Kovats, R., & Lachowycz, K. (2007). Heat-related and cold-related deaths in England and Wales: Who is at risk? *Occupational and Environmental Medicine*, 64(2), 93–100. doi:10.1136/oem.2006.029017.

Hashizume, M., Wagatsuma, Y., Hayashi, T., Saha, S., Streatfield, K., & Yunus, M. (2009). The effect of temperature on mortality in rural Bangladesh—A population-based time-series study. *International Journal of Epidemiology*, 38(6), 1689–1697. doi:10.1093/ije/dyn376.

Hong Kong Observatory. (2015). *Hong Kong is a warming world*. Retrieved from www.hko.gov.hk/climate_change/climate_change_e.pdf.

Höppe, P. (1999). The physiological equivalent temperature—A universal index for the biometeorological assessment of the thermal environment. *International Journal of Biometeorology*, 43(2), 71–75. doi:10.1007/s004840050118.

Hsiao, Y., & Cheng, S. (2013). Is there a disparity in the hospital care received under a universal health insurance program in Taiwan? *International Journal for Quality in Health Care*, 25(3), 232–238. doi:10.1093/intqhc/mzt029.

Huynen, M., Martens, P., Schram, D., Weijenberg, M., & Kunst, A. (2001). The impact of heat waves and cold spells on mortality rates in the Dutch population. *Environmental Health Perspectives, 109*(5), 463–470. doi:10.2307/3454704.

Inglis, S. C., Clark, R. A., Shakib, S., Wong, D. T., Molaee, P., Wilkinson, D., & Stewart, S. (2008). Hot summers and heart failure: Seasonal variations in morbidity and mortality in Australian heart failure patients (1994–2005). *European Journal of Heart Failure, 10*(6), 540–549. doi:10.1016/s1567-4215(08)60059-4.

Intergovernmental Panel on Climate Change [IPCC]. (2007). *Climate change 2007: Impacts, adaptation and vulnerability. Contribution of Working Group II to the Fourth Assessment Report of the Intergovernmental Panel on Climate Change* [M. L. Parry, O. F. Canziani, J. P. Palutikof, P. J. van der Linden, & C.E. Hanson (Eds.)]. Cambridge, UK: Cambridge University Press.

Kan, H., Jia, J., & Chen, B. (2003). Temperature and daily mortality in Shanghai: A time-series study. *Biomedical Environmental Sciences, 16*(2), 133–139.

Kan, H., London, S., Chen, H., Song, G., Chen, G., Jiang, L., ... Chen, B. (2007). Diurnal temperature range and daily mortality in Shanghai, China. *Environmental Research, 103*(3), 424–431. doi:10.1016/j.envres.2006.11.009.

Kim, H., Ha, J.-S., & Park, J. (2006). High temperature, heat index, and mortality in 6 major cities in South Korea. *Archives of Environmental & Occupational Health, 61*(6), 265–270. doi:10.3200/aeoh.61.6.265-270.

Kysely, J., Pokorna, L., Kyncl, J., & Kriz, B. (2009). Excess cardiovascular mortality associated with cold spells in the Czech Republic. *BMC Public Health, 9*(19). doi:10.1186/1471-2458-9-19.

Leung, Y., Yip, K., & Yeung, K. (2008). Relationship between thermal index and mortality in Hong Kong. *Meteorological Applications, 15*(3), 399–409. doi:10.1002/met.82.

Lin, S., Luo, M., Walker, R., Liu, X., Hwang, S., & Chinery, R. (2009). Extreme high temperatures and hospital admissions for respiratory and cardiovascular diseases. *Epidemiology, 20*(5), 738–746. doi:10.1097/ede.0b013e3181ad5522.

McMichael, A. J., Wilkinson, P., Kovats, R. S., Pattenden, S., Hajat, S., Armstrong, B., ... Nikiforov, B. (2008). International study of temperature, heat and urban mortality: The "ISOTHURM" project. *International Journal of Epidemiology, 37*(5), 1121–1131. doi:10.1093/ije/dyn086.

McMurray, J., & Pfeffer, M. (2005). Heart failure. *The Lancet, 365*(9474), 1877–1889. doi:10.1016/s0140-6736(05)66621-4.

Milo-Cotter, O., Setter, I., Uriel, N., Kaluski, E., Vered, Z., Golik, A., & Cotter, G. (2006). The daily incidence of acute heart failure is correlated with low minimal night temperature: Cold immersion pulmonary edema revisited? *Journal of Cardiac Failure, 12*(2), 114–119. doi:10.1016/j.cardfail.2005.09.006.

Ng, E., & Cheng, V. (2012). Urban human thermal comfort in hot and humid Hong Kong. *Energy and Buildings, 55*, 51–65. doi:10.1016/j.enbuild.2011.09.025.

Ng, E., Liang, C., Wang, Y. N., & Yuan, C. (2012). A study on the cooling effects of greening in high-density city: An experience from Hong Kong. *Building and Environment, 47*, 256–271.

Pirard, P., Vandentorren, S., Pascal, M., Laaidi, K., Le Tertre, A., Cassadou, S., & Ledrans, M. (2005). Summary of the mortality impact assessment of the 2003 heat wave in France. *Eurosurveillance, 10*(7), 153–156. doi:10.2807/esm.10.07.00554-en.

Qiu, H., Yu, I. T., Tse, L. A., Tian, L., Wang, X., & Wong, T. W. (2013). Is greater temperature change within a day associated with increased emergency hospital admissions for heart failure? *Circulation: Heart Failure*, 6(5), 930–935. doi:10.1161/circheart failure.113.000360.

Revich, B., & Shaposhnikov, D. (2008). Excess mortality during heat waves and cold spells in Moscow, Russia. *Occupational and Environmental Medicine*, 65(10), 691–696. doi:10.1136/oem.2007.033944.

Saez, M., Sunyer, J., Castellsagué, J., Murillo, C., & Antó, J. (1995). Relationship between weather temperature and mortality: A time series analysis approach in Barcelona. *International Journal of Epidemiology*, 24(3), 576–582. doi:10.1093/ije/24.3.576.

Simon, N. W. (2006). *Generalized additive models: An introduction with R.* Boca Raton, FL: Chapman & Hall.

Smargiassi, A., Goldberg, M., Plante, C., Fournier, M., Baudouin, Y., & Kosatsky, T. (2009). Variation of daily warm season mortality as a function of micro-urban heat islands. *Journal of Epidemiology & Community Health*, 63(8), 659–664. doi:10.1136/jech.2008.078147.

Stewart, S., McIntyre, K., Capewell, S., & McMurray, J. J. V. (2002). Heart failure in a cold climate: Seasonal variation in heart failure-related morbidity and mortality. *Journal of the American College of Cardiology*, 39(5), 760–766. doi:10.1016/S0735-1097(02)01685-6.

Tan, J., Zheng, Y., Song, G., Kalkstein, L., Kalkstein, A., & Tang, X. (2007). Heat wave impacts on mortality in Shanghai, 1998 and 2003. *International Journal of Biometeorology*, 51(3), 193–200. doi:10.1007/s00484-006-0058-3.

Tan, J., Zheng, Y., Tang, X., Guo, C., Li, L., Song, G., … Chen, H. (2010). The urban heat island and its impact on heat waves and human health in Shanghai. *International Journal of Biometeorology*, 54(1), 75–84. doi:10.1007/s00484-009-0256-x.

United Nations Development Programme [UNDP]. (2006). *Human development report 2006: Beyond scarcity: Power, poverty and the global water crisis.* New York: Author. Retrieved from www.undp.org/content/dam/undp/library/corporate/HDR/2006%20 Global%20HDR/HDR-2006-Beyond%20scarcity-Power-poverty-and-the-global-water-crisis.pdf.

Vandentorren, S., Bretin, P., Zeghnoun, A., Mandereau-Bruno, L., Croisier, A., Cochet, C., … Ledrans, M. (2006). August 2003 heat wave in France: Risk factors for death of elderly people living at home. *European Journal of Public Health*, 16(6), 583–591. doi: 10.1093/eurpub/ckl063.

Wong, E. L. Y., Coulter, A., Cheung, A. W. L., Yam, C. H. K., Yeoh, E.-K., & Griffiths, S. (2013). Item generation in the development of an inpatient experience questionnaire: A qualitative study. *BMC Health Services Research*, 13(1), 265. doi:10.1186/1472-6963-13-265.

Xie, H., Yao, Z., Zhang, Y., Xu, Y., Xu, X., Liu, T., … Ma, W. (2013). Short-term effects of the 2008 cold spell on mortality in three subtropical cities in Guangdong Province, China. *Environmental Health Perspectives*, 121(2), 210–216. doi:10.1289/ehp. 1104541.

Zeileis, A., Kleiber, C., & Jackman, S. (2008). Regression models for count data in R. *Journal of Statistical Software*, 27(8). doi:10.18637/jss.v027.i08.

9 Temperature impact on general and communicable disease-related morbidities

Although extensive evidence exists to highlight the temperature–mortality impact, due to lack of comprehensive, comparable citywide hospital databases in most middle- and low-income communities, the temperature–morbidity patterns remain only partially understood in Asia (Kovats, Hajat, & Wilkinson, 2004; Nitschke, Tucker, & Bi, 2007). Hong Kong has recorded one of the highest urban ambient temperature increase and income disparity globally. With its citywide hospital database covering 83% of hospital admissions, a number of studies related to temperature and morbidity were published to examine a number of major disease burdens and socio-demographic patterns of the health impact in this metropolis. This chapter shares the research results on the overall impact of temperature on disease burden and how it might have impacted hospitalisation. Communicable disease study outcomes such as pneumonia, hand, foot, and mouth disease, rotavirus/Norwalk virus infection, and *Salmonella*-related in-hospital burden are discussed.

Communicable diseases: vector-borne, food-borne, and water-borne diseases

Among common communicable diseases, vector-borne diseases are associated with environmental and climate changes. Transmission of vector-borne diseases depends on factors such as climate, altitude, population density, and specific environmental requirements of the various mosquito species. Climate and environmental changes have shifted the geographic distribution and seasonal patterns of vector-borne disease transmission. Warmer temperatures occurring earlier in the year and extending for a longer time may prolong the disease transmission periods (Yang et al., 2012). Increased survivability and prolonged breeding season of mosquito species *Anopheles*, *Aedes aegypti*, and *Aedes albopictus* with warmer ambient environment and human biting frequency of the mosquitos will also increase risks of disease transmission. Moreover, seasonal variation will occur. Warmer temperatures during summer may become too hot for the survival of malaria-transmitting mosquito genus *Anopheles*; the malaria burden may decrease in epidemic potential during the summer but increase during spring and fall seasons with warmer ambient temperature.

Vector-borne diseases

Disease vectors are sensitive to climate conditions, and in general, higher temperature and heavier rainfall create favourable conditions for the vector to survive and transmit diseases in urban context. The population in Hong Kong is susceptible to vector-borne diseases (VBDs) such as dengue fever, Japanese encephalitis, malaria, scrub typhus, and spotted fever (Department of Health of the Government of the Hong Kong Special Administrative Region, Centre for Health Protection (CHP), 2016a). Although there is currently no research data available for understanding the impact of weather changes on the various aspects of vector-borne diseases in Hong Kong, published research results in mainland China, based on 670 locations evenly distributed across the country, indicated that environmental variables suitable for malaria transmission had shifted northwards, whereas transmission intensity in the central part of the country had increased due to prolonged suitable periods (Wong et al., 2014; Yang et al., 2012).

In Hong Kong, it has been projected that there will be less rainfall from February to May and more rainfall from June to November, and higher possibility of extremely low rainfall (below 100 mm) and extreme high rainfall (above 800 mm) (Cheung, Hart, & Peart, 2015). Such changes in rainfall pattern, together with projected rise in temperatures, are bound to push up the number of vector-borne infection cases in Hong Kong. In fact, the number of dengue fever cases in Hong Kong has been on the increase in the last 5 years, from 30 cases in 2011 to 114 cases in 2015 (a 280% rise) (Department of Health of the Government of the Hong Kong Special Administrative Region, CHP, 2016b).

Food-borne and water-borne diseases

Food-borne diseases may be caused by ingestion of foodstuffs contaminated with microorganisms (e.g. *Salmonella*) or chemicals (e.g. pesticides), and are mostly associated with gastrointestinal symptoms (e.g. diarrhoea) (World Health Organization [WHO], 2016). Similarly, water-borne diseases are caused by ingestion of water contaminated by pathogens, or through other faecal-oral routes (e.g. cholera) (Wong et al., 2014). Environmental effects of climate change may affect the level of pathogens and chemicals in food and water, e.g. warm weather encourages growth of *Salmonella* in food and planktonic organisms in water, heavy rainfall leads to contamination of the drinking water system (Vardoulakis & Heaviside, 2012). The most important mechanisms to prevent them are to have the relevant and appropriate surveillance and response system in place. Currently, there are limited scientific reports on the impact of how climate change might have affected food/water-borne disease patterns in Hong Kong. Urgent review of data and evidence is needed to examine how current health protection measures and programmes in Hong Kong (such as the Prevention and Control of Disease Ordinance (Cap 599), the *Salmonella* Surveillance Programme of the Department of Health, and the Food Surveillance

Programme of the Centre for Food Safety) should be enhanced to support preparedness and emergency response for the potential but imminent health threats in the decades to come.

Temperature and hospital admissions

Evidence from European and American cities indicates high ambient temperature may increase hospitalisation (Fish, Bennett, & Millard, 1985; Fleury, Charron, Holt, Allen, & Maarouf, 2006; Kovats et al., 2004; Mastrangelo et al., 2007; Nitschke et al., 2007; Tai, Lee, Shih, & Chen, 2007). At-risk disease categories include respiratory, renal diseases (Kovats et al., 2004), cerebro-vascular accidents, transient ischemic attacks, subarachnoid haemorrhage, and infectious diseases (both vector- and food-borne) (Bangs, Larasati, Corwin, & Wuryadi, 2006; Checkley et al., 2000; D'Souza, Becker, Hall, & Moodie, 2004; Hashizume et al., 2007; Thammapalo, Chongsuwiwatwong, McNeil, & Geater, 2005; Paz, 2006; Yé, Louis, Simboro, & Sauerborn, 2007). In addition, those who are critically ill (Stéphan et al., 2005), of extremes of age, of low socio-economic status (Jones et al., 1982), with pre-existing medical conditions, with mental health medication (Chan et al., 2018), being healthcare workers, being pregnant women (Luton, Alran, Fourchotte, Sibony, & Oury, 2004), in institutional care, living alone, and having poor mobility are found to be at high risk.

A retrospective ecological study was conducted to understand the relationship among temperature, pollution, and routine hospital admissions during 1998–2009 (Chan, Goggins, Yue, & Lee, 2013). Meteorological variables, including mean daily temperatures, mean relative humidity, mean wind speed, total solar radiation, and total daily rainfall were obtained from the Hong Kong Observatory (HKO). Pollution levels of daily means were calculated from hourly concentrations of nitrogen dioxide (NO_2), sulphur dioxide (SO_2), ozone (O_3), and particulate matter $\leq 10\,\mu m$ (PM_{10}) were obtained from the 11 general environmental collection stations of the Environmental Protection Department (EPD). Routine hospital admissions data were solicited from the Hong Kong Hospital Authority (HA). Variables included age, gender, district of residence, admitted hospital, admission and discharge dates, cause of hospitalisation, total length of hospital stay, and discharge status. Principal diagnosis data were retrieved using International Statistical Classification of Diseases and Related Health Problems (ICD-9), and the health outcomes examined were regarded as "hospitalisations", which refer to various causes of hospital admissions resulted from various medical reasons. The medical causes of hospitalisation examined in this study included unintentional injuries (including injuries of external causes ICD-9: 800–957; and accidents ICD-9: E800–E949), intentional injuries (including intentional self-harm ICD-9: E950–E959; and assaults ICD-9: E960–E969), infectious disease (ICD-9: 001–139; 320–323; 614–616), renal failure (ICD-9: 584–586), diabetes (ICD-9: 249–250), cirrhosis (ICD-9: 571.5, 571.6, 571.8, and 571.9), cancer (ICD-9: 140–239), as well as circulatory and respiratory diseases (ICD-9: 390–459 and 460–519, respectively). For the demographics, age was classified as: 75 years or over, 60–74 years, 15–59 years, and 0–14 years.

Poisson generalised additive models (GAMs) were built to examine the association between daily mean temperature and daily hospital admissions of various causes as described above. Due to the different lagged effect associated with temperature and hospitalisation patterns, two separate seasonality-based analyses, namely Hot (June–September) and Cold (November–March) were conducted. Results indicated the average hot season daily mean air temperature over the study period was 28.4°C, with a median of 28.6°C, and a range from 22.2°C to 31.8°C. For the cool season, the mean, median, and range of temperatures were 18.7°C, 19.0°C, and 8.2–26.9°C, respectively.

Table 9.1a summarises the routine hospital admissions data during the cool season (November–March) and summer (June–September) from 1998 to 2009 by causes of hospitalisation. Table 9.1b describes the demographics characteristics of sampled population with comparison to the Hong Kong 2009 Census. A total of 7,869,661 cases were admitted to the hospitals in Hong Kong during this period, among them 33.1% were admitted during summer. Of the health outcomes selected for analysis during the study period, respiratory diseases contributed to the highest number of admissions (17.1%), followed by cancer (16.1%) and circulatory diseases (15.1%). A total of 10% of admissions were due to unintentional injuries, 0.3% for intentional injuries, and 5.1% for infectious diseases during the study period.

Table 9.1a Descriptions of causes of hospitalisation in Hong Kong during November–March (cool season) and June–September (hot season), 1998–2009*

Causes of hospitalisation	November–March (cool season)		June–September (hot season)	
	Cases	%	Cases	%
Unintentional injuries	334,291	10.0	270,942	10.4
Intentional injuries	7,921	0.2	7,038	0.3
Infectious diseases	165,959	5.0	132,647	5.1
Chronic diseases				
Respiratory diseases	620,073	18.6	444,628	17.1
Circulatory diseases	544,027	16.3	393,495	15.1
Cancer	501,898	15.1	419,058	16.1
Renal failure	345,166	10.4	267,804	10.3
Diabetes	80,190	2.4	62,477	2.4
Cirrhosis	6,984	0.2	5,195	0.2
All other causes	725,727	21.8	601,857	23.1
Total	3,332,203	100.0	2,605,141	100.0

Table 9.1b Descriptions of demographic characteristics of people admitted to the hospitals in Hong Kong 1998–2009 and Hong Kong census population*

Demographic characteristics	n	%	HK population (2009)	%
Gender (N=2,605,139)				
Male	1,354,965	52.0	3,698,181	53.0
Female	1,250,174	48.0	3,279,519	47.0
Age (N=2,604,951)				
0–14 years	232,725	8.9	851,279	12.2
15–59 years	971,686	37.3	4,863,457	69.7
60–74 years	677,791	26.0	809,413	11.6
≥75 years	722,749	27.7	446,573	6.4
Area of residence (N=2,605,141)				
Hong Kong Island	538,421	20.7	1,283,897	18.4
Kowloon	887,899	34.1	2,058,422	29.5
New Territories	1,166,240	44.8	3,635,382	52.1
Unknown	12,581	0.5	–	–
Days of hospitalisation (N=2,605,141)				
≤1 day	972,969	37.3	–	–
2–3 days	587,930	22.6	–	–
4–5 days	316,169	12.1	–	–
6–10 days	353,811	13.6	–	–
11–30 days	286,794	11.0	–	–
≥31 days	87,468	3.4	–	–

Source: Census and Statistics Department of the Government of the Hong Kong Special Administrative Region.

Notes
* Source of data: Made available by Hong Kong Hospital Authority in 2011. Principal diagnosis data were retrieved using International Statistical Classification of Diseases and Related Health Problems (ICD-9), and the health outcomes examined included unintentional injuries (including injuries of external causes ICD-9: 800–957; and accidents ICD-9: E800–E949), intentional injuries (including intentional self-harm ICD-9: E950–E959; and assaults ICD-9: E960–E969), infectious disease (ICD-9: 001–139; 320–323; 614–616), renal failure (ICD-9: 584–586), diabetes (ICD-9: 249–250), cirrhosis (ICD-9: 571.5, 571.6, 571.8, and 571.9), cancer (ICD-9: 140–239), as well as circulatory and respiratory diseases (ICD-9: 390–459 and 460–519, respectively).

Hot season analyses

This final study model indicated that higher temperatures above 29°C were significantly (p = 0.003) associated with more hospitalisations. A 1°C rise above this threshold was associated with a 4.5% (95% confidence interval (CI): 2.1%, 7.0%) increase in hospitalisations. RH with a lag of 0 to 10 days ($RH_{(0-10)}$) remained non-linearly and significantly (p < 0.001) associated with hospitalisations. Higher NO_2 levels were positively and significantly associated with more hospitalisations, while lower MWS with a lag of 0 to 10 days ($MWS_{(0-10)}$) and higher GSR with a lag of 0 to 10 days ($GSR_{(0-10)}$) were non-significantly associated with more hospitalisations (p = 0.18 and 0.64, respectively).

For the subgroup analyses of the causes of hospitalisation, respiratory diseases, infectious diseases, and unintentional injury were associated with temperature rising above 28.5°C (see Table 9.2). No significant association with hot temperature was found for other natural hospitalisation causes, including cancer, circulatory diseases, diabetes mellitus, renal failure, and cirrhosis; no significant increase was found during very hot weather. For respiratory diseases, the initial model showed an increase in hospitalisations for MDT with a lag of 0 to 10 days ($MDT_{(0-10)}$) above 28.5°C, while $RH_{(0-10)}$ showed a pattern similar to that for all natural cause hospitalisations. The results of the subsequent model indicated that higher temperatures above 28.5°C were significantly ($p < 0.001$) associated with more respiratory disease hospitalisations with a 1°C rise above this threshold being associated with a 7.6% (95% CI: 5.1%, 10.2%) increase in hospitalisations. $RH_{(0-10)}$ remained non-linearly and significantly ($p < 0.001$) associated with hospitalisations. A 10 mg/m^3 increase in mean lags 0–4 O_3 was associated with a 1.6% (95% CI = 0.7%, 2.4%, $p = 0.0002$) increase in RD hospitalisation while NO_2 became non-significant once O_3 was controlled for. Higher $GSR_{(0-10)}$ was significantly ($p = 0.003$) associated with more hospitalisations, with a 5 MJ/m^2 (approximately equal to the interquartile range for this variable) higher level being associated with a 3.2% (1.2%, 5.2%) rise in RD hospitalisations (see Table 9.2).

For infectious diseases, the initial model showed that $MDT_{(0-10)}$ had a significant ($p = 0.01$) association with hospitalisations increasing above 28.5°C. $RH_{(0-10)}$ also had a significant ($p = 0.0003$) S-shaped association with hospitalisations rising between 73% and 84%, which is similar to the pattern for other non-injury-based hospitalisation. $GSR_{(0-10)}$ was not significantly associated with infectious disease hospitalisations. The subsequent model indicated that temperatures above 28.5°C were significantly ($p < 0.001$) associated with more infectious disease hospitalisations with a 1°C rise above this threshold being associated with a 4.5% (95% CI: 2.2%, 6.9%) increase in hospitalisations. $MWS_{(0-10)}$ was also significantly and negatively associated with infectious disease hospitalisations ($p = 0.006$), while humidity remained significantly associated with it ($p < 0.001$). Among causes in the infectious disease category, *Salmonella* hospitalisations were particularly sensitive to hot weather, with each 1°C rise in mean temperature accompanied by an 11.4% rise in *Salmonella* hospitalisations ($p < 0.001$) over the same day and the following 14 days.

For injury-related admissions, findings also indicated that a 1°C rise in temperatures above 28.5°C was associated with a significant ($p = 0.006$) increase of 1.9% (95% CI = 0.6%, 3.2%) in unintentional injury hospitalisations. Moreover, hospitalisations due to intentional injuries (self-harm or harm to others) were not significantly affected by hot weather. No significant gender difference was observed for either disease outcomes (see Table 9.2). For respiratory disease hospitalisations, the increase in hospitalisations during hot weather was found to be greater for children (0–14 years) and young adults (15–59 years), when compared with that of people aged 60–74 years and above 75 years. For infectious disease hospitalisations, the increase in hospitalisations during hot weather was found to be greater for people older than 75 years when compared with those of the younger groups.

Table 9.2 Summary of results of selected subgroup analysis by gender, age groups, of respiratory disease, and infectious disease hospitalisations of Hong Kong, 1998–2009 (hot season)*

	Respiratory diseases		Infectious diseases	
	% increase** (95%CI)	p	% increase** (95%CI)	p
Gender				
Male	7.5 (5.0–10.0)	<0.0001	3.0 (0.1–6.0)	0.0410
Female	7.5 (4.4–10.6)	<0.0001	6.0 (3.0–9.0)	0.0002
Age group				
0–14 years	19.5 (12.9–26.4)	<0.0001	3.7 (0.2–7.4)	0.0380
15–59 years	8.2 (4.0–12.6)	0.0001	0.9 (−2.7–4.1)	0.6000
60–74 years	7.1 (3.4–11.1)	0.0002	2.6 (−2.0–7.3)	0.2600
≥75 years	4.9 (1.9–8.0)	0.0014	9.6 (5.6–13.8)	0.0001

*Source of data: Made available by Hong Kong Hospital Authority in 2011.

Notes
** % increase in hospitalisations for each 1°C rise in temperature above 28.5°C.
Age was classified as: 75 years or over, 60–74 years, 15–59 years, and 0–14 years.

Cool season analyses

The cool season model indicated that cooler temperatures were significantly ($p < 0.0001$) associated with more hospitalisations across the range of temperature (8.2–26.9°C) observed in the cool season with a 1°C drop from the top end of the range (26.9°C) being associated with a 1.4% (95% CI: 0.9%, 1.8%) increase in hospitalisations. A $10 mg/m^3$ increase in NO_2 lagged by 0 and 1 days ($NO_{2(0-1)}$) was on average associated with a 1.2% (95% CI = 0.8%, 1.5%, $p = 0.0015$) increase.

Subgroup analyses by cause of admission indicated that the models with linear terms for $NO_{2(0-1)}$ and MDT with a lag of 0 to 21 days ($MDT_{(0-21)}$), and without other pollutants or GSR with a lag of 0 to 21 days ($GSR_{(0-21)}$) were also appropriate for the infectious disease (ID) hospitalisation. For infectious disease, a 1°C drop on average from 26.9°C was associated with a 1.0% (95% CI: 0.4%, 1.6%, $p = 0.002$) increase in hospitalisations, while a $10 \mu g/m^3$ increase in $NO_{2(0-1)}$ was on average associated with a 0.9% (95% CI = 0.4%, 1.5%) increase.

For respiratory diseases (RD), linear terms were used for $MDT_{(0-21)}$, $NO_{2(0-1)}$, and mean lags 0–1 O_3, while smooth terms were used for MWS with a lag of 0 to 21 days ($MWS_{(0-21)}$) and RH with a lag of 0 to 21 days ($RH_{(0-21)}$). From this model, a 1°C drop in $MDT_{(0-21)}$ on average from 26.2°C was associated with a 4.3% (95% CI: 3.6%, 4.7%) increase in hospitalisations, while a $10 \mu g/m^3$ increase in $NO_{2(0-1)}$ was on average associated with a 0.5% (95% CI = 0.03%, 1.0%, $p = 0.035$) increase, and a $10 \mu g/m^3$ increase in O_3 was associated with a 2.2% (95% CI = 1.7%, 2.7%, $p < 0.0001$) increase in hospitalisation. $MWS_{(0-21)}$ was also highly significantly ($p < 0.0001$) associated with RD hospitalisations, sharply decreasing for increases from 10 to 20 km/hr, rising slightly from 20 to 24 km/hr, which roughly corresponds to the interquartile range, then decreasing sharply again from 24 to 40 km/hr.

For cardiovascular diseases, linear terms were appropriate for $MDT_{(0-21)}$, $RH_{(0-21)}$, and $NO_{2(0-1)}$, while $MWS_{(0-21)}$ and $GSR_{(0-21)}$ were dropped. From this model a 1°C drop on average was associated with a 2.1% (95% CI: 1.6%, 2.5%, $p < 0.0001$) increase in hospitalisations, while a 10 μg/m^3 increase in $NO_{2(0-1)}$ was on average associated with a 1.6% (95% CI = 1.1%, 2.0%, $p < 0.0001$) increase, and a 10% rise in mean $RH_{(0-21)}$ was associated with a 1.6% (95% CI = 0.3%, 2.9%, $p = 0.014$) increase. Although no significant associations between temperature and hospital admissions for renal disease or cancer was found, increases in $NO_{2(0-1)}$ were significantly associated with more admissions of these diseases.

Subgroup analyses by age and gender were carried out for hospital admissions for respiratory, infectious, and cardiovascular diseases (see Table 9.3). Respiratory disease hospitalisations among children and those over 75 were more sensitive to cold temperatures, while for infectious diseases and cardiovascular admissions those over 75 were the most sensitive. Strong effect modification by gender was not evident.

Hospitalisations due to accidental causes were not associated with temperature during the cool season but were found to be significantly positively associated with same day higher wind speeds and NO_2 levels, but negatively associated with higher rainfall amounts. Higher same day mean temperature was significantly associated with more hospitalisations due to intentional injuries (assaults and attempted suicides) with a 1°C higher temperature from the lower end of the range (8.2°C) being associated with 2.4% (95% CI = 1.6%, 3.1%, $p < 0.0001$) higher admissions.

This study indicated that temperature thresholds for hospital admission were 0.3–0.8°C higher (28.5–29.0°C) than the mortality threshold (28.2°C) found in a previous mortality study (Chan et al., 2013). Overall, hospitalisations increased on average by 4.5% for each 1°C increase above 29.0°C and rose by 1.4% for each 1°C decrease over the range of temperatures (8.2–26.9°C) observed in the cool season. The findings imply that although Hong Kong, with its subtropical climate, has a significantly higher temperature threshold for morbidity, they also show that the overall per 1°C impact of cooler days on annual morbidity is higher.

In subgroup analyses, although the hot season was associated with higher hospitalisation for respiratory, infectious diseases, and accidents, the cold season exhibited another pattern. The model indicated respiratory, infectious, and cardiovascular disease hospitalisations were sensitive to cold temperatures. There was no evidence of a gender difference in sensitivity to high temperatures but age was found to be an important effect modifier. Studies from London have shown that risk factors for heat-related morbidity include being over 75 years of age for respiratory conditions, and being under age 5 for respiratory and renal diseases (Johnson et al., 2005; Kovats et al., 2004). For respiratory diseases, age extremes were at risk in cooler temperatures, but children (aged 0–14) were more vulnerable to high temperatures than adults. Infectious disease admissions were more significantly associated among older old (75 years or above) in both temperature extremes.

Relative humidity (RH) was found to be strongly associated with non-injury-based hospitalisations in the hot season and for most subgroups, with an

Table 9.3 Summary of results of selected subgroup analysis by gender, age groups, broad areas of residence, and median household income of districts of residence of respiratory disease and infectious disease hospitalisations of Hong Kong, 1998–2009 (cool season)*

	Respiratory diseases		Infectious diseases		Cardiovascular diseases	
	% increase** (95% CI)	p	% increase** (95% CI)	P	% increase* (95% CI)	p
Gender						
Male	4.1 (3.6, 4.7)	<0.0001	1.2 (0.5, 2.0)	0.0021	1.7 (1.1, 2.3)	<0.0001
Female	4.7 (4.1, 5.3)	<0.0001	0.9 (0.2, 1.6)	0.0070	2.2 (1.6, 2.7)	<0.0001
Age group						
0–14 years	5.0 (4.0, 6.1)	<0.0001	1.3 (0.3, 2.3)	0.0150	1.1 (−0.4, 2.5)	0.1400
15–59 years	2.2 (1.3, 3.1)	<0.0001	0.7 (0.0, 1.5)	0.0550	0.2 (−0.6, 1.0)	0.6000
60–74 years	3.7 (3.1, 4.4)	<0.0001	0.1 (−0.7, 0.8)	0.8400	0.9 (0.3, 1.6)	0.0048
≥75 years	5.1 (4.6, 5.6)	0.0001	3.4 (2.4, 4.4)	0.0001	3.8 (3.3, 4.4)	<0.0001

*Source of data: Made available by Hong Kong Hospital Authority in 2011.

Notes

** % increase in hospitalisations for each 1°C drop in mean lag 0–21 temperatures over the cooler temperatures ranges (8.2–26.9°C).

Age was classified as: 75 years or over, 60–74 years, 15–59 years, and 0–14 years.

increasing trend for RH between about 72% and 85% and declines above 85%. It should be noted that RH values < 72% are unusual in Hong Kong in the summer, and that values above 85% usually only occur on cooler days, below the heat thresholds of 28.5–29°C. Therefore, results are mostly consistent with higher RH exacerbating the effects of high temperatures on health. The decline above 85% may represent the possible beneficial effects of high humidity when temperatures are cooler. Higher wind speeds were generally associated with fewer hospitalisations for infectious disease admissions in the hot season and fewer respiratory diseases in the cool season. The latter finding was unexpected as the high winds can exacerbate the physiological effects of cold temperatures. One possible explanation for the former finding is that higher winds may lessen the physiological impact of high temperatures by helping the body's natural cooling processes. A possible partial explanation for both findings is that stronger winds may help clear pollutants from high concentration areas such as roadsides. Thus for a given measured pollutant level actual exposure may be less on days with high winds. A published study found low wind speeds in hot days (mean temperature above 29°C) were significantly associated with higher daily mortality and the associations were stronger in areas with a high urban heat island index (UHII) (Goggins, Chan, Ng, Ren, & Chen, 2012).

Hand, foot, and mouth disease (HFMD)

Hand, foot, and mouth disease (HFMD) is an emerging enterovirus-induced infectious disease for which the environmental risk factors promoting disease circulation remain inconclusive. It has been frequently reported worldwide since its discovery in 1957 (Ang et al., 2009; Chen, Chang, Wang, Cheng, & Yang, 2007; Duff, 1968; Nguyen et al., 2014), primarily affecting children aged 5 years and younger. Predominantly transmitted through person-to-person contact, respiratory droplets, or contaminated objects, HFMD is most commonly caused by *Coxsackievirus* A16 (CA16) and enterovirus 71 (EV71) (World Health Organization Regional Office for the Western Pacific, 2011). Clinical manifestations of HFMD includes fever, sore throat and mouth, small vesicles, ulcers and rashes on the skins and mucous membranes of the oral cavity. Most patients recover within 7–10 days without any clinical attention due to its typically mild and self-limiting nature. However, EV71 infections are usually associated with systemic complications, including aseptic meningitis, acute flaccid paralysis, brainstem encephalitis, pulmonary oedema or haemorrhage, and acute heart failure. Asian countries have seen an increasing number of HFMD epidemics in recent years. A total of 2,819,581 newly diagnosed HFMD cases, and 394 fatalities, were reported in China in 2014 (WHO, 2016). In addition, the largest ever outbreak of HMD in Singapore, resulting in 29,686 cases and one death, was observed in 2008 (Wu et al., 2010). Global efforts are still ongoing to identify the mechanism facilitating the continuous HFMD outbreaks observed in recent years.

A relationship between meteorological factors and the incidence of various infectious diseases has been frequently observed (Chong, Goggins, Zee, &

Wang, 2015; Fan et al., 2014). Evidence of the seasonality of HFMD has been found in studies from many locations (Blomqvist et al., 2010; Chua & Kasri, 2011; Hii, Rocklov, & Ng, 2011; Li, Yang, Di, & Wang, 2014; Onozuka & Hashizume, 2011). For countries with relatively higher latitudes, such as Finland (Blomqvist et al., 2010) and Japan (Onozuka & Hashizume, 2011), a single peak of HFMD has been seen, during the summer, and autumn months, respectively. However, two annual peaks have been observed in regions with subtropical and tropical climates including Taiwan, Hong Kong, Malaysia, Singapore, and parts of mainland China. In addition to temperature, other weather factors, such as precipitation (Chen et al., 2014; Cheng et al., 2014; Hii et al., 2011; Wang et al., 2011), wind speed (Ma, Lam, Wong, & Chuang, 2010; Wang et al., 2011), and sunshine (Wu, Yunus, Streatfield, & Emch, 2014) have been investigated as well. There are several plausible mechanisms whereby these meteorological factors could affect the breeding, growth, and transmission of pathogens, as well as human behaviour.

Using modern regression methods and controlling for multiple environmental factors, long-term trends, and seasonality, a time-series study model of daily counts of HFMD public hospital admissions from 2008 through 2011 in Hong Kong was regressed on daily mean temperature, relative humidity, wind speed, solar radiation, and total rainfall, using a combination of negative binomial generalised additive models and distributed lag non-linear models, adjusting for trend, season, and day of week (Wang, Goggins, & Chan, 2016). A positive association pattern between temperature and HFMD, with increasing trends from 8 to 20°C and above 25°C with a plateau in between was identified. A hockey-stick relationship of relative humidity with HFMD was found, with markedly increasing risks over 80%. Moderate rainfall and stronger wind and solar radiation were also found to be associated with more admissions. The study provides quantitative evidence that short-term meteorological variations could be used as early indicators for potential HFMD outbreaks. Climate change is likely to lead to a substantial increase in severe HFMD cases in this subtropical city in the absence of further interventions.

Rainfall, temperature, and *Salmonella*

Globally, it has been estimated that 93.8 million gastroenteritis cases and 155,000 associated deaths occur annually worldwide (Majowicz et al., 2010). Salmonellosis, non-typhoidal *Salmonella* infection, typically caused by *Salmonella* species other than *Salmonella* Typhi and *Salmonella* Paratyphi, is one of the most widespread food-borne diseases (faecal-oral transmission can also occur) with millions of cases occurring annually all over the world (WHO, 2018). Studies of associations between *Salmonella* and meteorological variables have focused on temperature (Akil, Ahmad, & Reddy, 2014; Britton, Hales, Venugopal, & Baker, 2010; Fleury et al., 2006; Jiang et al., 2015; Lake et al., 2009; Uejio, 2017; Zhang, Bi, & Hiller, 2010). Higher temperatures have consistently been found to be associated with higher incidence of *Salmonella* infection, although association magnitudes and lengths of lagged effects have varied. In contrast, the association of *Salmonella* infection with relative humidity (RH) and rainfall has been less well studied. A few studies from Australia have examined rainfall, with conflicting results reported (Stephen & Barnett, 2016; Zhang, Bi, & Hiller, 2008; Zhang et al., 2010): positive associations were reported for Brisbane and Townsville (Zhang et al., 2010) and Queensland (Stephen & Barnett, 2016) while a negative association was found in Adelaide (Zhang et al., 2008). A United States study found that exposure to extreme precipitation 90th percentile was associated with a 5.6% increase in the risk of salmonellosis (Jiang et al., 2015) and in Asia, a Singaporean study reported a 1% increase in the mean RH was associated with a 1.3% decrease in reported cases 6 weeks later. However, no cumulative association was assessed and the use of weekly data might not capture the true lag dependency (Aik et al., 2018).

A study was conducted to investigate associations between hospitalisations for non-typhoidal salmonellosis and RH, rainfall, and temperature in Hong Kong (Wang, Goggins, & Chan, 2018b). With negative binomial distribution assumed, time-series regression models adjusting for season and time trend were constructed employing distributed lag non-linear models and generalised additive models. Meteorological variables including mean temperature, RH, and daily total rainfall as well as indicator variables including day of the week and public holiday were incorporated in the models.

Results indicated that higher temperature was strongly associated with more hospitalisations over the entire range of temperatures observed. A relative risk of hospitalisation of 6.13 (95% CI = 3.52–10.67) was found at a temperature of 30.5°C, relative to 13°C, with lag 0–16 days. Positive associations were found for RH above 60% and rainfall between 0 and 0.14 mm. Extreme high humidity (96%) and trace rainfall (0.02 mm) were associated with 2.06 (95% CI = 1.35–3.14), lag 0–17 days, and 1.30 (95% CI = 1.01–1.67), lag 0–26 days, relative risks of hospitalisations, relative to 60% and no rain, respectively. In summary, high temperatures, high relative humidity, and light rainfall are positively associated with *Salmonella* hospitalisations. The very strong association with temperatures implies that hotter days will lead to increases in *Salmonella* morbidity in the absence of other changes, and the public health implications of this could be exacerbated by global climate change.

Rotavirus and norovirus

Diarrhoea is one of the top three leading causes of children's mortality globally (GBD 2013 Mortality and Causes of Death Collaborators, 2015; Lozano et al., 2012) and environmental factors were found to contribute to diarrhoea diseases (Chou et al., 2010; Hashizume et al., 2007; Phung et al., 2015; Wu et al., 2014). In Hong Kong, a subtropical city, evidence has shown that rotavirus and norovirus were the most common viruses introducing diarrhoeal hospitalisations among children under 18, of which 87% were children aged 0–5 years (Biswas, Lyon, Nelson, Lau, & Lewindon, 1996; Li, Chan, & Tang, 2009).

Evidence showed the seasonality of rotavirus infection and concluded that a 1 cm increase in mean monthly rainfall was associated with 1% and 0.3% reduction in the incidence, respectively (Jagai et al., 2012; Levy, Hubbard, & Eisenberg, 2009; Wang, Goggins, & Chan, 2018a). Time-series regression, one from Spain (Hervás et al., 2014) and one from Great Britain and the Netherlands (Atchison et al., 2010), found no evidence of an independent association between rain and rotavirus disease.

More consistent results have been reported for norovirus infection. A systematic review of the global seasonality of norovirus (Ahmed, Lopman, & Levy, 2013) reported a positive association between norovirus outbreaks and average rainfall in the wettest months. And both higher incidence of norovirus outbreaks and higher loads of microbial in beach waters have been observed with heavy antecedent rainfall in studies from Australia (Bruggink & Marshall, 2010), Norway (Eregno et al., 2016), and Louisiana of the United States (Wang & Deng, 2016). Nonetheless, except for the study in Australia reporting a 90-day lag between peak average rainfall and norovirus epidemic (Bruggink & Marshall, 2010), the delayed effect of precipitation on both rotavirus and norovirus remains unclear.

Other meteorological factors investigated previously include temperature and relative humidity (RH). Generally, cool and dry weather conditions were associated with higher rotavirus incidence while the association between temperature and norovirus infection remains inconclusive. Studies from England and Wales (Lopman, Armstrong, Atchison, & Gray, 2009) and Toronto of Canada (Greer, Drews, & Fisman, 2009) found every 1°C increase in air temperature was statistically significantly associated with a 15% reduction and an 8% increase in the risk of norovirus infection, respectively.

Overall, the impact of rainfall on diarrhoeal diseases in the urban metropolis remains inconclusive. A study examines the association between short-term variation in rainfall, temperature, and humidity, and rotavirus and norovirus hospitalisations among young children in Hong Kong (Wang et al., 2018a). Generalised additive negative binomial regression models were created with distributed lag non-linear terms fit with daily counts of hospital admissions due to rotavirus and norovirus infection as the outcomes and daily total rainfall and other meteorological variables as predictors, adjusting for seasonality and trend. Findings indicated that greater rainfall was inversely associated with fewer rotavirus, but more norovirus-related hospitalisations. Extreme precipitation (99.5 mm, 99th percentile) was found to be associated with 0.40 (95% CI = 0.20–0.79) and 1.93 (95% CI = 1.21–3.09) times the risk of hospitalisation due to rotavirus and norovirus infection respectively, relative to trace rainfall. Seasonal variation was found with stronger associations observed in winter for rotavirus and in summer for norovirus. Moreover, rotavirus was notably found to have a longer duration impact than norovirus. Overall, higher temperatures were found to be associated with fewer hospitalisations for both rotavirus and norovirus infection, while higher relative humidity was generally associated with more norovirus, but fewer rotavirus, hospitalisations. Meanwhile, with the introduction of the rotavirus vaccine, norovirus is likely to become a greater health threat than rotavirus and thus greater precipitation may become more clearly associated with more childhood diarrhoea.

Conclusion

This chapter describes research findings that demonstrate how the temperature–hospitalisation pattern varies with different types of communicable diseases in Hong Kong. Change in temperature was also found to be a stronger marker for hospital admissions in Taiwan (Tai et al., 2007) and ambulance transport in South Australia (Nitschke et al., 2007). With a set of compatible databases in daily meteorological variables, pollution, and Hong Kong hospital admission information spanning more than a decade, study findings have contributed to a better understanding of how temperature may affect communicable diseases related to hospitalisation in this Chinese city of densely populated living environment. Research evidence also suggests that there are long-term effects of heat-related illnesses. With the potential climate change implications on urban ambient temperature, findings might be useful for clinical service planning and emergency contingency response in time periods with prolonged elevated temperature. Health risk awareness, self-protection education, community resources empowerment, and coordinated multidisciplinary and sectoral response planning should be developed. Surge capacity consideration and implication on scheduled clinical visits of chronic disease patients might also be affected.

References

Ahmed, S. M., Lopman, B. A., & Levy, K. (2013). A systematic review and meta-analysis of the global seasonality of norovirus. *PLOS ONE*, 8, Article e75922. doi: 10.1371/journal.pone.0075922.

Aik, J., Heywood, A. E., Newall, A. T., Ng, L. C., Kirk, M. D., & Turner, R. (2018). Climate variability and salmonellosis in Singapore—a time series analysis. *Science of the Total Environment*, 639, 1261–1267.

Akil, L., Ahmad, H. A., & Reddy, R. S. (2014). Effects of climate change on *Salmonella* infections. *Foodborne Pathogens and Disease*, 11(12), 974–980.

Ang, L. W., Koh, B. K., Chan, K. P., Chua, L. T., James, L., & Goh, K. T. (2009). Epidemiology and control of hand, foot and mouth disease in Singapore, 2001–2007. *Annals of the Academy of Medicine of Singapore*, 38(2), 106–112. pmid:19271036.

Atchison, C. J., Tam, C. C., Hajat, S., Pelt, W. V., Cowden, J. M., & Lopman, B. A. (2010). Temperature-dependent transmission of rotavirus in Great Britain and The Netherlands. *Proceedings of the Royal Society B: Biological Sciences*, 277(1683), 933–942. doi:10.1098/rspb.2009.1755.

Bangs, M. J., Larasati, R. P., Corwin, A. L., & Wuryadi, S. (2006). Climatic factors associated with epidemic dengue in Palembang, Indonesia: Implications of short-term meteorological events on virus transmission. *Southeast Asian Journal of Tropical Medicine and Public Health*, 37(6), 1103–1116.

Biswas, R., Lyon, D. J., Nelson, E. A., Lau, D., & Lewindon, P. J. (1996). Aetiology of acute diarrhoea in hospitalized children in Hong Kong. *Tropical Medicine & International Health*, 1, 679–683.

Blomqvist, S., Klemola, P., Kaijalainen, S., Paananen, A., Simonen, M., Vuorinen, T., & Roivainen, M. (2010). Co-circulation of coxsackieviruses A6 and A10 in hand, foot and mouth disease outbreak in Finland. *Journal of Clinical Virology*, 48(1), 49–54. doi:10.1016/j.jcv.2010.02.002.

Britton, E., Hales, S., Venugopal, K., & Baker, M. G. (2010). Positive association between ambient temperature and salmonellosis notifications in New Zealand, 1965–2006. *Australian and New Zealand Journal of Public Health*, 34(2), 126–129.

Bruggink, L. D., & Marshall, L. A. (2010). The incidence of norovirus-associated gastroenteritis outbreaks in Victoria, Australia (2002–2007) and their relationship with rainfall. *International Journal of Environmental Research and Public Health*, 7, 2822–2827. doi:10.3390/ijerph7072822.

Chan, E. Y., Goggins, W. B., Yue, J. S., & Lee, P. (2013). Hospital admissions as a function of temperature, other weather phenomena and pollution levels in an urban setting in China. *Bulletin of the World Health Organization*, 91(8), 576–584. doi:10.2471/blt.12.113035.

Chan, E. Y. Y., Lam, H. C. Y., So, S. H. W., Goggins, III, W. B., Ho, J. Y., Liu, S., & Chung, P. P. W. (2018). Association between ambient temperatures and mental disorder hospitalizations in a subtropical city: A time-series study of Hong Kong Special Administrative Region. *International Journal of Environmental Research and Public Health*, 15, 754. doi:10.3390/ijerph15040754.

Checkley, W., Epstein, L. D., Gilman, R. H., Figueroa, D., Cama, R. I., & Patz, J. A. (2000). Effects of El Niño and ambient temperature on hospital admissions for diarrhoeal diseases in Peruvian children. *The Lancet*, 355, 442–450.

Chen, C., Lin, H., Li, X., Lang, L., Xiao, X., Ding, P., ... Liu, Q. (2014). Short-term effects of meteorological factors on children hand, foot and mouth disease in Guangzhou, China. *International Journal of Biometeorology*, 58(7), 1605–1614. doi:10.1007/s00484-013-0764-6.

Chen, K. T., Chang, H. L., Wang, S. T., Cheng, Y. T., & Yang, J. Y. (2007). Epidemiologic features of hand-foot-mouth disease and herpangina caused by enterovirus 71 in Taiwan, 1998–2005. *Pediatrics*, 120(2), e244–252. pmid:17671037.

Cheng, J., Wu, J., Xu, Z., Zhu, R., Wang, X., Li, K., ... Su, H. (2014). Associations between extreme precipitation and childhood hand, foot and mouth disease in urban and rural areas in Hefei, China. *Science of the Total Environment*, 497–498, 484–490. doi:10.1016/j.scitotenv.2014.08.006.

Cheung, C. C., Hart, A. M., & Peart, M. R. (2015). Projection of future rainfall in Hong Kong using logistic regression and generalized linear model. Paper presented at the 5th International Workshop on Climate Informatics, 24–25 September 2015, Boulder, United States.

Chong, K. C., Goggins, W., Zee, B. C., & Wang, M. H. (2015). Identifying meteorological drivers for the seasonal variations of influenza infections in a subtropical city—Hong Kong. *International Journal of Environmental Research and Public Health*, 12(2), 1560–1576. pmid:25635916.

Chou, W., Wu, J., Wang, Y., Huang, H., Sung, F., & Chuang, C. (2010). Modeling the impact of climate variability on diarrhea-associated diseases in Taiwan (1996–2007). *Science of the Total Environment*, 409(1), 43–51. doi:10.1016/j.scitotenv.2010.09.001.

Chua, K. B., & Kasri, A. R. (2011). Hand foot and mouth disease due to enterovirus 71 in Malaysia. *Virologica Sinica*, 26(4), 221–228. pmid:21847753.

Department of Health of the Government of the Hong Kong Special Administrative Region, Centre for Health Protection [CHP]. (2016a). Vector-borne diseases [online]. Retrieved from www.chp.gov.hk/en/content/9/24/34622.html.

Department of Health of the Government of the Hong Kong Special Administrative Region, Centre for Health Protection [CHP]. (2016b). Number of notifiable infectious diseases by month [online]. Retrieved fromwww.chp.gov.hk/en/data/1/10/26/43/3829. html.

D'Souza, R. M., Becker, N. G., Hall, G., & Moodie, K. B. (2004). Does ambient temperature affect foodborne disease? *Epidemiology*, 15(1), 86–92.

Duff, M. F. (1968). Hand-foot-and-mouth syndrome in humans: Coxsackie A10 infections in New Zealand. *British Medical Journal*, 2(5606), 661–664. pmid:5658411.

Eregno, F. E., Tryland, I., Tjomsland, T., Myrmel, M., Robertson, L., & Heistad, A. (2016). Quantitative microbial risk assessment combined with hydrodynamic modelling to estimate the public health risk associated with bathing after rainfall events. *Science of the Total Environment, 548–549*, 270–279. doi:10.1016/j.scitotenv.2016. 01.034.

Fan, J., Lin, H., Wang, C., Bai, L., Yang, S., Chu, C., … Liu, Q. (2014). Identifying the high-risk areas and associated meteorological factors of dengue transmission in Guangdong Province, China from 2005 to 2011. *Epidemiology & Infection, 142*(03), 634–643. doi:10.1017/s0950268813001519.

Fish, P. D., Bennett, G. C., & Millard, P. H. (1985). Heatwave morbidity and mortality in old age. *Age and Ageing, 14*(4), 243–245. doi:10.1093/ageing/14.4.243.

Fleury, M., Charron, D. F., Holt, J. D., Allen, O. B., & Maarouf, A. R. (2006). A time series analysis of the relationship of ambient temperature and common bacterial enteric infections in two Canadian provinces. *International Journal of Biometeorology, 50*(6), 385–391. doi:10.1007/s00484-006-0028-9.

GBD 2013 Mortality and Causes of Death Collaborators. (2015). Global, regional, and national age–sex specific all-cause and cause-specific mortality for 240 causes of death, 1990–2013: A systematic analysis for the Global Burden of Disease Study 2013. *The Lancet, 385*(9963), 117–171. doi:10.1016/s0140-6736(14)61682-2.

Goggins, W. B., Chan, E. Y. Y., Ng, E., Ren, C., & Chen, L. (2012). Effect modification of the association between short-term meteorological factors and mortality by urban heat islands in Hong Kong. *PLOS ONE, 7*(6), e38551.

Greer, L., Drews, S. J., & Fisman, D. N. (2009). Why "winter" vomiting disease? Seasonality, hydrology, and norovirus epidemiology in Toronto Canada. *Ecohealth, 6*, 192–199. doi:10.1007/s10393-009-0247-8.

Hashizume, M., Armstrong, B., Hajat, S., Wagatsuma, Y., Faruque, A. S., Hayashi, T., & Sack, D. A. (2007). Association between climate variability and hospital visits for non-cholera diarrhoea in Bangladesh: Effects and vulnerable groups. *International Journal of Epidemiology, 36*(5), 1030–1037. doi:10.1093/ije/dym148.

Hervás, D., Hervás-Masip, J., Rosell, A., Mena, A., Pérez, J. L., & Hervás, J. A. (2014). Are hospitalizations for rotavirus gastroenteritis associated with meteorologic factors? *European Journal of Clinical Microbiology & Infectious Diseases, 33*(9), 1547–1553. doi:10.1007/s10096-014-2106-y.

Hii, Y. L., Rocklov, J., & Ng, N. (2011). Short term effects of weather on hand, foot and mouth disease. *PLOS ONE, 6*(2), e16796. pmid:21347303.

Intergovernmental Panel on Climate Change [IPCC]. (2007). *Climate change 2007: Impacts, adaptation and vulnerability: Contribution of Working Group II to the Fourth Assessment Report of the Intergovernmental Panel on Climate Change.* (M. L. Parry, O. F. Canziani, J. P. Palutikof, P. J. van der Linden, & C. E. Hanson, Eds.) Cambridge, United Kingdom: Cambridge University Press.

Jagai, J. S., Sarkar, R., Castronovo, D., Kattula, D., Mcentee, J., Ward, H., ... Naumova, E. N. (2012). Seasonality of rotavirus in South Asia: A meta-analysis approach assessing associations with temperature, precipitation, and vegetation index. *PLOS ONE, 7*(5). doi:10.1371/journal.pone.0038168.

Jiang, C., Shaw, K. S., Upperman, C. R., Blythe, D., Mitchell, C., Murtugudde, R., ... Sapkota, A. (2015). Climate change, extreme events and increased risk of salmonellosis in Maryland, USA: Evidence for coastal vulnerability. *Environment International, 83,* 58–62. doi:10.1016/j.envint.2015.06.006.

Johnson, H., Kovats, R. S., McGregor, G., Stedman, J., Gibbs, M., Walton, H., & Cook, L. (2005). The impact of the 2003 heat wave on mortality and hospital admissions in England. *Health Statistics Quarterly, 25,* 6–11. doi:10.1097/00001648-200407000-00323.

Jones, T. S., Liang, A. P., Kilbourne, E. M., Griffin, M. R., Patriarca, P. A., Wassilak, S. G., ... Thacker, S. B. (1982). Morbidity and mortality associated with the July 1980 heat wave in St Louis and Kansas City, MO. *JAMA, 247*(24), 3327–3331.

Kovats, R. S., Hajat, S., & Wilkinson, P. (2004). Contrasting patterns of mortality and hospital admissions during hot weather and heat waves in Greater London, UK. *Occupational and Environmental Medicine, 61*(11), 893–898. doi:10.1136/oem.2003.012047.

Lake, I. R., Gillespie, I. A., Bentham, G., Nichols, G. L., Lane, C., Adak, G. K., & Threlfall, E. J. (2009). A re-evaluation of the impact of temperature and climate change on foodborne illness. *Epidemiology and Infection, 137*(11), 1538–1547. doi:10.1017/s0950268809002477.

Levy, K., Hubbard, A. E., & Eisenberg, J. N. (2009). Seasonality of rotavirus disease in the tropics: A systematic review and meta-analysis. *International Journal of Epidemiology, 38,* 1487–1496, doi:10.1093/ije/dyn260.

Li, C. S., Chan, P. K., & Tang, J. W. (2009). Prevalence of diarrhea viruses in hospitalized children in Hong Kong in 2008. *Journal of Medical Virology, 81,* 1903–1911. doi:10.1002/jmv.21611.

Li, T., Yang, Z., Di, B., & Wang, M. (2014). Hand-foot-and-mouth disease and weather factors in Guangzhou, southern China. *Epidemiology & Infection, 142*(8), 1741–50. pmid:24267476.

Lopman, B., Armstrong, B., Atchison, C., & Gray, J. J. (2009). Host, weather and virological factors drive norovirus epidemiology: Time-series analysis of laboratory surveillance data in England and Wales. *PLOS ONE, 4,* Article e6671. doi:10.1371/journal.pone.0006671.

Lozano, R., Naghavi, M., Foreman, K., Lim, S., Shibuya, K., Aboyans, V., ... Murray, C. J. (2012). Global and regional mortality from 235 causes of death for 20 age groups in 1990 and 2010: A systematic analysis for the Global Burden of Disease Study 2010. *The Lancet, 380*(9859), 2095–2128. doi:10.1016/s0140-6736(12)61728-0.

Luton, D., Alran, S., Fourchotte, V., Sibony, O., & Oury, J. (2004). Paris heat wave and oligohydramnios. *American Journal of Obstetrics and Gynecology, 191*(6), 2103–2105. doi:10.1016/j.ajog.2004.05.090.

Ma, E., Lam, T., Wong, C., & Chuang, S. K. (2010). Is hand, foot and mouth disease associated with meteorological parameters? *Epidemiology & Infection, 138*(12), 1779–1788. pmid:20875200.

Majowicz, S. E., Musto, J., Scallan, E., Angulo, F. J., Kirk, M., O'Brien, S. J., ... Hoekstra, R. M. (2010). The global burden of nontyphoidal *Salmonella* gastroenteritis. *Clinical Infectious Diseases, 50*(6), 882–889. doi:10.1086/650733.

Mastrangelo, G., Fedeli, U., Visentin, C., Milan, G., Fadda, E., & Spolaore, P. (2007). Pattern and determinants of hospitalization during heat waves: An ecologic study. *BMC Public Health, 7*(1), 200. doi:10.1186/1471-2458-7-200.

Nguyen, N. T., Pham, H. V., Hoang, C. Q., Nguyen, T. M., Nguyen, L. T., Phan, H. C., ... Minh, N. N. (2014). Epidemiological and clinical characteristics of children who died from hand, foot and mouth disease in Vietnam, 2011. *BMC Infectious Diseases, 14*(1). doi:10.1186/1471-2334-14-341.

Nitschke, M., Tucker, G. R., & Bi, P. (2007). Morbidity and mortality during heatwaves in metropolitan Adelaide. *The Medical Journal of Australia, 187*(11–12), 662–665.

Onozuka, D., & Hashizume, M. (2011). The influence of temperature and humidity on the incidence of hand, foot, and mouth disease in Japan. *Science of the Total Environment, 410–411*, 119–125. pmid:22014509.

Paz, S. (2006). The West Nile Virus outbreak in Israel (2000) from a new perspective: The regional impact of climate change. *International Journal of Environmental Health Research, 16*(1), 1–13.

Phung, D., Huang, C., Rutherford, S., Chu, C., Wang, X., Nguyen, M., ... Nguyen, T. H. (2015). Association between climate factors and diarrhoea in a Mekong Delta area. *International Journal of Biometeorology, 59*(9), 1321–1331. doi:10.1007/s00484-014-0942-1.

Stéphan, F., Ghiglione, S., Decailliot, F., Yakhou, L., Duvaldestin, P., & Legrand, P. (2005). Effect of excessive environmental heat on core temperature in critically ill patients. An observational study during the 2003 European heat wave. *British Journal of Anaesthesia, 94*(1), 39–45.

Stephen, D. M., & Barnett, A. G. (2016). Effect of temperature and precipitation on salmonellosis cases in South-East Queensland, Australia: An observational study. *BMJ Open, 6*(2). Article e010204.

Tai, C., Lee, C., Shih, C., & Chen, S. (2007). Effects of ambient temperature on volume, specialty composition and triage levels of emergency department visits. *Emergency Medicine Journal, 24*(9), 641–644. doi:10.1136/emj.2006.045310.

Thammapalo, S., Chongsuwiwatwong, V., McNeil, D., & Geater, A. (2005). The climatic factors influencing the occurrence of dengue hemorrhagic fever in Thailand. *Southeast Asian Journal of Tropical Medicine and Public Health, 36*(1), 191–196.

Uejio, C. K. (2017). Temperature influences on *Salmonella* infections across the continental United States. *Annals of the American Association of Geographers, 107*(3), 751–764.

Vardoulakis, S., & Heaviside, C. (Eds.). (2012). *Health effects of climate change in the UK 2012: Current evidence, recommendations and research gaps.* UK: Health Protection Agency. Retrieved from https://assets.publishing.service.gov.uk/government/uploads/system/uploads/attachment_data/file/371103/Health_Effects_of_Climate_Change_in_the_UK_2012_V13_with_cover_accessible.pdf.

Wang, J., & Deng, Z. (2016). Modeling and prediction of oyster norovirus outbreaks along Gulf of Mexico coast. *Environmental Health Perspectives, 124*, 627–633. doi:10.1289/ehp.1509764.

Wang, P., Goggins, W. B., & Chan, E. Y. Y. (2016). Hand, foot and mouth disease in Hong Kong: A time-series analysis on its relationship with weather. *PLOS ONE, 11*(8), e0161006. doi:10.1371/journal.pone.0161006.

Wang, P., Goggins, W. B., & Chan, E. Y. Y. (2018a). A time-series study of the association of rainfall, relative humidity and ambient temperature with hospitalizations for rotavirus and norovirus infection among children in Hong Kong. *Science of the Total Environment, 643,* 414–422. doi:10.1016/j.scitotenv.2018.06.189.

Wang, P., Goggins, W. B., & Chan, E. Y. Y. (2018b). Associations of *Salmonella* hospitalizations with ambient temperature, humidity and rainfall in Hong Kong. *Environment International, 120,* 223–230. doi:10.1016/j.envint.2018.08.014.

Wang, Y., Feng, Z., Yang, Y., Self, S., Gao, Y., Longini, I. M., ... Yang, W. (2011). Hand, foot, and mouth disease in China. *Epidemiology, 22*(6), 781–792. doi:10.1097/ede.0b013e318231d67a.

Wong, P. P., Losada, I. J., Gattuso, J. P., Hinkel, J., Khattabi, A., McInnes, K. L., ... Sallenger, A. (2014). *Climate change 2014: Impacts, adaptation, and vulnerability. Part A: Global and sectoral aspects. Contribution of Working Group II to the Fifth Assessment Report of the Intergovernmental Panel on Climate Change* (pp. 361–409). Cambridge, United Kingdom and New York, NY: Cambridge University Press. Retrieved from www.ipcc.ch/report/ar5/wg2//.

World Health Organization [WHO]. (2016). Foodborne diseases [online]. Retrieved from www.who.int/topics/foodborne_diseases/en/.

World Health Organization [WHO]. (2018). *Salmonella* (non-typhoidal) [online]. Retrieved from www.who.int/en/news-room/fact-sheets/detail/salmonella-(non-typhoidal).

World Health Organization Regional Office for the Western Pacific. (2011). *A guide to clinical management and public health response for hand, foot and mouth disease (HFMD)*. Manila, the Philippines: Author. Retrieved from http://iris.wpro.who.int/bitstream/handle/10665.1/5521/9789290615255_eng.pdf.

Wu, J., Yunus, M., Streatfield, P. K., & Emch, M. (2014). Association of climate variability and childhood diarrhoeal disease in rural Bangladesh, 2000–2006. *Epidemiology & Infection, 142,* 1859–1868.

Wu, Y., Yeo, A., Phoon, M., Tan, E., Poh, C., Quak, S., & Chow, V. T. (2010). The largest outbreak of hand, foot and mouth disease in Singapore in 2008: The role of enterovirus 71 and coxsackievirus A strains. *International Journal of Infectious Diseases, 14*(12). doi:10.1016/j.ijid.2010.07.006.

Yang, G., Tanner, M., Utzinger, J., Malone, J. B., Bergquist, R., Chan, E. Y., ... Zhou, X. (2012). Malaria surveillance-response strategies in different transmission zones of the People's Republic of China: Preparing for climate change. *Malaria Journal, 11*(1). doi:10.1186/1475-2875-11-426.

Yé, Y., Louis, V. R., Simboro, S., & Sauerborn, R. (2007). Effect of meteorological factors on clinical malaria risk among children: An assessment using village-based meteorological stations and community-based parasitological survey. *BMC Public Health, 7,* 101.

Zhang, Y., Bi, P., & Hiller, J. E. (2008). Climate variations and salmonellosis transmission in Adelaide, South Australia: A comparison between regression models. *International Journal of Biometeorology, 52*(3), 179–187.

Zhang, Y., Bi, P., & Hiller, J. E. (2010). Climate variations and *Salmonella* infection in Australian subtropical and tropical regions. *Science of the Total Environment, 408*(3), 524–530.

10 Temperature and non-communicable disease hospitalisation

Non-communicable diseases (NCDs) are usually presented as diseases chronic or long-term in nature. Although NCD patients may be aware or unware of their disease status, they typically require long-term investment and commitment of healthcare systems to support and maintain health and well-being eventually. This chapter describes the impact of temperature on a number of non-communicable conditions namely, COPD, asthma, injury, mental health, myocardial infarction, stroke, and heart failure.

Impact of weather on air quality

Weather conditions may significantly affect air quality. Warmer temperature increases atmospheric concentrations of ground-level ozone and particulate matter (PM) (Crimmins et al., 2016) and may pose higher risks of cardiovascular and respiratory illnesses to the affected community. Stagnant air also means worsening of air quality due to lower dispersion effect. A study on the Pearl River Delta region in China predicts that air stagnation is likely to lead to higher frequency of severe air pollution (Cheung & Yim, 2015).

Impact of pollution on cardiovascular- and respiratory-related health

Research in Hong Kong indicated that higher daily ozone levels were strongly associated with higher short-term mortality in Hong Kong. Specifically, among various non-communicable disease-related mortalities, respiratory and cardiovascular mortalities are most significantly associated (Goggins, Chan, Yang, & Chong, 2013; refer also to Chapter 8). For hospitalisation, heart disease hospitalisation in Hong Kong rose by 1.1% with a 10 ppb increase in nitrogen dioxide (NO_2) level (Goggins, Chan, & Yang, 2013). Cardiorespiratory fitness of children in high pollution districts was significantly poorer than that in low pollution districts, with the situation slightly more serious for girls (Gao, Chan, Zhu, & Wong, 2013).

Study on the lung functions of local children found that lung functions of primary-school-age boys in high pollution districts were significantly lower than those in low pollution districts, e.g. 8.4% lower as measured by forced expiratory flow at 75% of forced vital capacity. Particulate matter (PM_{10}) was the primary pollutant found to be responsible for the lung function deficit (Gao, Chan, Li, He, & Wong, 2013). Further research has confirmed certain adverse health effects on local children's respiratory systems from long-term exposure to ambient air pollution, in particular significantly higher risk for coughing at night and phlegm without cold for girls, marginal significance for elevated risk for asthma, wheezing, and phlegm without cold for boys (Gao, Chan, Li, Lau, & Wong, 2014).

Impact of temperature on cardiovascular- and respiratory-related health

COPD and pneumonia

Pneumonia and chronic obstructive pulmonary diseases (COPD) are the commonest causes of respiratory hospitalisation among older adults. According to the World Health Organization (WHO), there are more than 65 million people suffering from moderate to severe COPD, while about 450 million people are affected by pneumonia each year (WHO, n.d.). COPD and pneumonia each accounted for about 5% of overall global deaths in 2012 and were the third and the fourth leading causes of death, respectively (WHO, 2016). Both diseases have been reported to be associated with ambient temperature. Extreme high and extreme low ambient temperature has been reported to be associated with COPD and pneumonia, potentially due to the increased risk of respiratory infections and decreased lung function during periods of extreme temperature (Donaldson, Seemungal, Jeffries, & Wedzicha, 1999; Tang, 2009).

Even in regular temperature ranges, variation of ambient temperatures has been reported to be associated with COPD hospitalisation, emergency room visits, and outpatient clinic visits, although the nature of associations reported was inconsistent, possibly due to the different climates and study designs (Donaldson et al., 1999; Hajat et al., 2016; Liang, Liu, & Kuo, 2009; Lim, Hong, & Kim, 2012; Lin et al., 2009; Qiu et al., 2013; Sauerzapf, Jones, & Cross, 2009; Song et al., 2008; Tseng et al., 2013; Vaneckova & Bambrick, 2013; Wang & Lin, 2014, 2015). Studies from Sydney in Australia, New York in the United States, and Norfolk in the United Kingdom have reported higher COPD risks during high temperature (Lin et al., 2009; Sauerzapf et al., 2009; Vaneckova & Bambrick, 2013), while studies from London, Taiwan, and England have reported increased risk at low temperature (Donaldson et al., 1999; Hajat et al., 2016; Liang et al., 2009; Tseng et al., 2013; Wang & Lin, 2014). Another study from Taiwan has reported a U-shaped association (Wang & Lin, 2015). Previous studies have reported different temperature–pneumonia associations. A study from Japan reported higher pneumonia risk at high temperatures (Onozuka, Hashizume, & Hagihara, 2009) and a Shanghai study reported increased risks at low temperatures (Liu et al., 2014), while studies from Hong Kong and Beijing have reported U-shaped associations (Qiu, Sun, Tang, Chan, & Tian, 2016; Su et al., 2014).

Although COPD is non-communicable while pneumonia is infectious, both conditions affect older people the most. About 50% of pneumonia deaths and 89% of COPD deaths in 2012 were among people aged ≥ 60 years old (WHO, 2016). Although older people may be more vulnerable to extreme high and low temperature in general due to thermoregulation impairment, reduced immune function, higher prevalence of co-morbidities, and longer history of diseases (Guo, Barnett, & Tong, 2012; Kim & Joh, 2006; Yu et al., 2012). With the ageing population, understanding the associating factors of hospitalisation of older people is important for lowering disease burdens by building up surge capacity and decreasing attributed risks. Revealing the similarities and differences of associations with meteorological variables between COPD and pneumonia morbidities may enhance the health protection capacity of authorities for service and policy planning. A study of COPD and pneumonia hospitalisation in Sydney during extreme hot temperature (Vaneckova & Bambrick, 2013) was published but the association with cold temperature and the associated lagged effect were not reported. A study from Brazil has found negative association between relative humidity, wind speed, and outpatient visits for pneumonia (Souza, Fernandes, Pavão, Lastoria, & Albrez, 2012), while another study from Germany found a significant protective effect of solar radiation on COPD ambulatory visits (Ferrari et al., 2012).

A study was conducted in Hong Kong to evaluate and compare the associations of ambient temperature and other environmental factors with pneumonia and COPD admissions among adults ≥ 60 years old in a retrospective time-series approach with seasonality, long-term trend, and holiday adjusted (Lam, Chan, & Goggins, 2018). Daily cause-specific hospitalisation counts in Hong Kong during 2004–2011 were regressed on daily meteorological variables using distributed lag non-linear models. Associations were compared between diseases by ratio of relative risks. Analyses were stratified by season and age group (60–74 years old versus ≥ 75 years old). In hot season, high temperature (>28°C) and high relative humidity (>82%) were statistically significantly associated with more pneumonia in lagged 0–2 and lagged 0–10 days, respectively. Pneumonia hospitalisations among the older people (≥ 75 years old) also increased with high solar radiation and high wind speed. During the cold season, consistent hockey-stick associations with temperature and relative humidity were found for both admissions and both age groups. The minimum morbidity temperature and relative humidity were at about 21–22°C and 82%. The lagged effects of low temperature were comparable for both diseases (lagged 0–20 days). The low-temperature–admissions associations with COPD were stronger and were strongest among older people. This study found elevated pneumonia and COPD admissions risks among adults ≥ 60 during periods of extreme weather conditions, and the associations varied by season and age group. Vulnerable groups should be advised to avoid exposures, such as staying indoors and maintaining satisfactory indoor conditions, to minimise risks.

Asthma

According to WHO, asthma is among the most common chronic respiratory diseases and there are currently over 235 million people with the disease worldwide (WHO, 2013). Asthma is characterised by chronic airway inflammation and high sensitivity to various triggers. Once triggered, the inflamed airway swells further, the muscle of the airway wall tightens and extra mucus is secreted, leading to the common symptoms of asthma, including coughing, wheezing, shortness of breath, and chest tightness. Although the fundamental causes of asthma are still unclear, some factors that trigger asthma have been identified, including environmental factors (such as pollens, pollutants, and tobacco smoke, and chemical irritants at the workplace), host factors (such as respiratory infections), and psychological factors (such as fear and anger). Asthma cannot be cured but can be controlled by medicines and by avoiding exposure to risk factors.

Previous studies have assessed the environmental risk factors for asthma and some have reported that high and low ambient temperatures were associated with higher asthma morbidity (Babin et al., 2007; Delamater, Finley, & Banerjee, 2012; Guo et al., 2012; Li et al., 2014; Mireku, Wang, Ager, Reddy, & Baptist, 2009; Son, Bell, & Lee, 2014; Wang & Lin, 2015; Xu et al., 2013; Zhang et al., 2014). However, likely due to differences in climate, socio-economic development, and genetic characteristics, the nature of these associations varied across studies in different geographic locations. A study from Australia (Xu et al., 2013) reported a positive association between childhood asthma morbidity and temperature, while a study from Shanghai (Guo, Jiang et al., 2012) reported higher numbers of admissions during periods of low temperature. In Hong Kong, large diurnal temperature ranges were found to be associated with more emergency hospital admissions for asthma (Qiu et al., 2015).

Thermoregulation ability, co-morbidity prevalence, lung function, responsiveness to rescue medicines, and disease severity are different among children, adults, and older people (Jenkins et al., 2003; Reed, 2006; Son, Lee, Anderson, & Bell, 2012; Yang et al., 2013). Age is thus regarded as a possible effect modifier of the asthma–temperature association. Several studies have reported on associations in different age groups (Abe et al., 2009; Son et al., 2014; Wang & Lin, 2015). However, only one study from Korea compared associations among children, adults, and older people from the same population (Son et al., 2014). It reported a higher risk for children under 15 than for adults or older people at low temperatures, but did not report on differences between age groups for other environmental variables.

A study examined associations between asthma hospitalisations and ambient temperatures and other environmental factors in Hong Kong using a time-series approach (Lam, Li, Chan, & Goggins, 2016). In addition, subgroup analyses by age group and season were done to assess potential effect modification by these variables. Previous studies have found associations between meteorological variables and asthma hospitalisations but the nature of these associations varied and few studies have been done in subtropical areas or evaluated effect modification by age. This study aimed to evaluate associations between asthma hospitalisations and meteorological factors and to assess effect modification of these associations by age and season in Hong Kong. Poisson generalised additive models combined with distributed lag non-linear models and piecewise linear models were used to model associations between daily asthma hospitalisations from 2004 to 2011 and meteorological factors and air pollutants, adjusting for day of week, seasonality, and trend. Subgroup analyses by age and season were performed. In the hot season, hospitalisations were lowest at 27°C, rose to a peak at 30°C, then plateaued between 30°C and 32°C. The cumulative relative risk for lags 0–3 days (RRlag0–3) for 30°C versus 27°C was 1.19 (95% confidence interval (CI): 1.06–1.34). In the cold season, temperature was negatively associated with asthma hospitalisations. The cumulative RRlag0–3 for 12°C versus 25°C was 1.33 (95% CI: 1.13–1.58). Adult admissions were most sensitive to temperatures in both seasons while admissions among children under 5 were least associated. Higher humidity and ozone levels in the hot season and low humidity in the cold season were also associated with more asthma admissions. People with asthma should avoid exposure to adverse conditions by limiting outdoor activities during periods of extreme temperatures, combination of high humidity and high temperature, combination of low humidity and low temperature, and high ozone levels.

Impact of temperature on asthma readmissions

Asthma can be triggered by various factors due to different etiologies. Environmental factors remain a common trigger of asthma, especially amongst children, and such ambient exposures can be harder to avoid when compared with behavioural triggers. As such, the contribution of environmental factors may be enhanced when considering repeat asthma cases when compared with initial presentations. A study examined asthma-related readmissions with daily asthma hospitalisations among children aged 0–5 years in Hong Kong during 2007–2011 (Lam et al., 2016). Study outcome was regressed with daily mean temperature using distributed lagged non-linear models, with adjustment for seasonal patterns, day-of-week effects, other meteorological factors, and air pollutants. Analyses were stratified by summer/winter and by type of admission (first admission and repeated admission) and found about 33% of the 12,284 asthma hospitalisations were repeat admissions.

Repeat admissions demonstrated higher sensitivity to high temperature in the summer. During this period, high temperatures were associated with increased risk of repeat admissions but not with first admissions: RR (95% CI) comparing 31°C versus 29°C across lags 0–15 days was 3.40 (1.26, 9.18) and 0.74 (0.31, 1.77) for repeat and first admissions respectively. In the cold season, all admissions increased with temperature decreases. A slightly stronger association was also found for repeat admissions when compared with first admissions: RR was 1.20 (1.00, 1.44) versus 1.10 (0.96, 1.26) respectively when comparing risk at 15°C versus 12°C across lags 0–5 days. A stronger association was found between ambient temperature and repeat asthma admissions when compared with first admissions. The higher sensitivity among those experiencing repeat admissions may allow for more personalised disease management. Given the substantial differences in associations by admission type, future studies of ambient exposures on asthma should consider analysing the two groups separately.

Heart failure

Heart failure (HF) is a syndrome in which the heart fails to meet the blood circulation needs with common causes including myocardial infarction and hypertension (McMurray & Pfeffer, 2005). Previous research has shown winter peaks for both hospitalisations and mortality from HF (refer also to Chapter 8), but few studies have examined the association between meteorological parameters and HF. A multi-country study showed temperature fluctuations were associated with acute HF, with more admissions found in warmer temperature with lag of 1–3 days and in colder temperature, with lag from 6 to 7 days (Das et al., 2014). A study examined daily HF admissions to Hong Kong public hospitals, which cover about 83% of total admissions, for 2002–2011 (Goggins & Chan, 2017). Poisson generalised additive regression models were used with daily HF admissions as outcomes and daily mean temperature, humidity, and wind speed as predictors, while controlling for pollutant levels, time trend, season, day of the week, and holiday. Non-linear distributed lag functions were used for predictors to allow for non-linear and delayed associations.

Study results indicated lower mean daily temperatures were strongly associated with increased HF admissions and mortality, with a cumulative (to 23 days) relative risk (RR) (95% CI) for HF admissions of 2.63 (2.43, 2.84) for an 11°C versus a 25°C day and cumulative (42 days) RR (95% CI) = 3.13 (1.90, 5.16) for HF mortality. The association with cold weather was stronger among older age groups and for new hospitalisations when compared with recurrent ones, while presence of co-morbidities did not modify the association. Both high and low relative humidity were modestly associated with more admissions. Both HF admissions and mortality in subtropical cities like Hong Kong were very strongly associated with cold temperatures. Reducing exposure to cold temperatures among those at risk for HF has the potential to reduce hospitalisations and mortality.

Myocardial infarction and diabetes mellitus

Due to progressive narrowing of coronary arteries of people with diabetes mellitus (DM) resulting in inadequate blood supply to the myocardium (Mendis et al., 2011), acute myocardial infarction (AMI) is the leading cause of death among people with DM (Leon & Maddox, 2015). These diseases have been found to occur more frequently with extreme temperatures. Mortality and morbidity from AMI have been found to increase with both high and low temperatures. Studies have shown increasing AMI mortality and morbidity during both high and low temperatures. Studies from Cuba (Rivero, Bolufé, Ortiz, Rodríguez, & Reyes, 2015), Sweden (Wichmann, Rosengren, Sjöberg, Barregard, & Sallsten, 2013), Massachusetts (Madrigano et al., 2014), Portugal (Vasconcelos, Freire, Almendra, Silva, & Santana, 2013), and Denmark (Wichmann, Ketzel, Ellermann, & Loft, 2012) found higher AMI risk at low temperatures, while studies from South Korea (Kwon et al., 2015; Lee et al., 2014) and England and Wales (Bhaskaran et al., 2010, 2012) have reported increased AMI risk at both extreme ends of temperatures.

Meanwhile, for diabetes mellitus, patients with DM have also been found to be more vulnerable than non-DM patients to other health problems during extreme temperatures. Positive associations between temperature and DM-related complications and mortality in studies from the United States (Basu, Pearson, Malig, Broadwin, & Green, 2012; Green et al., 2010; Schwartz, 2005) and Australia (Vaneckova & Bambrick, 2013). Studies from the Philippines (Seposo, Dang, & Honda, 2017) and China (Li et al., 2014; Yang et al., 2016) found increased DM mortality at both high and low temperatures. A worldwide meta-regression 30-country-based study found a positive association between glucose intolerance and outdoor temperature (Blauw et al., 2017). Few studies have been done on possible effect modification of this association by co-morbidity with DM, especially in warmer climates.

The temperature-sensitive natures of both DM and AMI and the higher vulnerability to other health problems among DM patients suggest the potential for a higher risk of temperature-related AMI admissions among DM patients. A German study examined the association between myocardial infarction occurrence and ambient temperatures and found that higher AMI occurrence was associated with lower temperatures but that there was no effect modification of this association by history of DM (Wolf et al., 2009). In Hong Kong, previous studies have also reported increased cardiovascular (Chan, Goggins, Yue, & Lee, 2013; Tian, Qiu, Sun, & Lin, 2016) and AMI hospital admissions (Goggins, Chan, & Yang, 2013) at low temperatures as well as higher excess risks of natural mortality among DM patients during periods of both low and high temperatures (Sun et al., 2016). The overall evidence points to a potential increased risk of AMI for DM patients during extremes of temperature.

A study compared the relative risks of AMI admissions during extreme temperatures between DM and non-DM patients in Hong Kong, a city with a subtropical climate, using a retrospective time-series approach (Lam, Chan, Luk, Chan, & Goggins, 2018). Adjusting for other meteorological variables and air pollutants, distributed lag non-linear models (DLNMs) were created to estimate the short-term association between daily mean temperature and AMI admissions (International Classification of Diseases 9th revision [ICD-9] code: 410.00–410.99), stratified by DM status (ICD-9: 250.00–250.99), to all public hospitals in Hong Kong from 2002 to 2011. Analyses were also stratified by season, age group, gender, and admission type (first admissions and readmissions) for a total of 53,769 AMI admissions during the study period (Lam, Chan, Luk, et al., 2018). Findings indicated AMI admissions among DM patients were linearly and negatively associated with temperature in the cold season (cumulative relative risk [cumRR] [95% confidence interval] in lag 0–22 days (12°C versus 24°C) = 2.10 [1.62–2.72]), while those among patients without DM only started increasing when temperatures dropped below 22°C with a weaker association (cumRR = 1.43 [1.21–1.69]). In the hot season, AMI hospitalisations among DM patients started increasing when the temperature dropped below or rose above 28.8°C (cumRR in lag 0–4 days [30.4 versus 28.8°C] = 1.14 [1.00–1.31]), while those among patients without DM showed no association with temperature.

The differences in sensitivity to temperature between patients with DM and without DM were most apparent in the group < 75 years old and among first-admission cases in the cold season. The main limitation of this study was the unavailability of data on individual exposure to ambient temperature. Overall, the analysis showed that DM patients had a higher increased risk of AMI admissions than non-DM patients did during extreme temperatures. AMI admissions risks among DM patients rise sharply in both high and low temperatures, with a stronger effect in low temperatures. Meanwhile, AMI risk among non-DM patients only increased mildly in low temperatures. Targeted health protection guidelines should be provided to warn DM patients and physicians about the dangers of extreme temperatures.

Mental health admissions

Mental illness is a global health burden accounting for 32.4% of years lived with disability (YLDs) and 13.0% of disability adjusted life years (DALYs) (Vigo, Thornicroft, & Atun, 2016). Mental disorders also have substantial impacts upon suicide rate (Chesney, Goodwin, & Fazel, 2014). The World Health Organization estimated the prevalence of lifetime mental disorder (including anxiety, mood, externalising, and substance use) to be within the inter-quartile ranges of 18.1%–36.1% (Kessler et al., 2009).

Climate change affects epidemiology of mental illness mainly through the impact of natural disasters (Berry, Bowen, & Kjellstrom, 2010; refer also to Chapter 3). Although a single disaster event, such as heavy storm or flooding, may lead to more significant impact on mental health when compared with a single heatwave or extreme high temperature event, increasing temperature is an unavoidable exposure for the global population. Studies from Shanghai and Toronto (Peng, Wang, Kan, Chen, & Wang, 2017; Wang, Lavigne, Ouellette-Kuntz, & Chen, 2014), two Northern Hemispheric cities located at higher latitudes above the Tropic of Cancer (23°26′12.9″), have reported higher relative risks of mental disorder admissions at warmer temperatures, but no association at low temperatures. A majority of other studies also reported a higher risk of mental disorders during warmer temperatures but they focused on hot seasons only (Vida, Durocher, Ouarda, & Gosselin, 2012; Williams et al., 2012), were conducted during heatwaves (Hansen et al., 2008; Nitschke et al., 2011; Trang, Rocklöv, Giang, Kullgren, & Nilsson, 2016), or looked at the effect of seasonality (Amr & Volpe, 2012; Trang, Rocklöv, Giang, & Nilsson, 2016). Suicide rate, which is closely relevant to mental disorders, has also been found to increase with warmer temperatures (Kim, Kim, & Kim, 2011; Töro et al., 2009; Tsai & Cho, 2012) in different regions.

Although several studies have reported the effects of temperature on mental disorders, analyses of mental health-related mortality or hospitalisation threshold temperatures, lagged effects, and relative risk were seldom included. The Chinese University of Hong Kong team has studied the temperature–health association in Hong Kong, a highly dense subtropical city, and found heterogeneous associations of high temperature with the risk of various health problems, including cardiovascular diseases (Goggins & Chan, 2017; Goggins, Woo, Ho, Chan, & Chau, 2012), respiratory diseases (Goggins, Chan, Yang, & Chong, 2013; Lam, Hajat, Chan, & Goggins, 2019), and infectious diseases (Wang, Goggins, & Chan, 2016), and overall hospitalisation and mortality (Chan, Goggins, Kim, & Griffiths, 2012; Chan et al., 2013; Goggins, Chan, Ng, Ren, & Chen, 2012). With increasing global average temperatures, understanding the potential impact of high temperatures on mental disorder hospitalisations will support the drafting of targeted population-based health policies that reduce the mental disease burden. This study aimed to evaluate the short-term association between ambient temperatures and mental disorder hospitalisations in a subtropical city with a mean annual temperature over 21°C.

Public hospital admissions data from the Hospital Authority of Hong Kong, which accounts for about 83% of the city's overall hospitalisations (Chan et al., 2013) and more than 99% cases for mental health-related hospitalisation are admitted to this public hospital system (Hospital Authority, Hong Kong SAR, 2018). The daily number of hospital admissions between 2002 and 2011 with principal diagnosis at discharge as mental disorders (MD) (International Classification of Diseases ICD-9-290.xx-319.xx) was obtained (ICD9Data.com, 2013). ICD-9 was used in this study as the clinical record system of the Hospital Authority in Hong Kong had kept records using ICD-9 during the study period. In addition to information on diagnosis, each admission record contained details on patient age and gender and all data were kept anonymous.

Daily meteorological records measured at the Hong Kong Observatory (HKO) were obtained for the study period, including mean temperature and mean relative humidity (RH), from the open-access data available on their website (www.hko.gov.hk/cis/climat_e.htm). The HKO data were selected because the website provides complete records for the required variables with no missing data during the study period and the monitoring station is located near the centre of Hong Kong, enabling recorded temperature to be representative of the general population. Aside from temperature, high levels of air pollutants have been reported to be associated with a higher risk of mental disorders (Chan et al., 2018). Daily air pollutants levels were also included in models to assess the associations and account for their potential confounding effects. Daily average level of air pollutants from all general air quality monitoring stations except Tap Mun were downloaded from the official website of the Environmental Protection Department of Hong Kong and averaged, including particulate matter (PM_{10}), sulphur dioxide (SO_2), nitrogen dioxide (NO_2), and ozone (O_3). Tap Mun station was excluded because it is located in a remote rural area with very low population density; thus the exposure might not be representative for the general population. Subgroup analyses by gender and age group (older people ≥75 years old, older adults 60–74 years old, adults 15–59 years old, and children < 15 years old) were performed to assess potential effect modification. Sub-disease classes including persistent mental disorders due to conditions classified elsewhere (ICD-9 294.xx), dementias (ICD-9 290.xx), schizophrenic disorders (ICD-9 295.xx), episodic mood disorders (ICD-9 296.xx), other nonorganic psychoses (ICD-9 298.xx), anxiety, dissociative and somatoform disorders (ICD-9 300.xx), depressive disorder, not elsewhere classified (ICD-9 311.xx), transient mental disorders due to conditions classified elsewhere (ICD-9 293.xx), drug-related mental disorders (ICD-9 292.xx and 305.xx), and alcohol-related mental disorders (ICD-9 291.xx and ICD-9 303.xx) were evaluated in subgroup analyses (ICD9Data.com, 2013). Cumulative relative risks (RR) were estimated by comparing the admission risk between extreme exposure and reference exposure. The extreme and reference points for comparisons were chosen based on the association found between exposure and overall admissions.

Results indicated that among the 7,150,288 all-cause admissions during the 10-year study period, there were 44,600 mental disorders admissions (0.62%) and the daily mean number of mental disorders admissions was 12.21. Among these, 52.45% were male, 36.19% were older people aged ≥75 years old, 16.39% were older adults aged 60–74 years old, 45.55% were adults aged 15–59 years old, and 1.87% were children aged below 15 years old. The median daily mean temperature during the study period was 24.6°C (interquartile range (IQR): 19.40, 27.80). For the four air pollutants examined in that study, only NO_2 showed a significant association with mental disorder admissions. No confounding effects by PM_{10}, SO_2, and ozone were observed and therefore NO_2 was the only air pollutant included in the final model. There was no significant seasonal trend for mental disorder admissions before and after adjustment of environmental factors.

Temperature showed a positive linear association with mental disorders and the association lasted for about 2 days. The RR increased significantly when temperature rose over 19.4°C (the lower quartile). The lagged 0–2 days RR at 28°C (temperature at the 75th percentile versus temperature at the 25th percentile at 19.4°C) was 1.09 (95% CI (1.03, 1.15)). Results in subgroup analyses showed that the linear association between temperature and overall mental disorders admissions was mainly contributed by the adult group 15–59 years old and the female group. Moreover, positive association for the 15–59 group became weaker when temperature was above 27°C (with the lower confidence interval of RR dropping below 1.00). Above the threshold at about 20°C, a strong association with warm temperature was exhibited by the older people group ≥ 75 years old and males. The lagged 0–2 days RR at 28°C (versus 19.4°C) for older people and adults were 1.20 (CI 1.09, 1.31) and 1.06 (CI 0.98, 1.15), respectively. The lagged 0–2 days RR at 28°C (versus 19.4°C) for males and females were 1.08 (CI: 1.01, 1.16) and 1.09 (CI 1.01, 1.18), respectively. It should be highlighted that in this study temperature showed no obvious effects on older adults and children.

In sub-disease analyses, transient mental disorders and episodic mood disorders showed a positive association with temperature while drug-related mental disorders demonstrated a positive association when temperature rose over a threshold of about 20°C. The association with transient mental disorders was strong and significant (RR 1.51 (CI 1.00, 2.27)), followed in strength by episodic mood disorders (RR 1.34 (CI 1.05, 1.71)) and then drug-related mental disorders (RR 1.13 (CI 1.00, 1.27)). Depressive disorder and other non-organic psychoses showed a significant lower risk at lower temperature while dementias and persistent mental disorders demonstrated a non-significant U-shaped association with temperature. No obvious association with temperature was observed for anxiety, dissociative, and somatoform disorders, schizophrenic disorders, and alcohol-related mental disorders. Temperature was positively associated with mental disorder admissions at lags 0–2 days. The association was mainly contributed by females and adults 15–59 years old. Transient mental disorders and episodic mood disorders demonstrated a robust positive association with temperature while drug-related mental disorders showed a positive association with temperature for temperature above 20°C.

The Hong Kong study results (Chan et al., 2018) were consistent with the two similar studies conducted at higher latitudes above the Tropic of Cancer. These studies, from Toronto (Wang et al., 2014) and Shanghai (Peng et al., 2017), found a higher relative risk of mental disorder admissions at warmer temperatures with short lagged effect (less than 1 week) and observed no cold effect. As a subtropical city below the Tropic of Cancer, the Hong Kong findings in this study demonstrated a linear relationship similar to Toronto but different from Shanghai, which had an obvious threshold. In contrast, a study from Germany found higher risks of all studied subtypes of mental disorders (ICD10 F00–F50) at lower temperatures (< 10°C) (Shiue, Perkins, & Bearman, 2016). A study from Egypt reported a positive correlation for mania, a negative correlation with depression, but no association for schizophrenia (Amr &Volpe, 2012).

Temperature might be associated with concentration of air pollutants and studies showed that extreme high levels of nitrogen dioxide were associated with higher risk of overall mental disorder admissions, in particular transient mental disorders, anxiety, dissociative and somatoform disorders, persistent mental disorders, and schizophrenic disorders (Becerra, Wilhelm, Olsen, Cockburn, & Ritz, 2013; Chan et al., 2018; Power et al., 2015). Previous studies have reported significant associations of ambient air pollutants with mental disorders and the sub-diseases. Nitrogen dioxide is one of the major air pollutants and nitrogen oxide, particulates, and ozone were found associated with higher odds of autism among children in California (Becerra et al., 2013; Volk, Lurmann, Penfold, Hertz-Picciotto, & McConnell, 2013). $PM_{2.5}$ was associated with anxiety among older female adults in the United States (Power et al., 2015).

Depression and related symptoms were found to be associated with exposure to high level of SO_2, PM_{10}, NO_2, ozone, and CO in Korea (Cho et al., 2014; Lim et al., 2012), exposure to high level of NO_2 in Barcelona (Vert et al., 2017) and Netherlands but was negatively associated with NO_2 in Norway (Zijlema et al., 2016). Particulates were associated with schizophrenia and coarse particulate with overall mental disorders in Beijing, China (Gao, Xu, Guo, Fan, & Zhu, 2017). Studies from Sweden also reported an association between PM_{10} and overall psychiatric emergency admissions in the warm season (Oudin et al., 2018) and found a positive association between NO_2 and psychiatric disorders in children and adolescents (Oudin, Brabäck, Aström, Strömgren, & Forsberg, 2016). The Hong Kong study agreed with most previous studies in finding that high NO_2 levels were associated with mental disorders (Chan et al., 2018). In particular, NO_2 has been reported to affect neurodegeneration (Yan, Yun, Ku, Li, & Sang, 2016) and this is consistent with the Hong Kong study findings that the association with NO_2 is most significant in the older age groups. However, particulates, another pollutant that was commonly reported in other studies as an associating factor of mental disorders as well as reduced cognitive function (Gatto et al., 2014), did not appear to be related to mental disorders in this study. More studies are needed to investigate the biological mechanisms.

Overall, evidence shows mental disorders to be positively associated with various diverse climatic regions. High temperature was significantly associated with an increased number of mental disorder hospitalisations in a subtropical urban city with average annual temperature above 21°C (Chan et al., 2018). The association was stronger among people above 75 years old. With the collective effect of global warming and an ageing population, the number of heat-related mental disorders may increase and may further intensify the disease burden across the public health, economic, and societal contexts. The significant positive trend between temperature and mental disorders demonstrated that the sensitivity of mental disorders to temperature is not lower than other commonly studied heat-related disease groups. Existing literature showed that admission risk of mental disorders or related problems mostly increased with temperature increases, regardless of geographic locations and latitude, and only a few studies have reported cold effects.

A review of literature may further explain how ambient temperature may affect risk of mental disorders in different ways. Temperature stress can affect physio-psychological functions directly by its effects on bio-chemicals. Heat stress is negatively associated with cognitive function and one of the plausible explanations is that it increases plasma serotonin that inhibits the production of dopamine, a neurotransmitter that is responsible for complex task performance (Taylor, Watkins, Marshall, Dascombe, & Foster, 2016). Previous studies also reported a correlation between high temperature and altered platelet serotonin that is associated with psychiatric disorders such as depression and schizophrenia (Ljubičić, Stipčević, Pivac, Jakovljević, & Mück-Šeler, 2007; Sarrias, Artigas, Martínez, & Gelpí, 1989). High ambient temperature may also worsen the adverse health impacts on substance use. Although patterns of substance use were not shown to change with temperature, a study from New York found higher mortality from cocaine use during hot days (>31.1°C) when compared with other days (Marzuk et al., 1998). The authors hypothesised that extra stress added to the cardiovascular system by high temperature might worsen the existing cardiovascular conditions caused by cocaine use. Other types of substance use that increase the cardiovascular load may cause similar effects and drive the number of hospital admissions. In addition, previous studies have found increased mortality and morbidity risks at high temperature among patients with mental and behavioural disorders (Page, Hajat, Sari Kovats, & Howard, 2012; Schmeltz & Gamble, 2017). People with reduced cognitive function may have less awareness of extreme environmental conditions and be less likely to apply self-protective measures, creating chances of higher personal exposures to high temperatures. Medications such as antipsychotics may also affect thermoregulation mechanisms like sweating, which may render patients with mental disorders more vulnerable to heat stress.

Furthermore, study showed that age was an effect modifier of the temperature–mental disorder admissions association. Mental disorder admissions among the older population were more sensitive to high temperature and high levels of NO_2 (Chan et al., 2018). The global ageing population will certainly increase the size of this vulnerable group. With the dual effect of global warming and ageing population, the burden of heat-related mental conditions will likely increase.

Healthcare professionals, patients, and caregivers should be advised to reduce exposure. Future studies for sub-diseases and understanding the biological mechanisms are warranted. Policies promoting reduced exposure to extreme high temperature such as reminders of using air conditioning and notifications to susceptible groups may be encouraged to lower the risk of mental disorder hospitalisations among adults and older people. Besides, NO_2 is one of the traffic-related air pollutants against which pollutant emission control would be feasible. Air-quality policies reducing or limiting the release of NO_2 should be promoted to protect the global population from over-excessive exposure to NO_2. The lagged effects identified in this study, 0–2 days for temperature and 0–8 days for NO_2, should also be considered by hospitals for capacity preparation.

Temperature, allergy, and health

Allergy, including asthma, rhinitis, eczema, conjunctivitis, urticaria, food allergy, and anaphylaxis, is a hypersensitivity reaction initiated by the immune system (WHO, 2003). According to the World Allergy Organization (WAO), estimated allergy prevalence by country ranged between 10 and 40% (Pawankar, Canonica, Holgate, Lockey, & Blasis, 2013). The prevalence is increasing particularly in developing regions and among children (Banac et al., 2013; Gupta, Sheikh, Strachan, & Anderson, 2007; Kim et al., 2016; Pawankar, 2014), which was possibly associated with "Westernized" lifestyles and urbanisations (Pawankar et al., 2013), despite the unclear effects of high temperature on existing allergic conditions.

While the impact of temperature and humidity on admission associated with allergy is uncertain, a study was conducted to examine the impact of high temperature on existing allergic symptoms among an adult population (Lam & Chan, 2018). The effects of high temperature on other non-allergic health outcomes were compared between adults with and without a history of allergic symptoms. A cross-sectional telephone survey study was conducted in Hong Kong 2 weeks after a heatwave in 2017. Socio-demographic information, history of allergic symptoms, non-allergic health symptoms, and self-reported changes of allergic symptoms during the study hot period were collected using multiple-choice questions. Of the 436 respondents, 24% had reported an allergic history. During the study hot period, 22.4% and 15.7% of those who had skin and nasal allergies reported worsened symptoms as compared with normal days. Comparing with people without an allergic history, those who reported having pre-existing allergic symptoms reported a higher rate of mucus secretions, mouth ulcers, poorer sleeping quality, and worsened mood during the study hot period. Pre-existing allergic symptoms were found associated with more adverse health effects and worse quality of life during hot days. A strategic health promotion policy should be planned to increase the awareness of the potential impacts of high temperature on allergy and the related health issues.

Injuries

Physical injuries are often resulted and associated with climate-related disasters or extreme weather events, e.g. drowning, and injuries sustained from walking or driving through floodwater, collapsed or damaged building, being crushed, cut, or struck during storms, and traffic accidents resulting from poor road conditions and landslides. In urban cities such as Hong Kong, major incidents with multiple casualties are likely to occur when extreme events happen to the high-density-based human habitat (e.g. a landslide occurs to residence near slopes) as well as to the population vulnerable to the secondary impacts of climate change (e.g. flooding post rainfall or fire post heatwave in its underground lifeline infrastructure like water and sewage, gas-pipes, and electricity and telecommunication lines). To protect the community from the expected increases of extreme weather events in the coming decades, better understanding of injuries patterns, health and service need estimations, relevant contingency plans, increase of health response surge capacity, and community resilience building towards emergency health impact would be necessary to minimise physical harm.

Conclusion

This chapter discusses studies that examine how temperature and various meteorological variables might affect non-death-related hospitalisation in a subtropical city. Overall, regardless of the clinical conditions examined, results of these studies show temperature variations and extremes may cause adverse implications on non-death human health outcomes and medical service utilisation. It is important to emphasise however that most of these adverse repercussions are avoidable if proactive measures are taken by authorities to remind and support patients with pre-existing medical conditions to protect themselves from potential risks. The next few chapters will explore the current understanding of how individuals living in urban communities might be further affected by meteorological impacts and how they might respond to warning and be supported in times of weather-related health-affecting context.

References

Abe, T., Tokuda, Y., Ohde, S., Ishimatsu, S., Nakamura, T., & Birrer, R. B. (2009). The relationship of short-term air pollution and weather to ED visits for asthma in Japan. *The American Journal of Emergency Medicine, 27*(2), 153.

Amr, M., & Volpe, F. M. (2012). Seasonal influences on admissions for mood disorders and schizophrenia in a teaching psychiatric hospital in Egypt. *Journal of Affective Disorders, 137*, 56–60.

Babin, S. M., Burkom, H. S., Holtry, R. S., Tabernero, N. R., Stokes, L. D., Davies-Cole, J. O., … Lee, D. H. (2007). Pediatric patient asthma-related emergency department visits and admissions in Washington, DC, from 2001–2004, and associations with air quality, socio-economic status and age group. *Environmental Health, 6*, 9. doi:10.1186/1476-069X-6-9.

Banac, S., Rožmanić, V., Manestar, K., Korotaj-Rožmanić, Z., Lah-Tomulić, K., Vidović, I., … Petrić, T. (2013). Rising trends in the prevalence of asthma and allergic diseases among school children in the north-west coastal part of Croatia. *Journal of Asthma, 50*(8), 810–814.

Basu, R., Pearson, D., Malig, B., Broadwin, R., & Green, R. (2012). The effect of high ambient temperature on emergency room visits. *Epidemiology, 23*(6), 813–820.

Becerra, T. A., Wilhelm, M., Olsen, J., Cockburn, M., & Ritz, B. (2013). Ambient air pollution and autism in Los Angeles County, California. *Environmental Health Perspectives, 121*, 380–386.

Berry, H. L., Bowen, K., & Kjellstrom, T. (2010). Climate change and mental health: A causal pathways framework. *International Journal of Public Health, 55*, 123–132.

Bhaskaran, K., Armstrong, B., Hajat, S., Haines, A., Wilkinson, P., & Smeeth, L. (2012). Heat and risk of myocardial infarction: Hourly level case-crossover analysis of MINAP database. *The BMJ, 345*, e8050.

Bhaskaran, K., Hajat, S., Haines, A., Herrett, E., Wilkinson, P., & Smeeth, L. (2010). Short term effects of temperature on risk of myocardial infarction in England and Wales: Time series regression analysis of the Myocardial Ischaemia National Audit Project. *The BMJ, 341*, 3823.

Blauw, L. L., Aziz, N. A., Tannemaat, M. R., Blauw, C. A., de Craen, A. J., Pijl, H., … Rensen, P. C. N. (2017). Diabetes incidence and glucose intolerance prevalence increase with higher outdoor temperature. *BMJ Open Diabetes Research & Care, 5*, e000317.

Chan, E. Y. Y., Goggins, W. B., Kim, J. J., & Griffiths, S. M. (2012). A study of intracity variation of temperature-related mortality and socioeconomic status among the Chinese population in Hong Kong. *Journal of Epidemiology and Community Health, 66*, 322–327.

Chan, E. Y. Y, Goggins, W. B., Yue, S. K., & Lee, P. (2013). Hospital admissions as a function of temperature, other weather phenomena and pollution levels in an urban setting in China. *Bulletin of the World Health Organization, 91*(8), 576–584.

Chan, E. Y. Y., Lam, H. C. Y., So, S. H. W., Goggins, W. B., Ho, J. Y., Liu, S., & Chung, P. P. W. (2018). Association between ambient temperatures and mental disorder hospitalizations in a subtropical city: A time-series study of Hong Kong Special Administrative Region. *International Journal of Environment Research and Public Health, 15*(4), 754. doi:10.3390/ijerph15040754.

Chesney, E., Goodwin, G. M., & Fazel, S. (2014). Risks of all-cause and suicide mortality in mental disorders: A meta-review. *World Psychiatry, 13*, 153–160.

Cheung, C. C., & Yim, S. H. L. (2015). Projecting the impacts of climate change on air quality using statistical downscaling of atmospheric stability indices: A case study in Pearl River Delta. In J. G. Dy, J. Emile-Geay, V. Lakshmanan, & Y. Liu (Eds.), *Proceedings of the 5th International Workshop on Climate Informatics*, Boulder, United States.

Cho, J., Choi, Y. J., Suh, M., Sohn, J., Kim, H., Cho, S. K., ... Shin, D. C. (2014). Air pollution as a risk factor for depressive episode in patients with cardiovascular disease, diabetes mellitus, or asthma. *Journal of Affective Disorders, 157*, 45–51.

Crimmins, A., Balbus, J., Gamble, J. L., Beard, C. B., Bell, J. E, Dodgen, D., ... Herring, S. C. (2016). *The impacts of climate change on human health in the United States: A scientific assessment*. Washington, DC: Global Change Research Program.

Das, D., Bakal, J. A., Westerhout, C. M., Hernandez, A. F., O'Connor, C. M., Atar, D., ... Ezekowitz, J. A. (2014). The association between meteorological events and acute heart failure: New insights from ASCEND-HF. *International Journal of Cardiology, 177*, 819–824.

Delamater, P. L., Finley, A. O., & Banerjee, S. (2012). An analysis of asthma hospitalizations, air pollution, and weather conditions in Los Angeles County, California. *Science of Total Environment, 425*, 110.

Donaldson, G. C., Seemungal, T., Jeffries, D. J., & Wedzicha, J. A. (1999). Effect of temperature on lung function and symptoms in chronic obstructive pulmonary disease. *European Respiratory Journal, 13*, 844–849.

Ferrari, U., Exner, T., Wanka, E. R., Bergemann, C., Meyer-Arnek, J., Hildenbrand, B., ... Fischer, R. (2012). Influence of air pressure, humidity, solar radiation, temperature, and wind speed on ambulatory visits due to chronic obstructive pulmonary disease in Bavaria, Germany. *International Journal of Biometeorology, 56*(1), 137–143.

Fisk, W. J. (2001). Estimates of potential nationwide productivity and health benefits from better indoor environments: An update. In J. Spengler, J. M. Samet, & J. F. McCarthy (Eds.), *Indoor air quality handbook* (pp. 1–36). New York, NY: McGraw Hill.

Gao, Q., Xu, Q., Guo, X., Fan, H., & Zhu, H. (2017). Particulate matter air pollution associated with hospital admissions for mental disorders: A time-series study in Beijing, China. *European Psychiatry, 44*, 68–75.

Gao, Y., Chan, E. Y. Y., Li, L. P., He, Q. Q., & Wong, T. W. (2013). Chronic effects of ambient air pollution on lung function among Chinese children. *Archives of Disease in Childhood, 98*(2), 128–135.

Gao, Y., Chan, E. Y. Y., Li, L. P., Lau, P. W. C, & Wong, T. W. (2014). Chronic effects of ambient air pollution on respiratory morbidities among Chinese children: A cross-sectional study in Hong Kong. *BMC Public Health*, *14*(1), 1.

Gao, Y., Chan, E. Y. Y., Zhu, Y., & Wong, T. W. (2013). Adverse effect of outdoor air pollution on cardiorespiratory fitness in Chinese children. *Atmospheric Environment*, *64*, 10–17.

Gatto, N. M., Henderson, V. W., Hodis, H. N., John, J. A. S., Lurmann, F., Chen, J.-C., & Mack, W. J. (2014). Components of air pollution and cognitive function in middle-aged and older adults in Los Angeles. *Neurotoxicology*, *40*, 1–7.

Goggins, W. B., & Chan, E. Y. Y. (2017). A study of the short-term associations between hospital admissions and mortality from heart failure and meteorological variables in Hong Kong: Weather and heart failure in Hong Kong. *International Journal of Cardiology*, *228*, 537–542. doi:10.1016/j.ijcard.2016.11.106.

Goggins, W. B., Chan, E. Y. Y., Ng, E., Ren, C., & Chen, L. (2012). Effect modification of the association between short-term meteorological factors and mortality by urban heat islands in Hong Kong. *PLOS ONE*, *7*, e38551.

Goggins, W. B., Chan, E. Y. Y., & Yang, C. Y. (2013). Weather, pollution, and acute myocardial infarction in Hong Kong and Taiwan. *International Journal of Cardiology*, *168*(1), 243–249.

Goggins, W. B., Chan, E. Y. Y., Yang, C. Y., & Chong, M. (2013). Associations between mortality and meteorological and pollutant variables during the cool season in two Asian cities with sub-tropical climates: Hong Kong and Taipei. *Environmental Health*, *12*(1), 59. doi:10.1186/1476-069X-12-59.

Goggins, W. B., Woo, J., Ho, S., Chan, E. Y. Y., & Chau, P. H. (2012). Weather, season, and daily stroke admissions in Hong Kong. *International Journal of Biometeorology*, *56*, 865–872.

Green, R. S., Basu, R., Malig, B., Broadwin, R., Kim, J. J., & Ostro, B. (2010). The effect of temperature on hospital admissions in nine California counties. *International Journal of Public Health*, *55*(2), 113–121.

Guo, Y., Barnett, A. G., & Tong, S. (2012). High temperatures-related elderly mortality varied greatly from year to year: Important information for heat-warning systems. *Scientific Reports*, *2*, 830. doi:10.1038/srep00830.

Guo, Y., Jiang, F., Peng, L., Zhang, J., Geng, F., Xu, J., … Shen, X. (2012). The association between cold spells and pediatric outpatient visits for asthma in Shanghai, China. *PLOS ONE*, *7*, e42232. doi:10.1371/journal.pone.0042232.

Gupta, R., Sheikh, A., Strachan, D. P., & Anderson, H. R. (2007). Time trends in allergic disorders in the UK. *Thorax*, *62*(1), 91–96. doi:10.1136/thx.2004.038844.

Hajat, S., Chalabi, Z., Wilkinson, P., Erens, B., Jones, L., & Mays, N. (2016). Public health vulnerability to wintertime weather: Time-series regression and episode analyses of National Mortality and Morbidity Databases to inform the cold weather plan for England. *Public Health*, *137*, 26–34. doi:10.1016/j.puhe.2015.12.015.

Hansen, A., Bi, P., Nitschke, M., Ryan, P., Pisaniello, D., & Tucker, G. (2008). The effect of heat waves on mental health in a temperate Australian city. *Environmental Health Perspectives*, *116*, 1369–1375.

Hospital Authority, Hong Kong SAR. (2018). *HA statistical report*. Retrieved from www.ha.org.hk/visitor/ha_visitor_index.asp?Content_ID=224130&Lang=ENG&Dimension=100&Parent_ID=10221&Ver=HTML.

Hussain, A., Wenbi, R., da Silva, A. L., Nadher, M., & Mudhish, M. (2015). Health and emergency-care platform for the elderly and disabled people in the smart city. *Journal of Systems and Software*, *110*, 253–263.

ICD9Data.com. (2013). Mental disorders 290-319 [online]. Retrieved from www.icd9 data.com/2013/Volume1/290-319/default.htm.

Jenkins, H. A., Cherniack, R., Szefler, S. J., Covar, R., Gelfand, E. W., & Spahn, J. D. (2003). A comparison of the clinical characteristics of children and adults with severe asthma. *Chest, 124*(4), 318.

Kessler, R. C., Aguilar-Gaxiola, S., Alonso, J., Chatterji, S., Lee, S., Ormel, J., ... Wang, P. S. (2009). The global burden of mental disorders: An update from the WHO World Mental Health (WMH) Surveys. *Epidemiology and Psychiatric Science, 18,* 23–29.

Kim, B. K., Kim, J. Y., Kang, M. K., Yang, M. S., Park, H. W., Min, K. U., ... Kang, H. R. (2016). Allergies are still on the rise? A 6-year nationwide population-based study in Korea. *Allergology International, 65*(2), 186–191.

Kim, Y., & Joh, S. (2006). A vulnerability study of the low-income elderly in the context of high temperature and mortality in Seoul, Korea. *Science of the Total Environment, 371*(1–3), 82–88.

Kim, Y., Kim, H., & Kim, D. S. (2011). Association between daily environmental temperature and suicide mortality in Korea (2001–2005). *Psychiatry Research, 186,* 390–396.

Kwon, B. Y., Lee, E., Lee, S., Heo, S., Jo, K., Kim J., & Park, M. S. (2015). Vulnerabilities to temperature effects on acute myocardial infarction hospital admissions in South Korea. *International Journal of Environmental Research and Public Health, 37,* 14571–14588.

Lam, H. C. Y., & Chan, E. Y. Y. (2018). *The impact of high temperature on existing allergic symptoms among an adult population* (CCOUC Working Paper Series). Hong Kong: Collaborating Centre for Oxford University and CUHK for Disaster and Medical Humanitarian Response.

Lam, H. C. Y., Chan, E. Y. Y., & Goggins, W. B. (2018). Comparison of short-term associations with meteorological variables between COPD and pneumonia hospitalization among the elderly in Hong Kong—A time-series study. *International Journal of Biometeorology, 62,* 1447. doi:10.1007/s00484-018-1542-2.

Lam, H. C. Y., Chan, J. C. N, Luk, A. O. Y., Chan, E. Y. Y., & Goggins, W. B. (2018). Short-term association between ambient temperature and acute myocardial infarction hospitalizations for diabetes mellitus patients: A time series study. *PLOS Medicine, 15*(7), e1002612. doi:10.1371/journal.pmed.1002612.

Lam, H. C. Y., Hajat, S., Chan, E. Y. Y., & Goggins, W. B. (2019). Different sensitivities to ambient temperature between first- and re-admission childhood asthma cases in Hong Kong: A time series study. *Environmental Research, 170,* 487–492.

Lam, H. C. Y., Li, A. M., Chan, E. Y. Y., & Goggins, W. B. (2016). The short-term association between asthma hospitalisations, ambient temperature, other meteorological factors and air pollutants in Hong Kong: A time-series study. *Thorax, 71,* 1097–1109.

Lee, S., Lee, E., Park, M. S., Kwon, B. Y., Kim, H., Jung, D. H., ... Rha, S. W. (2014). Short-term effect of temperature on daily emergency visits for acute myocardial infarction with threshold temperatures. *PLOS ONE, 9*(4).

Leon, B. M., & Maddox, T. M. (2015). Diabetes and cardiovascular disease: Epidemiology, biological mechanisms, treatment recommendations and future research. *World Journal of Diabetes, 6*(13), 1246. doi:10.4239/wjd.v6.i13.1246.

Li, S., Baker, P. J., Jalaludin, B. B., Guo, Y., Marks, G. B. Denison, L. S., & Williams, G. M. (2014). Are children's asthmatic symptoms related to ambient temperature? A panel study in Australia. *Environmental Research, 133,* 239–245.

Li, Y., Lan, L., Wang, Y., Yang, C., Tang, W., Cui, G., ... Jin, Y. (2014). Extremely cold and hot temperatures increase the risk of diabetes mortality in metropolitan areas of two Chinese cities. *Environmental Research*, *134*, 91–97. doi:10.1016/j.envres.2014. 06.022.

Liang, W. M., Liu, W. P., & Kuo, H. W. (2009). Diurnal temperature range and emergency room admissions for chronic obstructive pulmonary disease in Taiwan. *International Journal of Biometeorology*, *53*(1), 17–23. doi:10.1007/s00484-008-0187-y.

Lim, Y. H., Hong, Y. C., & Kim, H. (2012). Effects of diurnal temperature range on cardiovascular and respiratory hospital admissions in Korea. *Science of the Total Environment*, *417–418*, 55–60. doi:10.1016/j.scitotenv.2011.

Lin, S., Luo, M., Walker, R. J., Liu, X., Hwang, S. A., & Chinery, R. (2009). Extreme high temperatures and hospital admissions for respiratory and cardiovascular diseases. *Epidemiology*, *20*(5), 738–746.

Liu, Y., Kan, H., Xu, J., Rogers, D., Peng, L., Ye, X., ... Wang, W. (2014). Temporal relationship between hospital admissions for pneumonia and weather conditions in Shanghai, China: A time-series analysis. *BMJ Open*, *4*(7), e004961. doi:10.1136/ bmjopen-2014-004961.

Ljubičić, D., Stipčević, T., Pivac, N., Jakovljević, M., & Mück-Šeler, D. (2007). The influence of daylight exposure on platelet 5-HT levels in patients with major depression and schizophrenia. *Journal of Photochemistry and Photobiology B: Biology*, *89*, 63–69.

Madrigano, J., Mittleman, M. A., Baccarelli, A., Goldberg, R., Melly, S., von Klot, S., & Schwartz, J. (2014). Temperature, myocardial infarction, and mortality: Effect modification by individual- and area-level characteristics. *Epidemiology*, *24*(3), 439–446.

Marzuk, P. M., Tardiff, K., Leon, A. C., Hirsch, C. S., Portera, L., Iqbal, M. I., ... Hartwell, N. (1998). Ambient temperature and mortality from unintentional cocaine overdose. *The Journal of the American Medical Association*, *279*, 1795–1800.

McMurray, J. J. V., & Pfeffer, M. A. (2005). Heart failure. *The Lancet*, *365*, 1877–1889.

Mendis, S., Thygesen, K., Kuulasmaa, K., Giampaoli, S., Mahonen, M., Ngu Bkackett, K., & Lisheng, L. (2011). World Health Organization definition of myocardial infarction: 2008–09 revision. *International Journal of Epidemiology*, *40*(1), 139–146.

Mireku, N., Wang, Y., Ager, J., Reddy, R. C., & Baptist, A. P. (2009). Changes in weather and the effects on pediatric asthma exacerbations. *Annals of Allergy Asthma and Immunology*, *103*(3), 220–224.

Nitschke, M., Tucker, G. R., Hansen, A. L., Williams, S., Zhang, Y., & Bi, P. (2011). Impact of two recent extreme heat episodes on morbidity and mortality in Adelaide, South Australia: A case-series analysis. *Environmental Health*, *10*(42).

Onozuka, D., Hashizume, M., & Hagihara, A. (2009). Impact of weather factors on mycoplasma pneumoniae pneumonia. *Thorax*, *64*(6), 507–511.

Oudin, A., Åström, D. O., Asplund, P., Steingrimsson, S., Szabo, Z., & Carlsen, H. K. (2018). The association between daily concentrations of air pollution and visits to a psychiatric emergency unit: A case-crossover study. *Environmental Health*, *17*, 4.

Oudin, A., Brabäck, L., Aström, D. O., Strömgren, M., & Forsberg, B. (2016). Association between neighbourhood air pollution concentrations and dispensed medication for psychiatric disorders in a large longitudinal cohort of Swedish children and adolescents. *BMJ Open*, *6*, 1–12.

Page, L. A., Hajat, S., Sari Kovats, R., & Howard, L. M. (2012). Temperature-related deaths in people with psychosis, dementia and substance misuse. *British Journal of Psychiatry*, *200*, 485–490.

Pawankar, R. (2014). Allergic diseases and asthma: A global public health concern and a call to action. *World Allergy Organization Journal*, *7*(1), 12. doi:10.1186/1939-4551-7-12.

Pawankar, R., Canonica, G. W., Holgate, S. T., Lockey, R. F., & Blasis, M. S. (Eds.). (2013). *WAO white book on allergy: Update 2013*. Retrieved from www.worldallergy. org/UserFiles/file/WhiteBook2-2013-v8.pdf.

Peng, Z., Wang, Q., Kan, H., Chen, R., & Wang, W. (2017). Effects of ambient temperature on daily hospital admissions for mental disorders in Shanghai, China: A time-series analysis. *Science of the Total Environment, 590–591*, 281–286.

Power, M. C., Kioumourtzoglou, M. A., Hart, J. E., Okereke, O. I., Laden, F., & Weisskopf, M. G. (2015). The relation between past exposure to fine particulate air pollution and prevalent anxiety: Observational cohort study. *The BMJ, 350*, h1111.

Qiu, H., Sun, S., Tang, R., Chan, K. P., & Tian, L. (2016). Pneumonia hospitalization risk in the elderly attributable to cold and hot temperatures in Hong Kong, China. *American Journal of Epidemiology, 184*(8), 555–569. doi:10.1093/aje/kww041.

Qiu, H., Yu, I. T. S., Tse, L. A., Chan, E. Y. Y., Wong, T. W., & Tian, L. (2015). Greater temperature variation within a day associated with increased emergency hospital admissions for asthma. *Science of Total Environment, 505*, 508–513.

Qiu, H., Yu, I. T. S., Wang, Z., Tina, L., Tse, L. A., & Wong, T. W. (2013). Season and humidity dependence of the effects of air pollution on COPD hospitalizations in Hong Kong. *Atmospheric Environment, 76*, 74–80.

Reed, C. E. (2006). The natural history of asthma. *Journal of Allergy and Clinical Immunology, 118*(3), 543–548.

Rivero, A., Bolufé, J., Ortiz, P. L., Rodríguez, Y., & Reyes, M. C. (2015). Influence of climate variability on acute myocardial infarction mortality in Havana, 2001–2012. *MEDICC Review, 17*(2), 14–19.

Sarrias, M. J., Artigas, F., Martínez, E., & Gelpí, E. (1989). Seasonal changes of plasma serotonin and related parameters: Correlation with environmental measures. *Biology Psychiatry, 26*, 695–706.

Sauerzapf, V., Jones, P., & Cross, J. (2009). Environmental factors and hospitalisation for chronic obstructive pulmonary disease in a rural county of England. *Journal of Epidemiology and Community Health, 63*(4), 324–328. doi:10.1136/jech.2008.077024.

Schmeltz, M. T., & Gamble, J. L. (2017). Risk characterization of hospitalizations for mental illness and/or behavioral disorders with concurrent heat-related illness. *PLOS ONE, 12*, e0186509.

Schwartz, J. (2005). Who is sensitive to extremes of temperature? A case-only analysis. *Epidemiology, 16*(1), 67–72.

Seposo, X. T., Dang, T. N., & Honda, Y. (2017). How does ambient air temperature affect diabetes mortality in tropical cities? *International Journal of Environmental Research and Public Health, 14*(385).

Shiue, I., Perkins, D. R., & Bearman, N. (2016). Physically equivalent temperature and mental and behavioural disorders in Germany in 2009–2011. *Journal of Mental Health, 25*, 148–153.

Son, J. Y., Bell, M. L., & Lee, J. T. (2014). The impact of heat, cold, and heat waves on hospital admissions in eight cities in Korea. *International Journal of Biometeorology, 58*(9), 1893–1903.

Son, J. Y., Lee, J. T., Anderson, G. B., & Bell, M. L. (2012). The impact of heat waves on mortality in seven major cities in Korea. *Environmental Health Perspectives, 120*(4), 566–571.

Song, G., Chen, G., Jiang, L., Xhang, Y., Zhao, N., Chen, B., & Kan, H. (2008). Diurnal temperature range as a novel risk factor for COPD death. *Respirology, 13*(7), 1066–1069. doi:10.1111/j.1440-1843.2008.01401.x.

Souza, A. D., Fernandes, W. A., Pavão, H. G., Lastoria, G., & Albrez, E. A. (2012). Potential impacts of climate variability on respiratory morbidity in children, infants, and adults. *Journal Brasileiro de Pneumologia, 38,* 708–715.

Su, Q., Liu, H, Yuan, X., Xiao, Y., Zhang, X., Sun, R., … Zhao, X. (2014). The interaction effects of temperature and humidity on emergency room visits for respiratory diseases in Beijing, China. *Cell Biochemistry and Biophysics, 70*(2), 1377–1384. doi: 10.1007/s12013-014-0067-5.

Sun, S., Tian, L., Qiu, H., Chan, K. P., Tsang, H., Tang, R., … Wong, C. M. (2016). The influence of pre-existing health conditions on short-term mortality risks of temperature: Evidence from a prospective Chinese elderly cohort in Hong Kong. *Environmental Research, 148,* 7–14. doi:10.1016/j.envres.2016.03.012.

Tang, J. W. (2009). The effect of environmental parameters on the survival of airborne infectious agents. *Journal of Royal Society Interface,* 6, S737–S746.

Taylor, L., Watkins, S. L., Marshall, H., Dascombe, B. J., & Foster, J. (2016). The impact of different environmental conditions on cognitive function: A focused review. *Frontiers in Physiology,* 6, 1–12.

Tian, L., Qiu, H., Sun, S., & Lin, H. (2016). Emergency cardiovascular hospitalization risk attributable to cold temperatures in Hong Kong. *Circulation: Cardiovascular Quality and Outcomes,* 9(2), 135–142.

Töro, K., Dunay, G., Bartholy, J., Pongrácz, R., Kis, Z., & Keller, É. (2009). Relationship between suicidal cases and meteorological conditions. *Journal of Forensic and Legal Medicine,* 16, 277–279.

Trang, P. M., Rocklöv, J., Giang, K. B., Kullgren, G., & Nilsson, M. (2016). Heatwaves and hospital admissions for mental disorders in Northern Vietnam. *PLOS ONE, 11,* e0155609. doi:10.137/journal.pone.0155609.

Trang, P. M., Rocklöv, J., Giang, K. B., & Nilsson, M. (2016). Seasonality of hospital admissions for mental disorders in Hanoi, Vietnam. *Global Health Action,* 9, 32116b.

Tsai, J. F., & Cho, W. (2012). Temperature change dominates the suicidal seasonality in Taiwan: A time-series analysis. *Journal of Affective Disorders,* 136, 412–418.

Tseng, C. M., Chen, Y. T., Ou, S. M., Hsiao, Y. H., Li, S. Y., Wang, S. J., … Perng, D. W. (2013). The effect of cold temperature on increased exacerbation of chronic obstructive pulmonary disease: A nationwide study. *PLOS ONE,* 8(3), e57066. doi: 10.1371/journal.pone.0057066.

Vaneckova, P., & Bambrick, H. (2013). Cause-specific hospital admissions on hot days in Sydney, Australia. *PLOS ONE,* 8(2), e55459.

Vasconcelos, J., Freire, E., Almendra, R., Silva, G. L., & Santana, P. (2013). The impact of winter cold weather on acute myocardial infarctions in Portugal. *Environmental Pollution, 183,* 14–18. doi:10.1016/j.envpol.2013.01.037.

Vert, C., Sánchez-Benavides, G., Martínez, D., Gotsens, X., Gramunt, N., Cirach, M., … Gascon, M. (2017). Effect of long-term exposure to air pollution on anxiety and depression in adults: A cross-sectional study. *International Journal of Hygiene and Environmental Health, 220,* 1074–1080.

Vida, S., Durocher, M., Ouarda, T. B. M. J., & Gosselin, P. (2012). Relationship between ambient temperature and humidity and visits to mental health emergency departments in Québec. *Psychiatric Services,* 63(11), 1150–1153. doi:10.1176/appi.ps.201100485.

Vigo, D., Thornicroft, G., & Atun, R. (2016). Estimating the true global burden of mental illness. *Lancet Psychiatry,* 3, 171–178.

Volk, H. E., Lurmann, F., Penfold, B., Hertz-Picciotto, I., & McConnell, R. (2013). Traffic-related air pollution, particulate matter, and autism. *JAMA Psychiatry,* 70, 71.

Wang, P., Goggins, W. B., & Chan, E. Y. Y. (2016). Hand, foot and mouth disease in Hong Kong: A time-series analysis on its relationship with weather. *PLOS ONE, 11,* e0161006.

Wang, X., Lavigne, E., Ouellette-Kuntz, H., & Chen, B. E. (2014). Acute impacts of extreme temperature exposure on emergency room admissions related to mental and behavior disorders in Toronto, Canada. *Journal of Affective Disorders, 155,* 154–161.

Wang, Y. C., & Lin, Y. K. (2014). Association between temperature and emergency room visits for cardiorespiratory diseases, metabolic syndrome-related diseases, and accidents in metropolitan Taipei. *PLOS ONE, 9*(6), e99599. doi:10.1371/journal.pone.0099599.

Wang, Y. C., & Lin, Y. K. (2015). Temperature effects on outpatient visits of respiratory diseases, asthma, and chronic airway obstruction in Taiwan. *International Journal of Biometeorology, 59*(7), 815–825.

Wichmann, J., Ketzel, M., Ellermann, T., & Loft, S. (2012). Apparent temperature and acute myocardial infarction hospital admissions in Copenhagen, Denmark: A case-crossover study. *Environmental Health, 11,* 19.

Wichmann, J., Rosengren, A., Sjöberg, K., Barregard, L., & Sallsten, G. (2013). Association between ambient temperature and acute myocardial infarction hospitalisations in Gothenburg, Sweden: 1985–2010. *PLOS ONE, 8*(4), e62059. doi:10.1371/journal.pone.0062059.

Williams, S., Nitschke, M., Sullivan, T., Tucker, G. R., Weinstein, P., Pisaniello, D. L., … Bi, P. (2012). Heat and health in Adelaide, South Australia: Assessment of heat thresholds and temperature relationships. *Science of Total Environment, 414,* 126–133. doi: 10.1016/j.scitotenv.2011.11.038.

Wolf, K., Schneider, A., Breitner, S., von Klot, S., Meisinger, C., Cyrys, J., Hymer, H., … Peters, A. (2009). Temperature and the occurrence of myocardial infarction in Augsburg, Germany. *Circulation, 120,* 735–742. doi:10.1161/CIRCULATIONAHA.108.815860.

World Health Organization [WHO]. (n.d.). *Burden of COPD.* Retrieved from www.who.int/respiratory/copd/burden/en/.

World Health Organization. (2003). *Prevention of allergy and allergie asthma.* Retrieved from http://apps.who.int/iris/bitstream/handle/10665/68361/WHO_NMH_MNC_CRA_03.2.pdf;jsessionid=5240730BBCD60C2649029E8B0EA642D9?sequence=1.

World Health Organization. (2013). *Asthma fact sheet No 307.* Retrieved from www.who.int/mediacentre/factsheets/fs307/en/.

World Health Organization. (2016). *Global health estimates.* Retrieved from www.who.int/healthinfo/global_burden_disease/en/.

Xu, Z., Huang, C., Hu, W., Turner, L. R., Su, H., & Tong, S. (2013). Extreme temperatures and emergency department admissions for childhood asthma in Brisbane, Australia. *Occupational and Environmental Medicine, 70*(10), 730–735. doi:10.1136/oemed-2013-101538.

Yan, W., Yun, Y., Ku, T., Li, G., & Sang, N. (2016). NO_2 inhalation promotes Alzheimer's disease-like progression: Cyclooxygenase-2-derived prostaglandin E2 modulation and monoacylglycerol lipase inhibition-targeted medication. *Scientific Reports, 6,* 1–17.

Yang, J., Liu, H. Z., Ou, C. Q., Lin, G. Z., Zhou, Q., Shen, J. C., & Chen, P. Y. (2013). Impact of heat wave in 2005 on mortality in Guangzhou, China. *Biomedical and Environmental Sciences, 26,* 647.

Yang, J., Yin, P., Zhou, M., Ou, C. Q., Li, M., Liu, Y., ... Liu, Q. (2016). The effect of ambient temperature on diabetes mortality in China: A multi-city time series study. *Science of Total Environment*, 543(Pt A), 75–82.

Yu, W., Mengersen, K., Wang, X., Ye, X., Guo, Y., Pan, X., & Tong, S. (2012). Daily average temperature and mortality among the elderly: A meta-analysis and systematic review of epidemiological evidence. *International Journal of Biometeorology*, 56(4), 569–581. doi:10.1007/s00484-011-0497-3.

Zhang, Y., Peng, L., Kan, H., Xu, J., Chen, R., Liu, Y., & Wang, W. (2014). Effects of meteorological factors on daily hospital admissions for asthma in adults: A time-series analysis. *PLOS ONE*, 9, e102475. doi:10.1371/journal.pone.0102475.

Zijlema, W. L., Wolf, K., Emeny, R., Ladwig, K. H., Peters, A., Kongsgård, H., ... Rosmalen, J. G. (2016). The association of air pollution and depressed mood in 70,928 individuals from four European cohorts. *International Journal of Hygiene and Environmental Health*, 219(2), 212–219.

11 Climate Change Behavioural Adaptation I

Help-seeking and information-seeking behaviours under extreme climate events

To examine the mechanism and the extent that various climate change impacts might have on individual behaviour and public health burden, evidence is needed to understand community health and help-seeking behaviour (see also Chapter 2) in various extreme weather contexts. Limited studies have been carried out to examine predictors of individual help-seeking behaviour during elevated temperature. This chapter discusses studies that examined individual help-seeking behaviour during abnormal temperature and patterns of information-seeking behaviour exhibited by urban community during extreme temperature events.

Help-seeking behaviour in urban context

The adverse effect of extreme temperatures on human health has been well documented. The sensitivity of populations to temperature extremes, however, varies widely between different demographic groups. The older people are at the greatest risk of increased morbidity and mortality during heatwaves (Abrahamson et al., 2009; Chan, Goggins, Kim, & Griffiths, 2012; Chan, Goggins, Yue, & Lee, 2013; Curriero et al., 2002; Fouillet et al., 2006; Huyen, Martens, Schram, Weijenberg, & Kunst, 2001; Intergovernmental Panel on Climate Change [IPCC], 2007). A study in Hong Kong indicated that an average of 1°C increase in daily mean temperature above 28.2°C was associated with an estimated 1.8% increase in mortality over the same day (Chan et al., 2012). Subgroup analyses showed mortality of those who were aged over 75, women, unmarried, or living in densely populated areas such as Kowloon and those with unknown residence appeared to be more sensitive to high temperature effects. This suggests that there are intra-city differences in the association between temperature and mortality in urban areas (Chan et al., 2012) and in the potential public health strategies that could protect populations from the adverse health impact of elevated temperatures. At the same time, to develop appropriate heatwave-related harmful health effect prevention plans, it is important to understand the relationship between help-seeking behaviour and climate-related thresholds amongst population subgroups.

Although urban environment might contribute to the adverse health impact (via such phenomena as the heat island effect), individual behaviour may reduce the extent of morbidity and mortality during abnormal temperature context. However, how individuals seek help might not correlate with the temperature–mortality or temperature–morbidity pattern. A study examining help-seeking behaviour in Hong Kong was conducted by building a retrospective time-series Poisson generalised additive model (GAM) analysis (Chan, Goggins, Kim, Griffiths, & Mak, 2011). Using routine emergency help call data from the community call service agency during the warm seasons (June–September) between 1998 and 2007, a help-seeking-temperature relationship model was built.

The Senior Citizen Home Safety Association (SCHSA) of Hong Kong is a non-profit charitable organisation providing the "Personal Emergency Link" ("PE Link") Service to older citizens living alone and people in need. Although mostly for older population, the PE Link Service is open to applicants of all ages, home districts, and living environment with a residential telephone line. The 24-hour emergency hotline offers support to the emergency needs of callers and provides the necessary support services through referrals. In the event of an emergency, operators might (i) call the police or ambulance centre for medical assistance; (ii) call the emergency contact person for reporting the latest status of the user, including hospitalisation details; or (iii) fax the medical history to the accident and emergency department to facilitate rescue and medical care. If there is no response from the caller after 2 minutes of pressing the button, the centre will treat the case as an emergency and inform the fire service to undertake rescues accordingly.

Within the study period, 48,261 members enrolled in SCHSA. Over two-thirds of them enrolled as SCHSA members with the assistance of organisations such as the Social Welfare Department, the Housing Department, and SCHSA's Personal Emergency Link Charitable Programme, while the remaining paid on their own. The study model included meteorological data (i.e. daily weather variables including mean, maximum, and minimum temperatures, dew point temperatures, and mean humidity) from Hong Kong Observatory (HKO), pollution data (i.e. daily means calculated from hourly concentrations of nitrogen dioxide (NO_2), sulphur dioxide (SO_2), ozone (O_3), and PM_{10}—also known as respirable suspended particulates (RSP)) from the Hong Kong Environmental Protection Department (EPD), and underlying health needs patterns (i.e. average weekly consultation rates of influenza-like illnesses reported by general outpatient clinics and practitioners as a proxy indicator to control for the influence of influenza epidemics on mortality) from the Centre for Health Protection of Hong Kong SAR Government.

Results indicated a U-shaped association between daily emergency calls and daily *maximum* temperature (p = 0.034) and a ∩-shaped relationship with mean relative humidity (p = 0.011). There was also a U-shaped association between *mean* daily temperature and frequency of calls with a temperature threshold (at which calls started to increase) of 27–29°C. Subgroup analyses of the association between maximum temperature and the frequency of health-related calls indicated that females, those 75 years of age or older, and Hong Kong Island residents were more sensitive to high maximum temperatures, while males and Kowloon residents appeared more sensitive to lower maximum temperatures, i.e. "cool effects". Analysis of the emergency pattern showed 49% of calls were for explicit health-related reasons including dizziness, shortness of breath, and general pain.

Maximum temperature was statistically significantly associated with temperature above the threshold temperature of around 30–32°C, at which the frequency of health-related calls started to increase. Mean daily relative humidity (RH) demonstrated a significant U-shaped association with daily emergency health-related calls, with call frequency beginning to rise when RH was greater than 70–74% (10–25% of the RH distribution). Of note, heatwave durations and daily rainfall were not significantly associated with health-related calls. Maximum temperature was also found to be a stronger predictor of daily health-related calls than mean and minimum temperatures (both of which were non-significant when examined independently). Hence, maximum temperature was chosen for all subsequent modelling. Lagged effects of maximum temperature, diurnal temperature variation, and changes in temperature from the previous day were also not significant in the study model.

Findings also showed that during the warm seasons in Hong Kong, the volume of help-seeking calls at higher temperatures varies amongst demographic subgroups. Overall, the call volume dropped before the threshold temperature and rose again beyond this threshold to exhibit a U-shape distribution, but this presents different gender patterns. Call frequency among females appeared to be more sensitive to high temperatures, with a threshold of 28.5–30.5°C, while calls among males were more sensitive to cold temperatures (a threshold of 31.5–33.5°C). Results indicate differences in community help-seeking behaviour at elevated temperatures. Whilst the effect of extreme temperature was found to be particularly noticeable among older age groups and females (Johnson et al., 2005; Nitschke, Tucker, & Bi, 2007), few studies have examined the temperature threshold differences between demographic subgroups. A study that compared the differences in six major cities in South Korea found threshold temperatures for mortality varied between 27.0 and 29.7°C (Kim, Ha, & Park, 2006). Older people were found to be especially vulnerable, with lower threshold temperatures for mortality ranging from 24.5 to 28.5°C. Potential programmes or community outreach services should aim to protect vulnerable subgroups from the adverse health impact according to the behavioural pattern.

Geography and the issue with "cool temperature effects"

Help-seeking behaviour was more sensitive to elevated temperatures among women, those over 75 years of age, and people living in a wealthier part of Hong Kong (e.g. Hong Kong Island). While call volume from Kowloon was the highest overall, which is the most densely populated area of Hong Kong, the threshold temperature was also the highest compared to other areas. Thus, Kowloon residents were less likely to show an increase in help-seeking behaviour until temperatures were higher and were also more sensitive to "cool temperature" effects. Although this may be explained by physiological adaptation, it may also be influenced by a lack of knowledge (e.g. lower awareness of the potential adverse health implications and subsequent failure to seek help during high temperatures) and inappropriate behavioural practices (e.g. delaying or refusing to seek care). Future study would need to explore the underlying drivers and motivations of health and help-seeking behaviour in extreme temperature among different population subgroups.

Temperature variability

A study in Shanghai revealed that temperature variability may play an important role in heat-related health impact (Tan et al., 2007). The Shanghai study population included 6.3 million residents between 2001 and 2004 in suburban and urban areas and mortality was found to be strongly associated with diurnal temperature range (DTR) (i.e. within day variation in temperature). The DTR was found to be positively associated with mortality, particularly among those aged over 45. In the United States, higher risk of death was observed during summertime for cities with greater temperature variances (Braga, Zanobetti, & Schwartz, 2002). In Valencia, Spain, mortality increased in proportion to the range of temperatures varying between winters and summers (Ballester, Corella, Pérez-Hoyos, Sáez, & Hervás, 1997).

Moreover, study findings of community help-seeking behaviour were found to be comparable to the temperature-related mortality study in the same community, which found that 28.2°C was the critical threshold temperature for elevated mortality during the warm seasons (from May to October) in 1998–2006 (Chan et al., 2012). The Hong Kong study findings suggested that temperature extremes had a direct impact on help-seeking behaviour for health-related reasons and were sensitive to temperature. Morbidity studies also showed that hospital admissions rose with increased ambient temperature (Kovats, Hajat, & Wilkinson, 2004; Tai, Lee, Shih, & Chen, 2007). Policymakers may wish to consider plans incorporating temperature sensitivity and help-seeking behaviour to reduce hospital admissions during extreme temperatures.

Weather information acquisition

Weather information dissemination is significant for protecting the well-being of communities, especially during extreme climatic events. As part of community preparedness, community ability to acquire risk-related information and respond accordingly can enhance community resilience and minimise losses caused by hazards and their potential health impacts. Despite the global smart city movement, how weather information acquisition patterns may vary across community subgroups has not been extensively studied. Understanding of current and preferred weather information acquisition channels could inform the weather information providers to better meet user needs (Demuth et al., 2011). Since awareness is one of the prerequisites for public health action, a far-reaching weather information channel is crucial for the public, not only to receive weather information but also to promote their preparedness against weather hazards.

Extreme cold weather and use of mobile communication devices in Hong Kong

Hong Kong ranked fourth in global population density in 2017 (World Bank, 2018). With the recent rise in the intensity and frequency of extreme weather events (Hong Kong SAR Government Environment Bureau, 2015), the city is facing higher risks of health-related impacts. Located in a subtropical region, Hong Kong has an annual average temperature of 23.3°C. In January 2016, Hong Kong experienced its coldest winter in 59 years. A Cold Weather Warning was issued and the lowest temperature recorded by the Hong Kong Observatory (HKO) was 3.3°C on 24 January 2016 during a persisting cold surge period. The temperature on Tai Mo Shan, the highest peak in Hong Kong, dropped to a minimum of –6°C.

A cross-sectional telephone survey of Hong Kong residents ≥15 years old was conducted within 1 week after the 2016 cold spell (Chan, Huang, Mark, & Guo, 2017), which showed 73.1% of 1,008 respondents were using their preferred information acquisition channels to gauge their health risks as associated with temperature events. According to the study findings, 95.7% of the survey participants were aware of the Cold Weather Warning during the cold surge in the week before the survey. Among all respondents, 95.5% reported voluntarily keeping track of weather information. Female survey participants were more aware of the warning (96.5%) than male ones (94.6%). The youngest survey participants, in the 15–24 age group, had reported the lowest awareness of the warning (93.5%). Respondents were also asked about the minimum temperature on the interview day, and 69.0% of respondents indicated the corrected minimum temperature. A total of 371 participants could recall the temperature within a ±1°C error between the minimum actual temperature as recorded by HKO and the perceived temperature. Multiple linear regression was performed and found that male and higher actual minimum temperature were significant and strong predictors of large perceived temperature error, while smartphone application usage and age were non-significant in the multiple regression. The results indicated that female participants were associated with less perceived temperature error. One possible explanation could be that females paid more attention to detailed weather information because it remains common for females to assume a caregiver role. Given the high ownership and penetration of smartphones in Hong Kong, the number of survey participants who could recall the actual minimum temperature of the interview day was far lower than the number who claimed to know about the exact minimum temperature, even though almost all of the survey participants were aware of the Cold Weather Warning.

The study found that individual health protection measures were not widely adopted in the community despite the high dissemination rate of the Cold Weather Warning. A possible explanation may be that people failed to heed the information conveyed through the media/information channels they do not prefer, and perceptions or beliefs may need to be taken into account in determining compliance with official advice (Rubin, Amlôt, Page, & Wessely, 2009). Hence, individual uptake of health protection measures and the relationship with smartphone application use were further analysed. Smartphone application users were found more likely to use heaters and avoid prolonged exposure to wintry winds, but less likely to ensure adequate indoor air ventilation. In addition, χ^2 tests also found that survey participants who had a smaller difference between perceived and actual temperature (i.e. a more accurate temperature perception) were more likely to pay extra attention to the conditions of older people and people with chronic medical conditions (OR = 1.34, 95% confidence interval (CI): 1.03–1.74), and pay extra attention to children (OR = 1.45, 95% CI: 1.12–1.89) during the cold spell.

Health protection measures were generally more likely taken by mobile application users than non-users, except for ensuring adequate indoor air ventilation. Nevertheless, ventilation is crucial for maintaining better indoor air quality in winter because house dust mites may thrive under conditions of high relative humidity and allergies to them are more frequently found in mild humid winters (Daisey, Angell, & Apte, 2003). A low ventilation rate is also one of the factors that can lead to increased incidence of respiratory diseases caused by viruses (Brundage, Scott, Lednar, Smith, & Miller, 1988; Fisk, 2001). Future effort is required to provide tailored information to improve personal health protection. Moreover, significant differences in the change of behaviour between mobile application users and non-users were observed, especially with respect to appetite and mood. A higher proportion of mobile application users reported to have better appetite and mood during a Cold Weather Warning.

Channel of information-seeking behaviour

Analysis of information acquisition patterns showed that among those who were not currently using their preferred channel, 61.3% considered switching to smartphone application. Survey findings indicated that median temperature of which respondents claimed to start actively checking temperature–weather-related information was 32°C (30–33°C). When comparing between current and preferred channels of weather information acquisition of the respondents, 50.1% of respondents reported that television was the most popular channel used, followed by smartphone application (32.0%) and radio (8.4%). When asked about preferred channels, 45.6% indicated smartphone application is their preferred channel of information acquisitions. It should be noted that smartphone ownership was 86.6% among the survey participants. This is comparable to the smartphone penetration rate in Hong Kong, which was 85.8% in 2017 (Hong Kong SAR Government Census and Statistics Department, 2017). The proportion of weather information acquisition through smartphone application as the main channel was only 32.0%. It was found that smartphone ownership was inversely related to age. There was a clear willingness of respondents to use smartphone application for information acquisition. Smartphone application may be the dominant weather information acquisition channel in the near future, taking into consideration the high usage rate among young people and that this channel is more preferred by those aged 45–64.

The two-stage Stepwise Multiple Logistic Regression model was constructed to identify potential socio-demographic predictors for the information sources utilisation (Chan et al., 2017). Variables including gender, residential districts, education level, and history of chronic diseases were insignificant. Socio-demographic predictors associated with preferred/current use of new technology platforms (such as smartphone application) included age, education, and reported marital status. Television was the most widely used channel but most people would prefer smartphone application. Meanwhile, radio users were consistent in their usage pattern and did not seem to report many changes. Smartphone ownership was inversely related to age, although it may become the dominant source of information in the near future due to the high usage rate, especially among young people. For older people, issues with technology literacy and access to technology will be confounding factors for future application.

For a smart city aiming to enhance the performance of various traditional networks via the use of information and telecommunication technologies (Mohanty, Choppali, & Kougianos, 2016), public health significance of weather information dissemination channels can be amplified by coordinating with health monitoring systems and systems controlling healthcare service delivery (Boulos, Tsouros, & Holopainen, 2015; Hussain, Wenbi, da Silva, Nadher, & Mudhish, 2015). Meanwhile, those who exhibit less interest in or have no access to smartphone application should not be ignored. This is especially important since many of these people are among the most vulnerable (e.g. people of older age group and the less educated), they cannot access public services and resources, and they are susceptible to health risks. Weather information providers should disseminate relevant information through different channels to address the stratified information acquisition pattern identified.

Conclusion

Whilst the mortality threshold was found to be consistent among population subgroups (Chan et al., 2012), results indicated differences in community help-seeking and information-seeking behaviour in different temperature ranges. There is currently limited understanding of the effectiveness of population response to public warning of heat, especially among the high-risk population in urban communities. Policymakers and community outreach service providers should consider targeting more vulnerable subgroups to protect them from the adverse human health impact arising from elevated temperature.

References

Abrahamson, V., Wolf, J., Lorenzoni, I., Fenn, B., Kovats, S., Wilkinson, P., ... Raine, R. (2009). Perceptions of heatwave risks to health: Interview-based study of older people in London and Norwich, UK. *Journal of Public Health*, *31*(1), 119–126. doi: org/10.1093/pubmed/fdn102.

Ballester. F., Corella, D., Pérez-Hoyos, S., Sáez, M., & Hervás, A. (1997). Mortality as a function of temperature: A study in Valencia, Spain, 1991–1993. *International Journal of Epidemiology*, *26*(3), 551–561. doi:10.1093/ije/26.3.551.

Boulos, M. N. K., Tsouros, A. D., & Holopainen, A. (2015). Social, innovative and smart cities are happy and resilient: Insights from the WHO EURO 2014 International Healthy Cities Conference. *International Journal of Health Geographics*, *14*(1): Article No. 3.

Braga, A. L., Zanobetti, A., & Schwartz, J. (2002). The effect of weather on respiratory and cardiovascular deaths in 12 U.S. cities. *Environmental Health Perspectives*, *110*(9), 859–863. doi:10.1289/ehp. 02110859.

Brundage, J. F., Scott, R. M., Lednar, W. M., Smith, D. W., & Miller, R. N. (1988). Building-associated risk of febrile acute respiratory diseases in Army trainees. *JAMA*, *259*(14), 2108–2112.

Chan, E. Y., Goggins, W. B., Kim, J. J., & Griffiths, S. M. (2012). A study of intracity variation of temperature-related mortality and socioeconomic status among the Chinese population of Hong Kong. *Journal of Epidemiology and Community Health*, *66*(4), 322–327.

Chan, E. Y., Goggins, W. B., Kim, J. J., Griffiths, S., & Mak, T. K. (2011). Help-seeking behavior during elevated temperature in Chinese populations. *Journal of Urban Health*, *88*(4), 637–650.

Chan, E. Y. Y., Goggins, W. B., Yue, S. K., & Lee, P. Y. (2013). Hospital admissions as a function of temperature, other weather phenomena and pollution levels in an urban setting in China. *Bulletin of World Health Organization*, *91*(8), 576–584. doi:10.2471/ BLT.12.113035.

Chan, E. Y. Y., Huang, Z., Mark, C. K. M., & Guo, C. (2017). Weather information acquisition and health significance during extreme cold weather in a subtropical city: A cross-sectional survey in Hong Kong. *International Journal of Disaster Risk Science*, *8*(2), 134–144. doi:10.1007/s13753-017-0127-8.

Curriero, F. C., Heiner, K. S., Samet, J. M., Zeger, S. L., Strug, L., & Patz, J. A. (2002). Temperature and mortality in 11 cities of the eastern United States. *American Journal of Epidemiology*, *155*(1), 80–87. doi:10.1093/aje/155.1.80.

Daisey, J. M., Angell, W. J., & Apte, M. G. (2003). Indoor air quality, ventilation and health symptoms in schools: An analysis of existing information. *Indoor Air*, *13*(1), 53–64.

Demuth, J. L., Lazo, J. K., & Morss, R. E. (2011). Exploring variations in people's sources, uses, and perceptions of weather forecasts. *Weather, Climate, and Society*, *3*(3), 177–192.

Fisk, W. J. (2001). Estimates of potential nationwide productivity and health benefits from better indoor environments: An update. In J. Spengler, J. M. Samet, & J. F. McCarthy (Eds.), *Indoor air quality* handbook (pp. 1–36). New York, NY: McGraw Hill.

Fouillet, A., Rey, G., Laurent, F., Pavillon, G., Bellec, S., Guihenneuc-Jouyaux, C., ... Hémon, D. (2006). Excess mortality related to the August 2003 heat wave in France. *International Archives of Occupational and Environmental Health*, *80*(1), 16–24. doi:10. 1007/s00420-006-0089-4.

Hong Kong SAR Government Census and Statistics Department. (2017). *Thematic household survey report No. 62.* Retrieved from www.statistics.gov.hk/pub/B1130262 2017XXXXB0100.pdf.

Hong Kong SAR Government Environment Bureau. (2015). *Hong Kong climate change report 2015.* Retrieved from www.enb.gov.hk/sites/default/files/pdf/ClimateChangeEng. pdf.

Hussain, A., Wenbi, R., da Silva, A. L., Nadher, M., & Mudhish, M. (2015). Health and emergency-care platform for the elderly and disabled people in the smart city. *Journal of Systems and Software, 110,* 253–263.

Huynen, M. M., Martens, P., Schram, D., Weijenberg, M. P., & Kunst, A. E. (2001). The impact of heat waves and cold spells on mortality rates in the Dutch population. *Environmental Health Perspectives, 109*(5), 463–470. doi:10.1289/ehp. 01109463.

Intergovernmental Panel on Climate Change [IPCC]. (2007). *Climate change 2007: Synthesis report: Contribution of Working Groups I, II and III to the Fourth Assessment Report of the Intergovernmental Panel on Climate Change* [Core writing team, R. K. Pachauri, & A. Reisinger (Eds.)]. Geneva, Switzerland: Author. Retrieved from www.ipcc.ch/ publications_and_data/ar4/syr/en/contents.html.

Johnson, H., Kovats, R. S., McGregor, G., Stedman, J., Gibbs, M., Walton, H., … Black, E. (2005). The impact of the 2003 heat wave on mortality and hospital admissions in England. *Health Statistics Quarterly, 25,* 6–11.

Kim, H., Ha, J. S., & Park, J. (2006). High temperature, heat index, and mortality in 6 major cities in South Korea. *Archives of Occupational and Environmental Health, 61*(6), 265–270. doi:10.3200/AEOH.61.6.265-270.

Kovats, R. S., Hajat, S., & Wilkinson, P. (2004). Contrasting patterns of mortality and hospital admissions during hot weather and heat waves in Greater London, UK. *Occupational and Environmental Medicine, 61*(11), 893–898. doi:10.1136/oem.2003.012047.

Mohanty, S. P., Choppali, U., & Kougianos, E. (2016). Everything you wanted to know about smart cities: The Internet of things is the backbone. *IEEE Consumer Electronics Magazine, 5*(3), 60–70.

Nitschke, M., Tucker, G. R., & Bi, P. (2007). Morbidity and mortality during heatwaves in metropolitan Adelaide. *Medical Journal of Australia, 187,* 11–12.

Rubin, G. J., Amlôt, R., Page, L., & Wessely, S. (2009). Public perceptions, anxiety, and behaviour change in relation to the swine flu outbreak: Cross sectional telephone survey. *BMJ, 339*:b2651.

Tai, C. C., Lee, C. C., Shih, C. L., & Chen, S. C. (2007). Effects of ambient temperature on volume, specialty composition and triage levels of emergency department visits. *Emergency Medicine Journal, 24*(9), 641–644. doi:10.1136/emj.2006.045310.

Tan, J., Zheng, Y., Song, G., Kalkstein, L. S., Kalkstein, A. J., & Tang, X. (2007). Heat wave impacts on mortality in Shanghai, 1998 and 2003. *International Journal of Biometeorology, 51*(3), 193–200. doi:10.1007/s00484-006-0058-3.

World Bank. (2018). *Population density.* Retrieved from http://data.worldbank.org/ indicator/EN.POP.DNST?year_high_desc=true.

12 Climate Change Behavioural Adaptation II

Bottom-up approach of community risk perception and self-help behaviours under extreme climate events

As highlighted in the previous chapter, there might be specific socio-demographic patterns that community might seek help and information in weather- and extreme climate-related events. Community risk perception, health risk communication and behaviour strategies might affect the health outcomes of climate-related events. This chapter will discuss the general risk perceptions, knowledge, and behaviours associated with various impacts of climate change and highlight the potential.

General disaster risk perception in the community

In public health, there is a range of modelling methodologies for the study of community response, behaviour, and health outcome patterns. Regardless of the communication and behavioural theories adopted to develop the strategy, there are main prerequisites to ensure public health prevention action occurs (Chan & Shi, 2017; Last, 1998). These include awareness that (i) a problem exists, (ii) a sense that the problem matters, (iii) an understanding of what causes the problem, (iv) the capacity to influence, and (v) political will to influence the problem. This section discusses what is currently known about urban disaster risk perception.

Community might have understood health and disaster risks according to their experiences and perception. Studies conducted by Chan, Yue, Lee, and Wang (2016) showed the majority of urban dwellers (87.2%) did not perceive Hong Kong as a natural disaster-susceptible city. More than half (57.1%) reported beliefs that the local population had lower disaster awareness than other global cities. Infectious disease outbreak (74.0%), typhoon (12.9%), and fire (7.3%) were ranked as the most likely population-based disasters to occur. Only 1.2% perceived extreme weather as a potential threat (Chan et al., 2016). The risk perception among old people (≥65 years old) was significantly lower than other age groups (Chan et al., 2016). However, there is a knowledge gap in the relationship between risk perception and protective practices. Case Box 12.1 introduces a community preparedness study that describes how preparedness might be associated with impact.

Case Box 12.1 Is routine household typhoon preparedness enough for the future?

Typhoons, also known as cyclones or hurricanes depending on their location and strength, are the most common natural disaster in Southeast Asia (Doocy, Dick, Daniels, Kirsch, & Hopkins, 2013). In the past two decades, Hong Kong alone had on average 5–6 typhoons per year (Hong Kong Observatory (HKO), 2018), which subsequently also brought about landslides, torrential rain, and flooding. Reflecting findings from Doocy et al. (2013), the mortality rate due to typhoons has decreased in the past 70 years, while severe typhoons (T10, the highest level) have increased in frequency in the last decade. Between 1980 and 2010, only two T10 typhoons occurred yet three happened in the last decade (2012, 2017, 2018) (HKO, 2018). With the onset of climate change, more severe typhoons are expected and how densely populated urban cities can cope needs to be explored.

Typhoons are increasing in frequency and severity in Southeast Asia. The type and efficiency of household preparedness need to be explored. A population-based randomised telephone survey was conducted soon after Typhoon Mangkhut's landing in Hong Kong in September 2018. A total of 9.4% of respondents felt their home was at high risk of danger during typhoons despite 33.4% reporting some form of impact from Mangkhut (Chan et al., 2019). Over 70% reported doing at least one typhoon-specific preparedness measure. In spite of the high adaptation of preparedness measures, warranted by the frequent typhoons, Hong Kong residents were not adequately prepared for a severe typhoon. Unexpected effects such as flying air conditioners, commuters affected by roads blocked by debris, swaying buildings, and loss of power supply were not prepared for. Future preparedness for natural disasters, which will become more extreme due to climate change, needs to take into account unforeseen risks.

Heatwave as a health risk

Heatwaves present as one of the major climate change-related health risks to human population. These extreme weather events (EWEs) have a clear impact on society, including a rise in mortality and morbidity. These events increase strain on lifeline-supporting infrastructure (power, water, and transport), clothes and food retailing, tourism, and ecosystem services in a megacity context. It has been estimated that up to 70,000 people died because of the increased temperatures that struck Europe during the summer of 2003 (refer also to Chapter 4). While the effects of heat may be exacerbated in cities because of the heat island effect, the livelihoods and social well-being of non-urban communities can also be severely disrupted during and following periods of unusually hot weather.

The normal, healthy human body has a core temperature range of 36.1–37.8°C and can cope with temporarily increasing up to 38°C or 39°C without causing damage to health (Koppe, Kovats, Jendritzky, & Menne, 2004). Thermoregulation, the regulation and maintenance of core body temperature within these parameters, is managed by the hypothalamus through a careful and precise balance of heat generation and loss (Koppe et al., 2004; Matthies,

Bickler, Marín, & Hales, 2008). Thermoneutrality describes the parameters to maintain a healthy core body temperature and can be defined as the point at which metabolic activity is minimal. It varies around the circadian rhythm, sleep-wake cycles, and the menstrual cycle (Skinner, 2002). The heat remaining within the body is the difference between the heat generated and the heat lost. Heat is produced during and following activity since the body produces and releases heat through its use of energy (Koppe et al., 2004). Consequently, core body temperature will rise if generation exceeds loss and will drop if loss exceeds gain. Body temperature can also rise as a result of high external environmental temperature. Thermoreceptors, which are present throughout the skin, deep tissues, and organs, can immediately detect an increase of as little as 1°C (Matthies et al., 2008). They communicate with the hypothalamus (in the hypothalamic thermoregulatory centre), which, in turn, initiates the response to increase the physiological response of heat loss (Matthies et al., 2008). The human body loses heat via a number of routes, which include convection, conduction, radiation, and sweating. When the surrounding air temperature is higher than body temperature, heat loss via the convection route can be impaired and heat will be gained from the environment to the skin (Koppe et al., 2004). This will result in a raised core body temperature and the body will then initiate physiological responses such as sweating to aid in cooling (Koppe et al., 2004). Sweating is the most effective mechanism through which the body can lose heat and maintain thermoneutrality (Allen & Segal-Gidan, 2009; Koppe et al., 2004). The human body can produce up to 2 litres of sweat per hour (containing sodium, potassium, and water) and sweating can lead to dehydration and electrolyte imbalances if these substances are not replaced quickly enough (Koppe et al., 2004).

Meanwhile, it has also been argued that temperature alone is not a sufficient indicator of effect, and attention towards concurrent high humidity levels or a person's inability to sweat, as well as other physiological mechanisms (such as chronic illness, age, and medications) need to be taken into account (Hajat, O'Conner, & Kosatsky, 2010). High humidity and lack of sweating (anhydrosis) reduce the ability for heat to be released through evaporative cooling (Gupta et al., 2012; Hajat et al., 2010). However, it has been suggested that if a person is unable to sweat because of physical, pharmaceutical, or physiological reasons, then air movement will be of benefit to them if water is sprinkled onto their skin first (misting). High humidity has been proposed as one of the reasons why advice on fan use emanating from the United States (in certain areas of high humidity) often differs from that of Europe (generally areas of lower humidity) (Hajat et al., 2010).

Cooling interventions such as air-conditioning units might be unsustainable in a warming climate because of the positive feedback loop they create in the environment (their high energy consumption further adds to climate change by increasing GHG emissions), the increased risk of blackouts due to pressures on the energy grid, and their high operational cost. Furthermore, air conditioning might not be available to the most vulnerable members of society, because of costs. Therefore, in light of the increased risk of future heatwaves, the unsustainability of air conditioning, and the current uncertainty over the health effects of electric fans, there is a need for future research into their health impacts during heatwaves.

Health impacts resulting from raised body temperature range from mild heat-related illnesses to potentially severe consequences and death. Mild conditions include dehydration, heat cramps, heat oedema, heat syncope, and heat rash. Severe consequences include dehydration, heat exhaustion, heat stroke, cardiovascular and respiratory disease exacerbation, and death. The vulnerable populations include people with mental health illnesses, those on certain medications, older people (particularly the socially isolated and/or living alone and those residing in nursing/care homes), young children, and disabled and chronically ill people (particularly with cardiovascular and respiratory conditions) (see also Case Boxes 12.2 and 12.3).

The direct implication of heatwave might be heat stroke experience by affected individuals. Heat stroke may be divided into exertional and non-exertional (classic) heat stroke (Shahid, Hatle, Mansour, & Mimish, 1999). Exertional heat stroke, as its name suggests, occurs most often in healthy young people exercising, usually in hot and humid weather, probably without being acclimatised. Classic heat stroke occurs during extreme heatwaves with older people being particularly vulnerable (Grogan & Hopkins, 2002).

Case Box 12.2 Temperature and suicidal mortality in Hong Kong SAR, China

By Chao Luo, William Goggins, and Emily Ying Yang Chan

Previous studies of suicidal patterns exhibit seasonal spring peaks. Although suicidal seasonality might be triggered by meteorological factors, few studies have specifically examined the association between temperature and suicidal mortality in Asia. The findings of the studies are also contradictory. Therefore, our study aimed to explore the impacts of temperatures on daily suicidal mortality (Luo, Goggins, & Chan, 2017). Daily suicidal mortality data between 2000 and 2014 were obtained from the Hong Kong Census and Statistics Department, which were compiled from daily meteorological and air pollutants data obtained from the Hong Kong Observatory and the Environmental Protection Department, respectively. Generalised additive models were used to estimate the effects of daily mean temperature (°C) on daily suicidal mortality while controlling for other meteorological factors, air pollutants, day of the week, seasonality, and long-term trends. Lagged effects were also considered.

A total of 12,640 suicidal deaths were analysed. The highest suicide mortality rate was observed in April and May, with the lowest in December. Daily mean temperature was significantly associated with daily suicidal mortality above a threshold temperature of 12.5°C. Daily mean temperatures of 19.4°C (25th percentile) and 27.9°C (75th percentile) over lags 0–1 were associated with 24% higher (95% confidence interval (CI): 1.09, 1.41) and 64% higher (95% CI: 1.36, 2.00) suicidal risks when compared with 12.5°C, respectively.

The findings may contribute not only to a better understanding about the impacts of high temperature on suicide in Hong Kong, but may also provide evidence for policymakers to design preventive plans tackling increased suicidal rates under high temperature. However, more research is needed to identify the possible biological mechanisms behind how high temperature triggers suicidal behaviour.

Case Box 12.3 Temperature and falls-related hospital admissions in Hong Kong SAR, China

By Chao Luo, William Goggins, and Emily Ying Yang Chan

Previous studies have found increased falls incidences during winter months. However, most of the studies were conducted among older people only. Few studies have directly examined the impact of weather on the occurrence of falls. The findings of these studies are inconsistent as well. Therefore, our study aimed to explore the influences of weather variables on daily falls-related hospital admissions (Luo, Goggins, & Chan, 2018). Daily falls-related hospital admissions between 1998 and 2011 were obtained from the Hong Kong Hospital Authority, which were compiled from daily meteorological and air pollutants data obtained from the Hong Kong Observatory and the Environmental Protection Department, respectively. Generalised additive models were used to estimate the effects of daily mean temperature (°C) on daily falls-related hospital admissions while controlling for other meteorological factors, air pollutants, day of the week, seasonality, and long-term trends. Lagged effects were also considered.

A total of 400,737 falls hospitalisations were analysed. The highest falls incidence rate was observed in January, with the lowest in May. Below a threshold temperature of 28.5°C, daily mean temperature was significantly negatively associated with daily falls-related hospital admissions. Daily mean temperatures of 19.5°C (25th percentile) and 14.5°C (5th percentile) over lags 0–7 were associated with 11% higher (95% confidence interval (CI): 1.07, 1.15) and 21% higher (95% CI: 1.15, 1.21) falls hospitalisation risks when compared with 28.5°C, respectively. A negative association was found between ambient temperature and falls in the general population in the subtropical Asian city. Since falls are predicted to become the 17th leading cause of death globally by 2030, it is important to better understand the impacts of the changing climate on falls. Preventive measures such as providing proper heating may help decrease the risk of falls under low temperature.

Role of fans

One of the ways that people might try to get relief from the heat is to use an electric fan. The use of fans in a heatwave is to increase heat loss by increasing efficiency of all normal methods of heat loss—but particularly by evaporation and convection methods. Yet, increased sweating can lead to dehydration and electrolyte imbalances if not replenished quickly enough. Current evidence on the use of fans is limited. There are observational epidemiological studies

(Kaiser et al., 2001; Naughton et al., 2002) that have described varied effects of fan use on severe morbidity and mortality. Some studies have found no association between the use of electric fans and the onset of heat stroke; in other studies, fan use has been found to be slightly protective. For example, a meta-analysis conducted by Bouchama et al. (2007) found a protective association (for all-causes deaths during heatwaves) with the use of fans (odds ratio (OR) 0.60, 95% CI 0.4–1.1). However, this result was not statistically significant and the authors cautioned that the use of fans could not be justified by the evidence until further research is completed (Bouchama et al., 2007). The protocol for this review was accepted by the Gynaecological Cancer Group in April 2012 and published in The Cochrane Database of Systematic Reviews in May 2012 (Gupta et al., 2012). Semenza et al. (1996) compared 339 people who died during 14–17 July 1995 in Chicago, United States with 339 controls who were matched to the cases according to neighbourhood and age (Semenza et al., 1996). They report that "[w]e did not detect any reduction in mortality in association with the use of electric fans (data not shown)" (Semenza et al., 1996, p. 86) and conclude that "we did not find any evidence that the use of fans was protective, nor did we determine that any level of use of electric fans was associated with increased mortality" (Semenza et al., 1996, p. 89).

Kilbourne, Choi, Jones, and Thacker (1982) conducted their study during a heatwave in St Louis and Kansas City, United States during July and August 1980. They gathered questionnaire data for 156 people with heatstroke (severe heat illness with documented hyperthermia) and for 462 controls who matched by age, sex, and neighbourhood of residence. The data included the number of hours of home electric fan use per day and there was a lack of an association, which meant that electric fan use was not included in their regression analysis and, so, the relevant data are not reported in the paper. They also note that "[t]he distribution of fans was a prominent part of the emergency response to the 1980 heat wave" and that their finding "suggests that scarce relief resources should not be allocated in this manner in future heat waves" (Kilbourne et al., 1982, p. 3336). To identify evidence intervention that might reduce potential harm in the community, there is thus need for research to resolve the ongoing uncertainties about the potential beneficial and harmful effects of the use of electric fans during heatwaves.

Risk perception and utilisation of fans and air conditioners

The rising trend of heatwaves has resulted in much heat-related illness and death. Yet, people are not evenly affected by heatwaves. Previous studies have identified some risk and protective factors of the heat. Old people, those living alone, living in a place without a cooling device (e.g. an air conditioner, electric fan), living in urban areas, unable to care for oneself, confined to bed, not leaving home daily, with social deprivation, with pre-existing chronic diseases (such as cardiovascular, pulmonary, renal, and psychiatric illnesses), taking psychotropic medications, and drinking alcohol or caffeinated drinks are more vulnerable to heatwaves, whilst using air conditioners at home, visiting other air-conditioned places, using fans at home, taking extra baths/showers, wearing loose-fitting clothes, drinking extra water/fluid, having low-protein food, reducing normal activity levels, and avoiding going out in the hottest hours in a day may protect people during hot weather (Bouchama et al., 2007; Chan, Goggins, Kim, & Griffiths, 2012; Clements & Casani, 2009; Gupta et al., 2012; Hajat et al., 2010; Ibrahim, McInnes, Andrianopoulos, & Evans, 2012; Leung, Yip, & Yeung, 2008).

Even most cases of caused morbidity and mortality in heatwave are preventable: utilisation of air conditioners, as a cooling measure, has a strong protective effect and may be the leading protective factor against heat-related illness and death (Bouchama et al., 2007; Kenny, Yardley, Brown, Sigal, & Jay, 2010). A meta-analysis on six studies published before 2007 revealed that having air conditioners at home was associated with a relative risk reduction for heat-related death of 77% (OR = 0.23, 95% CI = 0.1–0.6) (Bouchama et al., 2007). The meta-analysis result was further confirmed by a later review on another two studies, with both ORs being 0.2 (Kenny et al., 2010). A study was conducted to investigate the ownership and utilisation of home cooling devices (consisting of electric fans and air conditioners) among general Hong Kong population aged 15 and above, identify related socio-demographic characteristics, and examine their associations with risk perception of climate change (Gao & Chan, 2019). Appropriate use of cooling devices can protect people from health impacts during heatwave. A population-based telephone survey was conducted during May–June 2012. Information like ownership and utilisation of home electric fans and air conditioners, risk perception of climate change, and socio-demographic characteristics was collected with a questionnaire. Univariate and multivariate analyses were performed to estimate associations of socio-demographic and other factors with the ownership and utilisation of the cooling devices. The final sample size of this study was 1,002, with an overall response rate of 63.0%.

This population-based telephone survey study found that the majority of the participants (final valid sample n = 1,002) owned electric fans (90.3%) or air conditioners (90.0%) at home. Of the owners, 91.5% usually used air conditioners and 95.1% usually used fans when feeling hot. Around half of the participants (54.3%) reported specific indoor temperature to switch on cooling devices, of whom 58.1% and 95.4% usually switched them on at or below 28°C and 31°C respectively. Older people, as well as those with lower education, with lower household income, unemployed/retired/housewives, living in public housing, and with chronic diseases were more likely to have no home air conditioners or not to switch them on even when feeling hot. Only living with vulnerable persons (aged < 15 or > 60 years old) had marginally significant relationship with use of fans in univariate analysis (0.05 < p < 0.10), whilst the risk of type of housing became marginally significant in the multivariable model, with those living in subsidised houses being more likely to use fans compared with those living in private houses. Overall, no statistically significant (p < 0.05) relationship between ownership and utilisation of fans was found with the studied socio-demographic factors.

Findings further indicated that low education level (OR = 3.97, 95% CI = 2.05–7.67, primary or below vs tertiary or above), unemployment status (OR = 2.52, 95% CI = 1.41–4.51, white collar jobs as reference), living in public housing (OR = 2.03, 95% CI = 1.21–3.39, private housing as reference), and low monthly household income (OR = 7.71, 95% CI = 2.99–19.9, household income >= HK$40,000 as reference) were risk factors for not using air conditioners, with household income having the strongest association with utilisation of home air conditioners. Each of the above-mentioned characteristics at least partly reflects poor socio-economic status of a person, suggesting in line with previous studies that financial conditions or financial considerations may be a major determinant of air conditioner use (Hansen et al., 2011). It may explain why the poor are at high risk for the health impact of heatwave observed from other studies (Chan et al., 2012; Hajat et al., 2010; Kenny et al., 2010).

Prices of electric fans, as low as HK$50 (US$6.44) for a second-hand working fan and HK$200 (US$25.8) for a new one, may be affordable even for the disadvantaged in Hong Kong (the median monthly household income in 2011 was HK$20,500, that is, US$2,640). In addition, previous studies indicated that older people and those with chronic diseases were more likely to use fans than air conditioners as ways for adapting to heat (Abrahamson et al., 2009; Sheridan, 2007; White-Newsome et al., 2011). Nearly 40% of the elderly (36.7%) did not turn air conditioners on when feeling hot, double of the proportion of not using fans (17.0%, $p < 0.001$). This result agrees with the previous studies (Abrahamson et al., 2009; Sheridan, 2007; White-Newsome et al., 2011) conducted in European cities. Similar patterns were also found in the participants with chronic diseases (26.9% of not using air conditioners vs 15.4% of not using fans, $p < 0.001$). It has been suggested that the use of air conditioners may be unsustainable in a warming climate because of the positive feedback loop they create through their high energy consumption (which will further add to climate change by increasing emissions), the increased risk of blackouts due to pressures on the energy grid, and their high operational cost (Gupta et al., 2012). Properly using electric fans might be a promising and sustainable alternative to reduce the health impact of heat. Thus, further studies should be focused on electric fan use during heatwaves.

Moreover, older people (≥65 years old) and those with chronic diseases were more likely not to use home air conditioners, which is consistent with most previous studies (Abrahamson et al., 2009; Hansen et al., 2011; Sheridan, 2007; White-Newsome et al., 2011). Personal perceptions of heat are crucial in shaping individual adaptive behaviours. When people perceived that adaptation to hot weather is unnecessary, they make few or no behaviour adjustments to prevent heat-related health risks (White-Newsome et al., 2011). The perception of heat among older people is diminished, which is a major barrier for them to take these actions (Hansen et al., 2011). Thermoregulatory impairment, chronic diseases, and dehydration and drug effects among older people further enhance their risk for heat (Koppe et al., 2004). In addition, chronic medical conditions significantly alter the body's physiologic response to heat load or the ability to tolerate changes in core body temperature (Allen & Segal-Gidan, 2009). Cardiovascular diseases, for example, are the most significant conditions that predispose to heat illness. Other chronic conditions include obesity, hyper-thyroidism, psychiatric disorders, and extensive skin diseases or damages (Allen & Segal-Gidan, 2009). Thus, it is of most importance to empower older people and those having chronic diseases by effective interventions to undertake adaptive behaviours during extreme heat to maintain thermal comfort and avoid heat stress.

Although more than half of the participants (57.7%) perceived climate change as a high risk to health, the level of risk perception had no significant relationship with ownership and utilisation of the cooling devices. It is also possible that the study may have missed other protective ways against heat undertaken by the participants (e.g. visit other air-conditioned places), which may result in the insignificant relationship. Yet, it is likely that though some people realise heatwaves are a health threat, they may not have moved from the "awareness" stage into the "practice" stage yet due to various reasons (e.g. insufficient knowledge about adaptive ways to heat and lack of intention to take actions). Nevertheless, comprehensive surveys focusing on both physiological and environmental factors during heatwaves would be helpful to reveal the relationship between risk perception and mitigation behaviours against heat. Findings suggested familial economic condition may be a major determinant to have and use air conditioners at home. Old people and those with chronic diseases are at high risk of climate change and therefore should be equipped with appropriate measures to use cooling devices. Though more than half of the Hong Kong general population recognised climate change as a threat, there are no signs showing that they have taken protective actions. Further studies should be conducted to identify risk factors of utilisation of electric fans and with a focus on disadvantaged people.

Heatwave: response to warning and personal heat protective measures

Following the European heatwave of 2003, some countries developed "heat health warning systems" to prevent heat-related morbidity and mortality (Kovats & Hajat, 2008). A study was conducted to understand the community's response to hot weather in terms of risk perception, awareness of warning signal, and personal protective measures taken for heat planning suggestions (Lam, Chan, & Man, 2018). A telephone survey was conducted 2 weeks after a heatwave in Hong Kong in August 2017, involving 436 respondents (≥ 15 years old). Socio-demographic characteristics, risk perception, awareness of the issue of Very Hot Weather Warning, and the uptake of personal protective measures during the study period (2017) were collected. Among all respondents, 45.3% believed heat would not affect their health at all and 28.8% among the above-65-year group thought the same. Around 87% were aware of the heat warning issued by the Hong Kong Observatory. During that period, 37.2–97.5% had applied at least one personal heat protective measure. The most common uptake measure was drinking more water (97.5%) and the least was the use of sunscreen (37.2%). Males were less likely to avoid the sun (OR 0.29 (95% CI 0.13, 0.65)) and put on sunscreen (OR 0.41 (95% CI 0.26, 0.64)) while people with a lower education level were less likely to use air conditioning (OR 0.22 (95% CI 0.05, 0.91)). The heat warning signal could reach most of the community. The uptake rate of the personal heat protective measures was high. Further study on understanding barriers of not applying measures among particular groups and evaluating effectiveness of health protective measures is needed. Awareness of heat-related health impacts should be raised among vulnerable groups.

Cold spell in subtropical urban context: risk perception, accuracy, and their association with personal health protection behaviours

With global climate change, more extreme temperature events may occur and such events are associated with adverse health impacts. Few prior studies have examined patterns of personal cold protection behaviours, especially among subtropical population. A 2-year prospective population-based cohort telephone survey was conducted in Hong Kong in 2016 (baseline after a colder cold wave) and 2017 (follow-up after a warmer cold wave) to assess health risk perception accuracy and the association with uptake of personal cold protection behaviours (Chan et al., in press). Adults aged 15 years old or above were surveyed with distribution of age, gender, and residential districts matched to the census data. Main study measures included socio-demographic information, self-reported health risk perception, and patterns of personal cold protection behaviours during cold waves. Among the 429 respondents, 45.0% were found to have a high underlying health risk but 63.7% of this subgroup had underestimated their health risks at low temperatures. Except for maintaining indoor ventilation, the self-reported personal cold protective measures uptake rate was higher during the more extreme 2016 cold wave. Those who had experienced adverse health effects during previous cold spells were more likely to put on more clothes (OR 5.48 (1.26–23.83)). Female (OR 1.93 (1.20–3.11)), those who felt cold at home during the study period (OR 3.72 (1.29–10.72)), and older groups (>24 years old vs 15–24 years old) (OR ranged from 3.35 to 4.04) were more likely to use heating equipment. Females were more likely to take up cold protective behaviours, which agreed with the findings from previous studies (Khare et al., 2015).

For health-seeking behaviour, males were found to be less willing to seek care or help than females (Doward, 2012). The higher rate of full-time workers and longer working hours among males, which may imply less time spent at home and less free time, may associate with the personal protective behaviours. Age was another factor associated with adoption of personal cold protective measure.

Although the effect of age on uptake of health protection behaviours is unclear, the differences in physiological conditions that affect the homeostatic process between age groups may explain the result. Young people have a higher metabolic rate and better thermoregulation (Barzilai, Huffman, Muzumdar, & Bartke, 2012; Frisard et al., 2007). Income, education level, risk perception, and risk perception accuracy were not found to be associated with uptake of personal protection behaviours during cold days.

The 2-year survey-based study has suggested the adaptation ability of the population to low temperature by implementing personal protective measures based on personal experiences. Study results also showed that personal cold protective behaviour changed according to the intensity of cold waves, age, gender, and past experiences, but not with risk perception and accuracy, income, or education level. A significant proportion of respondents did not consider themselves more vulnerable in extreme high temperatures regardless of their age and history of chronic diseases and similar results have been found in other cities in the United Kingdom and North America (proportions not reported) (Abrahamson et al., 2009; Sheridan, 2007). Self-risk perception and risk perception accuracy are both found not to be associated with health outcomes during cold waves but the findings did highlight the gap in health literacy and accuracy of self-risk perception. Targeted health education and service should be provided to vulnerable groups such as people with chronic disease and old people to reduce cold-related adverse health effects and complications.

It is noteworthy that with 80.2% (202/252) of respondents reporting owning heating equipment in Hong Kong, the uptake rate of using heating equipment (55%) was still low during severe cold waves in this subtropical city that has a daily mean temperature at about 19°C in the cold season. The pattern of warm-keeping behaviours may reflect acclimatisation as well as the low awareness of the adverse effects of cold waves among this subtropical population. This may increase the risk of health issues when a cold wave strikes. In the face of climate change, extreme temperature events may become more frequent. Heating equipment should be considered for households for health protection against the cold.

Special attention should also be paid to ensure indoor ventilation since poor ventilation may be associated with higher risk of infectious diseases. While the population were more likely to adopt keeping-warm measures such as the using of heating equipment, avoiding staying in windy areas, and wearing more clothes, they were less likely to manage indoor ventilation. This might reflect the concept of avoiding a significant drop in room temperature by keeping windows and doors closed. Central heating is not common in Hong Kong and the indoor temperature is thus usually similar to that of outdoors in winter, which may cause health issues during cold waves especially for older people who have compromised thermoregulation function. In contrast, it is important to point out that people in those areas that are affected by the heat island effect (e.g. those in Kowloon) are more likely to keep vigilant about indoor ventilation. Similar studies have been conducted in developed countries while the situations in developing countries, which have higher vulnerability due to the poorer living environment and information access, are unclear. Future study on the awareness and practices against extreme temperatures should be conducted in developing countries.

Impact of cold spell and heatwaves on physical activity in a subtropical urban population

Extreme temperatures are increasing due to climate change, however research on their impacts on health behaviour is rare. While cold winter temperatures have been identified as a barrier to physical activity, an increase of extremely hot temperatures due to climate change may also potentially affect frequency of physical activity. A study was conducted to estimate the change of self-reported frequency of outdoor physical activity (PA) during cold (2016) and heatwaves (2017) in a subtropical urban population and identify its predictors (Ho, Chan, Mo, & Lam, 2018). A prospective population-based cohort telephone survey study was conducted in an Asian subtropical city, a week after a 2016 cold spell and followed-up 1.5 years after, a week after a 2017 heatwave. Measures on self-reported changes in outdoor physical activities in heat and cold waves, socio-demographic variables, health status, warning awareness, temperature-related attitudes and knowledge, and protective behaviours were collected. Multivariable logistic regression analyses were carried out to assess predictors of change in outdoor PA over the two extreme temperature events.

Overall, more participants (53.3%, final n = 435) reported a decrease in PA in either or both the heat and cold waves, than reported an increase (10.3%), while 36.3% of participants maintained consistent PA in both the cold spells and heatwaves. Decreased PA was associated with females, worsened health status in winter, awareness of temperature, and certain protective behaviours, while increased PA was associated with students, those under 45, higher income, and better health status in summer. Study findings suggest a greater decrease of outdoor PA during cold spells and heatwaves and identify gender, age, income, health status, temperature-related awareness, and protective behaviours to be associated.

Community preparedness of health risks associated with the impact of climate change

Despite the dramatic growth of global dengue incidence and the serious health impacts caused by severe dengue fever, literatures describing the association between mosquito bite patterns and the adoption of mosquito-protective measures are limited. With climate change, vector-borne disease is likely to change its pattern and potential impact. It is important to understand community knowledge altitude and practices regarding the management of vector-borne diseases such as dengue fever. A population-based randomised telephone survey (n = 590) study was conducted 3 weeks after the government announcement of a local dengue outbreak in Hong Kong (Chan, Lo, Tsang, Man & Lam, 2018) in August 2018 to explore the awareness of a recent local dengue outbreak, knowledge of dengue fever, mosquito bite patterns, adoption rates of mosquito-protective measures, and the associating factors between mosquito bites and adoption of mosquito-protective measures among Hong Kong as a subtropical urban Asian community. Information was collected about awareness of the dengue outbreak, knowledge of dengue fever symptoms, mosquito bite patterns, and adoptions of mosquito-protective measures from adult Cantonese-speaking residents.

Most respondents were aware of the local outbreak (96.1%), could identify fever as a symptom of dengue (84.0%) and that it was a mosquito-borne disease (92.2%) but fewer could name other dengue symptoms (< 21%). About 40% of respondents claimed to be bitten by mosquitos in the study period. Transportation spots and places near water sources were high-risk spots for mosquito bites. Nearly 80% of the respondents claimed they had adopted at least one mosquito-preventive measure. Removing stagnant water (51.0%) and using mosquito repellent (39.8%) were the most common. The likelihood of adoptions of those measures was associated with the number of mosquito bites respondents experienced. As a high-risk community, most of the respondents adopted mosquito-protective measures during the high risk season but the effectiveness of the adopted measures remains uncertain. Insufficient knowledge of dengue symptoms may delay disease diagnosis and increase risk of outbreak. Effective policy against mosquito bites and dengue education should be developed to reduce risk of mosquito bites and the associated health impacts.

Conclusion

This chapter discusses how urban community perceived their health risks and corresponding actions that aim to protect health and well-being in urban context. While the discussion mostly focuses on the community perception and response to weather events, it is essential to understand the types of community behaviour that might mitigate climate change impact in a population.

References

Abrahamson, V., Wolf, J., Lorenzoni, I., Fenn, B., Kovats, S., Wilkinson, P., ... Raine, R. (2009). Perceptions of heatwave risks to health: Interview-based study of older people in London and Norwich, UK. *Journal of Public Health*, *31*(1), 119–126.

Allen, A., & Segal-Gidan, F. (2009). Heat related illness in the elderly. *Clinical Geriatrics*, *15*(17), 37–45.

Barzilai, N., Huffman, D. M., Muzumdar, R. H., & Bartke, A. (2012). The critical role of metabolic pathways in aging. *Diabetes*, *61*, 1315–1322. doi:10.2337/db11-1300.

Bouchama, A., Dehbi, M., Mohamed, G., Matthies, F., Shoukri, M., & Menne, B. (2007). Prognostic factors in heat wave related deaths: A meta-analysis. *Archives of Internal Medicine*, *167*, 2170–2176.

Chan, E. Y. Y., Goggins, W. B., Kim, J. J., & Griffiths, S. M. (2012). A study of intracity variation of temperature-related mortality and socioeconomic status among the Chinese population in Hong Kong. *Journal of Epidemiology and Community Health*, 66(4), 322–327.

Chan, E. Y. Y., Lam, H. C. Y., Huang, Z., Liu, S., Guo, C. L., & Goggins, W. B. (in press). Are risk perception and its accuracy associated with personal health protection behaviours against cold waves? *BMC Public Health*.

Chan, E. Y. Y., Lo, E. S. K., Tsang, S. N. S., Man, A. Y. T., & Lam, H. C. Y. (2018). *Dengue knowledge, mosquito bite patterns and the adoption of protective measures against mosquitos in a subtropical urban Asian community: A cross-sectional randomized telephone survey study* (CCOUC Working Paper Series). Hong Kong, China: Collaborating for Oxford University and CUHK for Disaster and Medical Humanitarian Response.

Chan, E. Y. Y., Man, A. Y. T., Lam, H. C. Y., Chan, G. K. W., Hall, B. J., & Hung, K. K. C. (2019). Is urban household emergency preparedness associated with short-term impact reduction after a super typhoon in subtropical city? *International Journal of Environmental Research and Public Health*, 16(3), 596.

Chan, E. Y. Y., & Shi, P. (2017). Health and risks: Integrating health into disaster risk reduction, risk communication, and building resilient communities. *International Journal of Disaster Risk Science*, 8(2), 107–108. doi:10.1007/s13753-017-0131-z.

Chan, E. Y. Y., Yue, J., Lee, P., & Wang, S. S. (2016). Socio-demographic predictors for urban community disaster health risk perception and household based preparedness in a Chinese urban city. *PLOS Currents Disasters*. doi:10.1371/currents.dis.287fb7fee6f9f4 521af441a236c2d519.

Clements, B. W., & Casani, J. A. P. (2009). *Disasters and public health: Planning and response*. Burlington, MA: Butterworth-Heinemann/Elsevier.

Doocy, S., Dick, A., Daniels, A., Kirsch, T. D., & Hopkins, J. (2013). The human impact of tropical cyclones: A historical review of events 1980–2009 and systematic literature review. *PLOS Currents Disasters*, 1, 1–25. doi:10.1371/currents.dis.2664354a55715120 63ed29d25ffbce74.

Doward, J. (2012). Men risk health by failing to seek NHS help, survey finds. Retrieved from www.theguardian.com/society/2012/nov/04/men-failing-seek-nhs-help.

Frisard, M. I., Broussard, A., Davies, S. S., Roberts, L. T., Rood, L., de Jonge, L., … Louisiana Healthy Aging Study. (2007). Aging, resting metabolic rate, and oxidative damage results from the Louisiana Healthy Aging Study. *Journals of Gerontology. Series A, Biological Sciences and Medical Sciences*, 62, 752–759. doi:10.1016/j.ijrobp. 2008.04.018.A.

Gao, Y., & Chan, E. Y. Y. (2019). Risk perception of climate change and utilization of fans and air conditioners in a representative population of Hong Kong. (CCOUC Working Paper Series). Hong Kong, China: Collaborating for Oxford University and CUHK for Disaster and Medical Humanitarian Response.

Grogan, H., & Hopkins, P. M. (2002). Heat stroke: Implications for critical care and anaesthesia. *British Journal of Anaesthesia*, 88(5), 700–707.

Gupta, S., Carmichael, C., Simpson, C., Clarke, M. J., Allen, C., Gao, Y., … Murray, V. (2012). Electric fans for reducing adverse health impacts in heatwaves. *Cochrane Database of Systematic Reviews*, 11(7). doi:10.1002/14651858.CD009888.pub2.

Hajat, S., O'Conner, M., & Kosatsky, T. (2010). Health effects of hot weather: From awareness of risk factors to effective health protection. *The Lancet*, 375(9717), 856–863.

Hansen, A., Bi, P., Nitschke, M., Pisaniello, D., Newbury, J., & Kitson, A. (2011). Perceptions of heat-susceptibility in older persons: Barriers to adaptation. *International Journal of Environmental Research and Public Health*, 8(12), 4714–4728.

Ho, J. Y., Chan, E. Y. Y., Mo, P. K. H., & Lam, H. C. Y. (2018). *Assessing the impact of cold and heat waves on physical activity in a sub-tropical urban population.* Paper presented at ISES-ISEE 2018 Joint Annual Meeting, 26–30 August, Ottawa, Canada.

Hong Kong Observatory. (2018). *Typhoon 5–6 (average number of tropical cyclones).* Retrieved from www.hko.gov.hk/education/article_e.htm?title=ele_00161.

Ibrahim, J. E., McInnes, J. A., Andrianopoulos, N., & Evans, S. (2012). Minimising harm from heatwaves: A survey of awareness, knowledge, and practices of health professionals and care providers in Victoria, Australia. *International Journal of Public Health, 57,* 297–304.

Kaiser, R., Rubin, C. H., Henderson, A. K., Wolfe, M. I., Kieszak, S., Parrott, C. L., & Adcock, M. (2001). Heat-related death and mental illness during the 1999 Cincinnati heat wave. *The American Journal of Forensic Medicine and Pathology, 22*(3), 303–307.

Kenny, G. P., Yardley, J., Brown, C., Sigal, R. J., & Jay, O. (2010). Heat stress in older individuals and patients with common chronic diseases. *Canadian Medical Association Journal, 182*(10), 1053–1060.

Khare, S., Hajat, S., Kovats, S., Lefevre, C. E., de Bruin, W. B. Dessai, S., & Bone, A. (2015). Heat protection behaviour in the UK: Results of an online survey after the 2013 heatwave. *BMC Public Health, 15,* 1–12. doi:10.1186/s12889-015-2181-8.

Kilbourne, E. M., Choi, K., Jones, T. S., & Thacker, S. B. (1982). Risk factors for heat-stroke: A case-control study. *Journal of the American Medical Association, 247,* 3332–3336.

Koppe, C., Kovats, S., Jendritzky, G., & Menne, B. (2004). *Heat-waves: Risks and responses* (Health and Global Environmental Change Series, No. 2). World Health Organization Regional Office for Europe.

Kovats, S., & Hajat, S. (2008). Heat stress and public health: A critical review. *Annual Review of Public Health, 29,* 41–55.

Lam, H. C. Y., Chan, E. Y. Y., & Man, A. Y. T. (2018). *Personal heat protective measures during the 2017 heatwave in Hong Kong: A telephone survey study.* Paper presented at the First Global Forum for Heat and Health, 19 December 2018, Hong Kong, China.

Last, J. M. (1998). *Dictionary of epidemiology.* UK: Oxford University Press.

Leung, Y. K., Yip, K. M., & Yeung, K. H. (2008). Relationship between thermal index and mortality in Hong Kong. *Meteorological Applications, 15,* 399–409.

Luo, C., Goggins, W. B., & Chan, E. Y. Y. (2017). Temperature and suicidal mortality in Hong Kong SAR, China. Paper presented at the Conference of International Society of Environmental Epidemiology (ISEE 2017), September, Sydney, Australia.

Luo, C., Goggins, W. B., & Chan, E. Y. Y. (2018). Temperature and falls-related hospital admissions in Hong Kong SAR, China. Paper presented at ISES-ISEE 2018 Joint Annual Meeting, 26–30 August, Ottawa, Canada.

Matthies, F., Bickler, G., Marín, N. C., & Hales, S. (2008). *Heat–health action plans.* World Health Organization Regional Office for Europe.

Naughton, M. P., Henderson, A., Mirabelli, M. C., Kaiser, R., Wilhelm, J. L., Kieszak, S. M., … McGeehin, M. A. (2002). Heat-related mortality during a 1999 heat wave in Chicago. *American Journal of Preventive Medicine, 22*(4), 221–227.

Semenza, J. C., Rubin, C. H., Falter, K. H., Selanikio, J. D., Flanders, A., Howe, H. L., & Wilhelm, J. L. (1996). Heat-related deaths during the July 1995 heat wave in Chicago. *New England Journal of Medicine, 335,* 84–90. doi:10.1056/NEJM199607113350203.

Shahid, M. S., Hatle, L., Mansour, H., & Mimish, L. (1999). Echocardiographic and Doppler study of patients with heatstroke and heat exhaustion. *International Journal of Cardiac Imaging, 15*(4), 279–285.

Sheridan, S. C. (2007). A survey of public perception and response to heat warnings across four North American cities: An evaluation of municipal effectiveness. *International Journal of Biometeorology, 52*(1), 3–15. doi:10.1007/s00484-006-0052-9.

Skinner, R. D. (2002). Temperature regulation during sleep. In T. L. Lee-Chiong, M. Sateia, & M. Carskadon (Eds.), *Sleep medicine* (pp. 71–76). Philadelphia, PA: Hanley & Belfus (Elsevier).

White-Newsome, J. L., Sanchez, B. N., Parker, E. A., Dvonch, J. T., Zhang, Z., & O'Neill, M. S. (2011). Assessing heat-adaptive among older, urban-dwelling adults. *Maturitas, 70*(1), 85–91.

13 Climate change mitigation, policies, research gaps, and next steps

This chapter has two sections. The first section discusses approaches in mitigation and health. Specifically, the concept of co-benefits and case studies of how community is approaching the idea will be explored. The second part of this chapter discusses how one of the latest global thematic research paradigms, namely health emergency disaster risk management (Health-EDRM) may support better building of mitigation programmes, policies, and strategies. Specifically, it will discuss how the potential research output generated by this paradigm might support the four major global policy agendas for 2015–2030, which include the Paris climate agreement, the Sendai Framework for Disaster Risk Reduction, Sustainable Development Goals (SDGs), and the New Urban Agenda.

Mitigation

Many climate mitigation strategies may not aim at improving health. However, well-designed mitigation policies should be multidisciplinary (see Case Box 13.1) and can bring co-benefits by improving health determinants across social, economic, and environmental systems. For example, forest conservation strategies for protecting *biodiversity* and *ecosystems* may also improve water quality and availability. Another typical example is the shift from private transport (e.g. cars) to public or active transport, which may result in air quality improvement and promotion of physical activity, such as walking and cycling. Climate-related mitigation actions may reduce greenhouse gas emissions by using new technologies and renewable energies. Mitigation can also be achieved by increasing the capacity of carbon sinks.

Overall, mitigation actions from non-health sectors can bring potential health co-benefits and co-harms to the health sectors. For mitigation actions that target air quality, *reduced mortality and morbidity associated with air pollution* is likely to be one of the most direct and immediate co-benefits of climate change mitigation actions particularly on cardiovascular and respiratory health. For instance, reducing emissions of methane and black carbon may avoid more than 2 million deaths per year. These potential health gains could offset the cost of mitigation actions (Intergovernmental Panel on Climate Change

---

Case Box 13.1   Multidisciplinary approach needed to deal with climate change and public health

By Christine Loh

Climate change is altering many types of risks associated with extreme weather. In subtropical Hong Kong, with more frequent and longer periods of high temperatures, and also short but very cold spells, temperature changes present a new threat to public health. Local research shows the effect of cold last longer and are greater than that of heat on people. Those over 75 are the most vulnerable to cold temperatures, while those between 65 and 74 are most vulnerable to heat (Yi & Chan, 2015). At-risk populations also include children, and the tens of thousands of people who live in substandard conditions. Hong Kong's general response to heat is air conditioning, and for those who do not have it, government community centres are open to them. Cold spells can be deadlier. As buildings and homes generally do not have heating, low temperatures can lead to hypothermia. Beyond temperature changes, severe typhoons often damage the homes of under-privileged communities, exposing them to higher overall risks.

Solutions to reduce climate-related risks require multidisciplinary approaches beyond treatment when illness or injury occurs. First, climate-ready emergency preparedness must include at-risk populations being informed and brought to safety when needed, and to encourage locally based action that may well depend on neighbours helping each other. Second, long-term transformation of the built environment is vital. Measures include siting buildings to minimise blockage to air ventilation, cooling the city through urban forestry, and using public funding to retrofit older dilapidated buildings that house low-income elderly and under-privileged families (CARe2018 Organising Committee, 2018).

[IPCC], 2015). *Reduced environmental health risks in communities and households* that may also bring about many indirect health benefits could arise from actions of the non-health sectors as well. For example, well-planned land use management may help prevent other environmental health risks, e.g. flooding, increased water run-off, and water contamination. Other *benefits to the health sector* including multidisciplinary climate mitigation strategies may create opportunities for other health protection in a community. These might include activities that (i) improve rural health facility infrastructure and access to energy for health facilities using renewable energy and environmentally friendly and disaster-resilient buildings; and (ii) reduce long-term energy, building, and operational costs of large urban healthcare centres and hospitals (World Health Organization [WHO] & World Bank, 2014). Table 13.1 shows examples of mitigation strategies that might bring co-benefits and harm to a community.

Table 13.1 Examples of mitigation strategies and co-benefits/co-harms

Sector	Mitigation strategies	Potential health drivers	Potential health co-benefits/co-harms
Energy	Reduce fossil fuel combustion	Air pollutants	Risk of cardiovascular and respiratory morbidity/mortality
	Increase biofuel production	Food availability Food prices	Food insecurity and malnutrition
	Carbon capture/ equestration	Water availability and quality	Risk of water-borne disease
Transport	Increase active transport	Urban air pollution Physical activity	Risk of CVDs, obesity and diabetes, depression
Agriculture	Reduce livestock production	Ozone and CO_2 production	Risk of CVDs and respiratory diseases
Land	Increase green space in cities	Physical activity Excessive heat exposure	Risk of CVDs and cancers

Source: Adapted from Remais et al. (2014).

Integrating health in mitigation strategies: health co-benefits

Mitigation policies with anticipated health co-benefits are likely to have widespread public support. However, in order to integrate "health" and "health co-benefits" in planning and implementing mitigation policies in non-health sectors, technical knowledge, strong political will, good multi-sectoral partnerships, and proactive leadership in the health and related sectors are required. Providing "health impact assessments" of climate change-related mitigation approaches may be an important method to characterise the potential health co-benefits from a planned strategy. Therefore, mitigation actions with the most benefits to health may be prioritised among other competing issues. Furthermore, cost-benefit assessments are also important for policy decision-making. In the assessments, health benefits should be considered as "offsets" or "trade-offs" from initial cost of mitigation investment. This is because a potential long-term mitigation cost is relatively small compared with anticipated cost-savings in health systems from the health benefits, such as prevented deaths, diseases, and disabilities. Thus proactive inclusion and engagement of the health sector is a key strategy to ensure how a fair assessment of cost may be conducted (WHO & World Bank, 2014).

The significant effect of individual lifestyles on both environmental change and health has drawn rapidly increasing attention in the research community recently (Hutchinson, Prady, Smith, White, & Graham, 2015). For instance, augmented physical activity as a result of walking and cycling to destinations instead of driving will not only reduce carbon emissions and air pollution, but also lower the risk of chronic diseases (Smith et al., 2015). Studies have provided evidence of co-benefits in areas of active travel (e.g. walking and cycling) (Wanner, Götschi, Martin-Diener, Kahlmeier, & Martin, 2012), public transport (Xia et al., 2015), food-related behaviours (e.g. vegetarian lifestyle, organic and locally sourced food, and plate waste) (VanDooren, Marinussen, Blonk, Aiking, & Vellinga, 2014), household energy use and waste management (Kurz, Gardner, Verplanken, & Abraham, 2015). In the United States, five categories of household actions can provide a behavioural wedge to reduce greenhouse gas (GHG) emissions rapidly: (i) home weatherisation and upgrades for heating and cooling equipment; (ii) energy-efficient vehicles and appliances; (iii) equipment maintenance; (iv) equipment adjustment; and (v) daily energy use behaviours (e.g. standby electricity and driving behaviour) (Dietz, Gardner, Gilligan, Stern, & Vandenbergh, 2009). However, co-benefits need to be adapted locally, as the benefits are largely contextual and affected by local practices, culture, lifestyle habits and so on (Ürge-Vorsatz, Herrero, Dubash, & Lecocq, 2014). In addition, there is currently a dearth of evidence on the patterns and predictors of such co-benefit practices. More evidence is urgently needed to understand the associations between the practices of healthy behaviours and demographical factors (Busch, VanStel, Schrijvers, & deLeeuw, 2013), or between environmental friendly behaviours and demographic factors (Fisher, Bashyal, & Bachman, 2012; Wiernik, Ones, & Dilchert, 2013), particularly in a densely populated urban context. Table 13.2 adapted from Chan et al. (2017) describes the patterns of 10 different co-benefit behaviours relevant to an Asian urban community and examines the relationship between demographics and the frequency of practising co-benefit behaviour (see also Case Box 13.2).

Table 13.2 Health and environmental benefits of 10 co-benefit behaviours

Category	Behaviour	Linkage	Health benefits	Environmental benefits
Active travel	Walk/cycle more	Reduce the use of motorised transportation, air pollutant emissions (e.g. particulate matter, ozone, volatile organic compounds), physical inactivity and risk factors (e.g. obesity) of non-communicable diseases	Reduce the risks of chronic diseases (e.g. cardiovascular diseases, diabetes, cancers), premature death, respiratory symptoms and illnesses (e.g. asthma, lung cancer), injuries from traffic accidents, depression and mental health problems	Improve air quality and reduce the operation of internal combustion engines and the emissions of greenhouse gases (GHG) and smog-forming VOCs and NO_x
Dietary-related behaviours	Buy more organic food	Reduce the exposure to additives, chemical fertilisers, or pesticides (e.g. insecticides, fungicides, rodenticides, pediculicides, and biocides) via inhalation, ingestion, dermal contact, or across the placenta	Reduce the risks of allergies, hay fever, cancer development (e.g. leukaemia), and neurodevelopmental delays in children, and triggers for multiple chemical sensitivity	Improve water and soil quality, and reduce soil degradation due to pesticides and the development of resistance in insects
	Consume less meat	Reduce GHGs produced by ruminant livestock (e.g. cows) and over-consumption of red meat, which usually contains more saturated fats	Reduce the risks of colorectal cancer, cardiovascular diseases, diabetes, and lung cancer potentially associated moderately with exposure to high temperature cooking	Reduce nitrogen and GHG emissions, and decrease land scarcity through less demand for cropland to grow animal feed
	Have one vegetarian meal a week	Reduce over-consumption of food with high fat content (e.g. saturated fats, trans-fats)	Reduce the risk of diseases (e.g. constipation, diverticular disease, gallstones, and appendicitis) and obesity, thereby lowering the risk of chronic diseases (e.g. coronary heart diseases)	Reduce GHG emissions and conserve water and energy since the vegetarian diet requires less water, primary energy, fertilisers, and pesticides than the non-vegetarian diet

Household conservation	Use less electricity	Alleviate air pollution from fossil fuel power plants (i.e. those burning coal, petroleum, and natural gas)	Reduce the risks of stroke, heart disease, lung cancer, and chronic lower respiratory tract diseases	Reduce GHG emissions, air pollution, and coal combustion waste, which could contaminate groundwater and soil if disposed improperly
	Use less air conditioning (AC)	Improve indoor air quality (IAQ) and increase indoor air exchange rate, air movement, and ventilation with open windows	Reduce the concentrations of indoor particle pollutants and VOCs, prevalence of sick building syndrome (SBS), and the risk of respiratory allergy	Reduce the release of anthropogenic heat, prevalence of urban heat island effect, and pollutants released from refrigerants
	Shower less than 5 minutes every day	Conserve limited water resources by reducing average household water consumption	Secure the local availability of clean water for drinking, cooking, and personal hygiene to reduce the risks of infectious diseases transmitted by water, food, and contact	Reduce the impacts of wastewater discharges on environmental water quality and conserve biodiversity

continued

Table 13.2 Continued

Category	Behaviour	Linkage	Health benefits	Environmental benefits
Waste management	Use less packaging and fewer disposable shopping bags	Reduce plastic waste and migration of chemicals from plastic bags and packaging materials	Reduce the risks of breast cancer and other disruptions to human reproductive functions potentially related to exposure to chemicals found in plastics (e.g. Bisphenol A)	Reduce the landfill burden, plastic debris in the marine or terrestrial environments and GHG emissions from plastic production and combustion
	Bring personal eating utensils when dining in restaurants or small eateries	Reduce plastic waste and exposure to harmful chemicals, and increase protection of hygiene	Protect personal hygiene and reduce potential risk of breast cancer, obesity, immune disorders, early puberty, reproductive harm, and other health disorders due to endocrine disruption from Bisphenol A	Reduce the landfill burden, plastic debris in the marine or terrestrial environments, and GHG emissions from plastic production and combustion
	Separate household waste	Reduce the amount of waste sent to landfills, particularly household hazardous waste	Reduce the risks of congenital anomalies, reproductive disorders, and the risk of cancer development	Increase the amount of material recovery and reduce the landfill burden, GHG emissions from primary material production, and leachate/migration of hazardous chemicals and other emissions (e.g. volatile organic compounds, particulate matter) into the surrounding environment of landfills

Source: Chan et al. (2017).

Case Box 13.2 Health and environmental co-benefit (HEC) behaviour patterns in Hong Kong

Climate change is known to pose risks to human health (IPCC, 2014; WHO, 2013). As human behaviour is regarded as a primary cause of climate change (IPCC, 2014), modifying it has been confirmed as one of the most efficient and low-cost methods to mitigate climate change (Abroms & Maibach, 2008). Climate change and human health are so closely linked that many mitigation measures naturally promote public health and environmental benefits at the same time, as captured in the concept of co-benefits. As defined by the IPCC and WHO, co-benefits involve "a climate change adaptation or mitigation strategy which has additional, positive effects on health or other areas" (Spickett, Katscherian, & Brown, 2015) and "health gains from strategies that are directed primarily at climate change, and mitigation of climate change from well-chosen policies for health advancement" (Smith et al., 2014). While co-benefits can be applied across a variety of sectors, the co-benefit behaviours this study investigates refer specifically to the behaviours that have positive effects on health and environment.

A population-based, stratified, and cross-sectional random-digit-dialling telephone survey was conducted between 28 January and 4 February 2016 (Chan et al., 2017). The survey was conducted in the Cantonese language, as 95.8% of the Hong Kong population are Cantonese speakers or are able to use Cantonese. The study population was the non-institutionalised population aged 15 years old or above residing in Hong Kong, including residents holding valid work or study visas. Exclusion criteria included (i) non-Cantonese-speaking respondents; (ii) children under the age of 15; (iii) overseas visitors holding tourist visas to Hong Kong or two-way permit holders from mainland China; and (iv) those unable to be interviewed due to medical reasons. A self-reported questionnaire was designed for data collection, which included information on the general socio-demographic background and practices of 10 different co-benefit behaviours of a respondent. The study was one of the key components of a larger climate change, extreme temperatures, and health survey. The socio-demographic background section comprised questions on gender, age, district of residence, marital status, education attainment, monthly household income, home ownership status, and type of housing. The 10 co-benefit behaviours were enquired through a common question: "In the past year, did you engage in the following lifestyle habits?" Behavioural frequencies of practising 10 co-benefit behaviours were reported on a 5-point Likert scale: never practised nor considered, never practised but considered, occasionally practised, practised at least once a week, and practised daily. The 10 co-benefit behaviours were chosen to address both the practices supported by scientific evidence as well as local community initiatives, such as showering less than 5 minutes every day. A backward-stepwise (likelihood ratio) multivariable logistic regression was performed to investigate the association between socio-demographic variables and the adoption of co-benefit behaviours.

A total of 1,017 respondents successfully completed the questionnaire, with a response rate of 63.6% (1,017/1,598). The most frequently practised co-benefit behaviour was "using less packaging and fewer disposable shopping bags", which was practised daily among 70.1% of the population. Several co-benefit behaviours had a daily practice among approximately 50% of the population, including walking/cycling more (54.8%), separating household waste (50.2%), using less electricity (48.3%), and using less air conditioning (44.1%). Those that were practised daily by around 30% of the population included consuming less meat (33.3%) and showering less than 5 minutes every day (23.7%). Behaviours that were practised daily by less than 10% of the population were having one vegetarian meal a week (5.8%), buying more organic food (4.3%), and bringing personal eating utensils when dining in restaurants or small eateries (4.0%). The results of multivariable logistic regression with backward-stepwise elimination indicated that the adoption of different types of co-benefit behaviours were associated with different socio-demographic variables. In general, females were more inclined to practise co-benefit behaviours, especially using less packaging and fewer disposable shopping bags (adjusted odd ratio (AOR) = 6.34, 95% confidence interval (CI): 2.75–14.60), having one vegetarian meal a week (AOR = 2.39, 95% CI: 1.79–3.18), buying more organic food (AOR = 2.19, 95% CI: 1.65–2.91), consuming less meat (AOR = 2.14, 95% CI: 1.60–2.87), separating household waste (AOR = 1.99, 95% CI: 1.49–2.66), using less electricity (AOR = 1.59, 95% CI: 1.19–2.14), using less air conditioning (AOR = 1.54, 95% CI: 1.11–2.13), and bringing personal eating utensils when dining in restaurants or small eateries (AOR = 1.53, 95% CI: 1.05–2.23).

Older people, both those between 45 and 64 and those 65 and above, were more likely to practise co-benefit behaviours daily when compared with younger people. Associations with older age were found in the following co-benefit behaviours: buying more organic food (age 45–64: AOR = 4.30, 95% CI: 2.54–7.29; age ≥65: AOR = 3.34, 95% CI: 1.83–6.10), consuming less meat (age 45–64: AOR = 3.44, 95% CI: 2.18–5.43; age ≥65: AOR = 3.32, 95% CI: 1.96–5.63), having one vegetarian meal a week (age 45–64: AOR = 2.36, 95% CI: 1.37–4.05; age ≥65: AOR = 1.88, 95% CI: 1.05–3.35), using less electricity (age 45–64: AOR = 1.73, 95% CI: 1.11–2.72; age ≥65: AOR = 2.27, 95% CI: 1.33–3.86), showering less than 5 minutes every day (age 45–64: AOR = 2.21, 95% CI: 1.39–3.51; age ≥65: AOR = 1.81, 95% CI: 1.08–3.04), and separating household waste (age 45–64: AOR = 2.97, 95% CI: 1.90–4.64; age ≥65: AOR = 2.80, 95% CI: 1.69–4.66).

Among the 10 co-benefit behaviours, education level was significantly associated with only bringing personal eating utensils when dining in restaurants or small eateries. The participants with post-secondary education level or above had 139% higher frequency of bringing their personal eating utensils than those who obtained primary or below education (AOR = 2.39, 95% CI: 1.18–4.84). Regarding the other socio-demographic predictors, marital status was significantly associated with active travel and having one vegetarian meal a week. Married participants were 96% more inclined to walk/cycle more in daily life (AOR = 1.96, 95% CI: 1.38–2.79) but 35% less inclined to have one vegetarian meal a week (AOR = 0.65, 95% CI: 0.47–0.91). Household income was significantly associated only with buying more organic food. Participants with household incomes of HK$40,000 or above per month were at least 66% more likely to buy more organic food daily (AOR = 1.66, 95% CI: 1.15–2.40). Compared with those living in public housing, respondents who lived in private permanent housing were less likely to use less air conditioning (AOR = 0.62, 95% CI: 0.43–0.90) but more willing to separate household waste (AOR = 1.46, 95% CI: 1.07–2.01), whereas those who lived in subsidised home ownership housing were also more willing to separate household waste (AOR = 2.19, 95% CI: 1.40–3.42).

In summary, among the 10 co-benefit behaviours, using less packaging and disposable shopping bags was practised daily by the highest proportion of people (70.1%). However, four behaviours were found to have been practised by less than half of the population, including bringing personal eating utensils when dining in restaurants or small eateries, showering less than 5 minutes, having one vegetarian meal a week, and buying more organic food. Multivariable logistic regression results showed that practising co-benefit behaviours was consistently associated with gender and age.

As indicated in the findings, urban population in Hong Kong showed a diverse pattern in the practice of health and environmental co-benefit (HEC) behaviours in their daily life. Using less packaging and fewer disposable shopping bags received the highest frequency in daily practice (70.1%), reflecting the success of the 2015 Plastic Shopping Bag Levy Scheme, a regulatory policy that requires a charge of HK$0.5 (US$0.06) for a plastic shopping bag (Environmental Protection Department of the Government of the Hong Kong Special Administrative Region, 2016). However, behaviours within the same categories also experienced a significant variation in self-reported practice frequency. The practices of having one vegetarian meal a week, bringing personal eating utensils when dining in restaurants or small eateries, and buying more organic food had a substantially lower proportion of daily practice than other behaviours in the same categories (4.0–5.8%). Although the behaviours of consuming less meat and having one vegetarian meal a week bear similar incentives as well as health and environmental benefits, the proportions of daily practice among the population differed significantly (daily practice of consuming less meat (33.3%) versus having one vegetarian meal a week (5.8%), $\chi2(4) = 27.681$, $p < 0.001$). This may be attributed to the perception and ease of the behaviour among the respondents, as it may be easier to reduce practising a behaviour than it is to schedule or regulate a specific dietary change. A similar situation can be found for the behaviours of using less packaging and fewer disposable shopping bags and bringing personal eating utensils when dining in restaurants or small eateries, whereby reducing the practice of a current behaviour (albeit with considerable policy support) was found among a significantly higher proportion of people (70.1%) than instilling the practice of a non-normative behaviour (4.0%) ($\chi2(4) = 140.685$, $p < 0.001$). Interestingly, in both cases, the patterns of socio-demographic associations were similar between the two behaviours despite differences in proportion of daily practice. In the case of buying organic food, the low proportion of daily practice (4.3%) can be attributed to a smaller share in the overall food market, complications around certification and labelling, and higher prices (Advisory Council on Food and Environmental Hygiene, 2013), as supported by the findings of an association with higher monthly income in this research.

Gender differences in the practice of co-benefit behaviours

Females consistently performed better than males across different co-benefit behaviours, which is consistent with the findings of previous studies on the gender associations of environmentally friendly behaviours. This study found that women are more inclined to use less electricity and air conditioning, use less packaging and fewer disposable shopping bags, bring personal eating utensils when dining in restaurants or small eateries, buy more organic food, and separate household waste. The associations found could potentially be due to the attitude and practices arising from traditional gender roles, where women are generally more involved in household affairs (e.g. shopping and cooking) than men (Women's Commission of the Government of the Hong Kong Special Administrative Region, 2010). Additionally, women were found to be more likely to have one vegetarian meal a week and consume less meat. The lower proportion of practising vegetarian-related behaviours by men could be associated with perceptions of meat consumption as a sign of masculinity (Rozin, Hormes, Faith, & Wansink, 2012; Schösle, deBoer, Boersema, & Aiking, 2015). Future promotion initiatives should confront traditional gender roles and stereotypes.

Age cohort differences in practising co-benefit behaviours

Contrary to a popular belief, study findings demonstrated that younger generations do not necessarily perform better in behaviours that benefit health and the environment. Instead, older people (age 45 or above) were more likely than younger people (age 44 or below) to practise co-benefit behaviours daily, especially for all dietary-related behaviours, reducing electricity and water usage, as well as separating household waste. These findings reveal a pattern similar to a meta-analysis of the relationship between age and pro-environmental variables, where older age was associated with more conservation behaviours (i.e. reducing use, avoiding waste, reusing, repurposing, and recycling). This may be attributable to a higher concern for frugality and conscientious behaviour among older people. In this study, those in the age cohort of 45 or above were born between the 1930s and 1960s, right around the period of wartime and post-war rapid industrialisation in Hong Kong, thus quite possibly growing up in a lifestyle of limited resources and conservation habits. Therefore, future promotion of conservation-related co-benefit behaviours should target and educate younger generations.

Variations in co-benefit practices with income and real estate ownership

Income and real estate ownership had diverse associations with the practice of different co-benefit behaviours. Those with higher household income were more likely to buy more organic food. A possible explanation could be that those with lower household income had a lower proportion of disposable income available for purchasing higher-priced organic food. Besides, respondents who lived in private permanent housing were less likely to use less air conditioning, while both they and those living in subsidised housing were more likely to separate household waste when compared with public housing residents. Generally, the residents in subsidised housing have a higher monthly income than the group who live in public housing, but lower than the group in private housing.

Policy implications

The local government has previously implemented a series of measures to promote co-benefit behaviours among the Hong Kong population. However, as supported by study findings, the impact of these measures varied. For example, the Plastic Shopping Bag Levy Scheme implemented in 2015, which charges HK$0.50

(US$0.06) per plastic shopping bag, was demonstrated to be relatively successful because 70.1% of participants self-reported to use less packaging and fewer disposable shopping bags daily—the most practised behaviour assessed in this study. Meanwhile, the Water Supplies Department organised a promotion initiative to conserve water by taking shorter showers through the Let's Save 10L Water campaign (Water Supplies Department of the Government of the Hong Kong Special Administrative Region, 2015), but research findings indicated nearly half of the residents never practised nor considered showering less than 5 minutes every day. More should be done to investigate the awareness and promote the practice of co-benefit behaviours, especially the behaviours with low frequency in daily practice. The role of community and healthcare practitioners to promote co-benefit practices should also be considered (see Case Box 13.3).

As illustrated by the study findings, a great variation in the frequency of practising co-benefit behaviours exists among an Asian urban population. Although over 70% of respondents reported using less packaging and fewer disposable shopping bags daily, four behaviours were found to have never been practised by more than half of the population, including bringing personal eating utensils when dining in restaurants or small eateries, showering less than 5 minutes every day, eating one vegetarian meal a week, and buying more organic food. More advocacy and policy implementation could be carried out to encourage the practice of these co-benefit behaviours, since these behaviours provide benefits for both health and the environment. Overall, women and older people were more inclined to practise co-benefit behaviours frequently in their daily lives, compared with men and younger people. Income and real estate ownership had mixed associations with co-benefit behaviours, since those more affluent were more likely to buy more organic food, separate household waste, and engage in active travel, but less likely to use less air conditioning.

The demographical trends found in this study are useful for targeted promotion, especially by multidisciplinary stakeholders of the health sector, government, and other civil society organisations in the community. Policymakers should incorporate concepts of co-benefits into account to ensure an optimal outcome, not only in terms of climate change and the environment, but also for the health of the population. In addition, this study provides a baseline of behaviour frequency, useful for further research on practice of co-benefit behaviours. Future research should examine if other factors (environmental policy) might be associated with the uptake of these co-benefit behaviours. Focus group study on community subgroups could also help provide qualitative insights to examine the potential enablers and barriers for promotion of related health programmes, policies, and strategies. To maximise limited resources for supporting both health protection and environmental sustainability, improving the understanding of causal pathways and predictors that might promote HEC behaviours should also be a high priority for further research in the coming decades.

Source: Chan et al. (2017)

Case Box 13.3 The role of family doctors and heat health

By Donald K. T. Li

Family doctors are the frontline of community health as they are usually the first medical practitioners people seek help from when unwell. At the First Global Forum on Heat and Health (2018), Dr Donald Li, President of the World Organization of Family Doctors (WONCA), talked about Working with Family Doctors: Opportunities for Global Impact (Global Heat Health Information Network, 2018). The role of family doctors should highlight community resilience and social accountability by advocating for patients' suffering during high temperatures and how that may impact chronic diseases and infectious diseases. As trusted medical professionals, family doctors are in a crucial position to monitor local issues (such as the effect of environmental variables in food systems) and provide tailored co-benefits to reduce personal environmental impact and improve human health (World Organization of Family Doctors [WONCA], 2017). Surrounding heatwaves and other disasters, this field of medicine is also fundamental to maintain regular medical services, provide community-level risk assessments, identify vulnerable groups, engage in recovery and rehabilitation, and, on a policy level, influence city-level disaster planning and advocate for health during multi-sectoral policy discussions.

Case Box 13.4 Students' knowledge and perception on climate change and disasters in two universities in Asia: a comparison

By Namgay Rinchen

Climate change and disasters are global concerns and form the key focus area of the Sustainable Development Goals (SDGs), Sendai Framework, and the Paris Agreement. Knowledge and perception on climate change and disasters of students in Khesar Gyalpo University of Medical Sciences of Bhutan and The Chinese University of Hong Kong were assessed and compared.

A cross-sectional study was conducted with retrospective analysis of two data sets collected by the Collaborating Centre for the Oxford University and The Chinese University of Hong Kong (CCOUC) in 2015 and 2017. Chi-square statistics were used and p-value < 0.05 was considered significant. There were a total of 727 valid responses. Only 9.6% of the participants scored 50% or more in the knowledge assessment and students from Bhutan fared better than Hong Kong counterparts (OR = 2.11, $p = 0.003$ and 95% CI 1.28–3.46). Less than 50% of the respondents perceived their place of residence is susceptible to disasters or that they are prepared for it. A majority of the students were aware of the impacts of climate change on health and there is a gender dimension to it.

Students' knowledge on disasters and climate change in these two Universities is suboptimal and they have low self-perceived disaster susceptibility and preparedness. Schools and universities should revisit their curricula to incorporate these topics and female participation in policy-making on climate change and health is crucial.

Source: Rinchen (2018)

Global policy implication of health emergency and disaster risk management (Health-EDRM) for climate change and health

There are a number of major global policies that might provide various frameworks for governments, policymakers, academics, and non-governmental agencies who are interested to examine and address the issues of climate in the health of the population. Health emergency and disaster risk management (Health-EDRM) is an umbrella paradigm aiming to identify scientific evidence and practice implications of research development to address knowledge gaps to address these policy attempts (see also Case Box 13.4). The following section describes Health-EDRM and the four major ones including the Paris climate agreement, the Sendai Framework for Disaster Risk Reduction, the New Urban Agenda (Habitat III), and the Sustainable Development Goals (SDGs).

Health emergency and disaster risk management

Disaster preparedness plays a critical role in mitigating the adverse health effects of natural disaster (Chan, 2017). Preparedness is defined by the United Nations International Strategy for Disaster Reduction (UNISDR, 2009, p. 21) as knowledge, capabilities, and actions of governments, organisations, community groups, and individuals "to effectively anticipate, respond to, and recover from, the impacts of likely, imminent or current hazard events or conditions". Preparedness efforts range from individual level activities (such as first aid training), to household actions (stockpiling of equipment and supplies), community efforts (training and field exercises), and governmental strategies (early warning systems, contingency plans, evacuation routes, and public information dissemination). Health emergency and disaster risk management (Health-EDRM) is a thematic research paradigm developed to address the various global policies described in the previous section. Health-EDRM is defined as *the systematic analysis and management of health risks surrounding emergencies and disasters by reducing the hazards and vulnerability along with extending preparedness, response, and recovery measures* (Lo et al., 2017; WHO & Public Health England [PHE], 2017). It concerns the management of health risks that might be associated with emergency and crisis. It is a research paradigm that resulted from the interest to address risks and highlighted in a number of global policies addressing disasters, climate change, sustainable development, and urbanisation. Fundamentally, Health-EDRM adopts and applies the hierarchy of prevention (refer also to Chapter 2) in conceptualising how risk might be categorised and tackled.

Paris climate agreement

WHO estimates that climate change will lead to an additional 250,000 potential deaths per year by 2030 due to malaria, malnutrition, diarrhoea, and heat stress alone, and calls climate change "the defining issue for the 21st century" (Chan, 2015). Adopted in 1992 with a membership of 197 parties, the United Nations Framework Convention on Climate Change (UNFCCC) is the most important international agreement to tackle climate change and has laid a solid foundation for future global development in this area. Article 1 of the UNFCCC clearly states that "adverse effects of climate change" include significant delete-rious effects on human health and Article 7 commits all parties to employ appropriate methods to minimise the effects of climate change on public health.

In 2015, international experts from a multidisciplinary background reached the conclusion that the effects of climate change "represent an unacceptably high and potentially catastrophic risk to human health" (Watts et al., 2015, p. 1861). In December 2015, the 21st Session of the Conference of the Parties (COP21) con-vened in Paris, France and the Paris Agreement was adopted. The central aim of the Paris climate agreement, which was agreed by 197 countries/parties, is to keep a global temperature rise for this century well below 2°C above pre-industrial levels and to drive efforts to limit the temperature increase even further to 1.5°C. It also aims to strengthen the ability of countries to deal with climate change impacts. The mobilisation of US$100 billion a year to help developing countries cope with climate change is to extend beyond 2020 and the figure will be con-sidered a floor until 2025. Under the agreement, each country has to set its own national cap for emissions, known as "nationally determined contributions" (NDCs). As for the Paris Agreement, adaptation efforts, which are highly relevant for reducing the health impact of climate-related disasters, featured prominently. Following the adoption of the Paris Agreement, the Second Global Conference on Health and Climate was hosted by the COP 21 presidency of France and the WHO in July 2016 (see also Case Box 13.5).

Case Box 13.5 Climate change in China

China has a population of over 1.3 billion and is the second largest economy in the world, with urban population increased from 29% in 1995 to 56% in 2015 (National Bureau of Statistics of China, 2016). By 2030, it is projected that over 1 billion people will be living in China's urban areas (World Bank & Development Research Centre of the State Council of China, 2014). The rapid urbanisation and economic growth in China has brought significant reductions in poverty, but also huge challenges in sustainable development. Climate change phenomena have been marked in China, with major implications for ecology and human health (National Development and Reform Commission of China, 2007).

Annual average air temperature in China has increased by 0.5–0.8°C over the past 100 years, with the warming trend more marked in western, eastern and northern China than in the south. Altered rainfall pattern has been observed with different trends among regions: little change in overall annual rainfall, decrease in annual rainfall in northern China, and significant increase in southern China and southwestern China. The sea level along China's coasts during the past 50 years has risen by 2.5 mm per year and more severe floods have occurred in the middle and lower reaches of the Yangtze River and southeastern China, with increasing droughts in northern and northeastern China.

A study examined the latest relevant publications in climate change and health in China (Chan, Ho, Hung, & Liu, in press). A total of 196 papers published post-millennium were considered and reviewed.

Findings indicated that the temperature–mortality association is the most extensively researched issue in China and both hot and cold temperatures increased mortality risk. Yet, most studies tend to focus on one indicator and typically under a 10-year time frame. Temperature-related morbidities are much less understood. Except for the already extensively researched outcome of cardio-vascular diseases, cause-specific morbidities should be given more attention, as it is important to inform targeted intervention for the vulnerable population. While mortalities from non-communicable diseases are well studied, infectious diseases are analysed mostly in terms of morbidity; leaving injuries, which are largely preventable, under-researched. Understanding on both mortality and morbidity is critical as the former can be applied to warning thresholds and policy planning, and the latter to health and related service planning. Building on the existing findings on temperature–mortality association, researchers should also consider conducting longer time trends and scenario-based projection studies on the health impacts of extreme temperatures to facilitate public health planning and risk reduction efforts.

No consistent association has been found for the effects of rainfall on infectious disease, while minimal studies were found on non-communicable diseases and injury. Studies rarely independently examined rainfall, humidity, or other meteorological factors, or health impacts other than those of infectious diseases. Yet, altered rainfall patterns will affect the trends of infectious diseases and occurrence of some extreme weather events like flooding. As rainfall distribution varies regionally, it is critical to develop further knowledge on the regional effects of rainfall variability on health for regional planning.

No research was identified to examine the health impact of sea-level rise in Chinese cities. According to the latest official data, sea-level rise occurred at an average rate of 3.2 mm per year between 1980 and 2016 and the average sea level along the Chinese coast in 2016 was 38 mm higher than that of 2015 (Xinhua, 2017). Major Chinese coastal cities including Shanghai and those in the river deltas like Hong Kong are facing inevitable challenge from a rising sea level and it is imminent to understand its health impact and implications on lifeline infrastructure support and fresh water supply.

Flooding is the extreme weather event that is highly relevant to China in terms of mortality, morbidity, and economic loss. Existing understanding on the health impact of floods is mainly limited to a few types of infectious diseases. Other outcomes should be considered, e.g. hepatitis A virus infection, malaria, injuries, mental health consequences (including anxiety and depression), and chronic disease complications. More attention should also be paid to the health impact of typhoon, especially in the context of rising sea level for the coastal cities. Projection studies for extreme weather events are also highly recommended.

As limited reviews have been conducted in the developing context, the above review highlights a wide range of topics and provides evidence to understand the development of climate and health research after the millennium. Rapid urbanisation is taking place in many developing countries in Asia and the experience of urban China is of significant reference for other places of similar latitude and socio-economic development. Based on the review findings, future climate change and health research in China or urban communities of middle-income countries should pay special attention to the following.

1   Health studies with sea-level rise, rainfall, or humidity as the main exposures;
2   Research on the specific climate change-related health needs among special populations in the urban areas in China, e.g. among urban migrant workers (percentage of urban employment rose from 28% to 52% between 1995 and 2015); and
3   More long-term studies over the health impact of climate change, inclusive of potential acclimatisation.

The Sendai Framework for Disaster Risk Reduction

Climate-related disasters, or extreme weather events, refer to "the occurrence of a value of a weather or climate variable above (or below) a threshold value near the upper (or lower) ends of the range of observed values of the variable" (IPCC, 2012, p. 5). While the frequency of natural disasters recorded in the Emergency Events Database (EM-DAT) of the Centre for Research on the Epidemiology of Disasters (CRED) increased almost three-fold between 2005 and 2014, the number of climate-related hydrological and meteorological events increased even more sharply during the same period (Thomas & López, 2015). Over the last decade, climate-related disasters accounted for more than 90% of all natural disasters, with hydrological disasters constituting over 50%, meteorological disasters about 30%, and climatological disasters around 10% (Guha-Sapir, Hoyois, & Below, 2016). Adopted by 187 Member States on 18 March 2015 at the third World Conference for Disaster Risk Reduction in Sendai of Japan to succeed the Hyogo Framework for Action (2005–2015) (Hyogo Framework) and chart the global direction in disaster risk reduction for the next decade, the Sendai Framework for Disaster Risk Reduction 2015–2030 (Sendai Framework) calls for a stronger role of national governments and all other stakeholders in reducing and managing disaster risks (United Nations Office for Disaster Risk Reduction, 2015). For the purpose of this chapter, the relationship between climate change and the Sendai Framework is the most relevant. As climate change is playing an increasing role in inducing and exacerbating natural hazards, e.g. flood, storm, and drought, it is considered one of the major drivers of disaster risk in the Sendai Framework and countries are urged to include climate change scenarios in their disaster risk assessments, with "climate change" mentioned 15 times in the Sendai Framework, mostly as a risk driver (Kelman, 2015). As a major disaster risk driver, research indicates that climate change discourse should be placed within the wider disaster risk reduction context (Kelman, 2017). The link between climate change and disaster risk is the most apparent through climate-related disasters.

While climate change has not been considered a necessary condition for climate-related hazards to occur, a changing climate leads to alternations in the frequency, intensity, spatial extent, duration, and timing of these events, including rising speed of tropical cyclones, more heatwaves, increased intensity of drought (IPCC, 2012). Apart from an increasing amount of evidence indicating that climate change is a significant driver of these events, there is research that finds the effect of climate change alone strong enough to cause extreme events to take place beyond natural variability (Herring et al., 2018). In fact, the United States National Academies of Sciences, Engineering, and Medicine (2016) concluded that it would no longer be an unqualified blanket statement to claim that individual climate event could not be attributable to climate change. Besides, climate change phenomenon could not be the only factor accounting for disaster losses, given the role played by factors related to exposure and vulnerability, e.g. urbanisation, population growth. An understanding of the health impact pathways of climate-related disasters and climate change is therefore crucial for developing strategies to reduce the health risks involved (Banwell, Rutherford, Mackey, & Chu, 2018) and to manage the simultaneous health impacts of climate change and natural hazards (Phalkey & Louis, 2016). As such, the concept of health emergency and disaster risk management (Health-EDRM) is highly relevant in the climate-related disaster setting. Health-EDRM refers to "the systematic analysis and management of health risks, posed by hazardous events, including emergencies and disasters, through a combination of hazard, exposure and vulnerability reduction to prevent and mitigate risks, preparedness, response, and recovery" (WHO & PHE, 2017, p.1). Health-EDRM is now a core component of general disaster risk reduction and is applicable to climate-related disasters specifically.

The health outcomes of climate-related disasters explained in the last section put a significant burden on the health system. A vulnerable health system that may be unable to absorb and cope with the impact of the disasters may exacerbate the negative health outcomes. This section will illustrate how Health-EDRM can be applied in a climate-related disaster context to minimise the negative health impact, through developing (i) health system resilience, (ii) community resilience, and (iii) an effective early warning system (WHO, 2017). All these strategies are espoused in the Sendai Framework.

The Sendai Framework is one of the core international documents guiding global developments for the coming 10 years, together with the 2030 Agenda for Sustainable Development (SDG), the Paris Agreement on Climate Change, and the New Urban Agenda. The expected outcome of the Sendai Framework is "[t]he substantial reduction of disaster risk and losses in lives, livelihoods and health and in the economic, physical, social, cultural and environmental assets of persons, businesses, communities and countries" (UNISDR, 2015, p. 12). To achieve this, the Sendai Framework calls for the strengthening of resilience to be brought about by prevention and reduction of hazard exposure and vulnerability, and increased preparedness for response and recovery. Reduction of disaster impact on health is clearly an explicit outcome of the Sendai Framework.

Four priorities were listed for action to ensure focused action by relevant actors, based on experience from the implementation of the Hyogo Framework.

Priority 1: *understanding disaster risk*

Priority 1 emphasises an understanding of disaster risk as the foundation for developing disaster risk management policies and practices. Disaster risk should be well understood from different aspects: vulnerability, capacity, exposure, hazard, and environment. A specific reference to health under this priority area is "[t]o systematically evaluate, record, share and publicly account for disaster losses and understand the economic, social, health, education, environmental and cultural heritage impacts, as appropriate, in the context of event-specific hazard-exposure and vulnerability information" (paragraph 24(b)). As highlighted in the earlier chapters, although health outcomes related to how climate and weather might affect population and individual well-being had been identified, the disaster risk awareness, literacy, preparedness, and response (refer to Chapters 11 and 12) might be limited in a developed urban community such as Hong Kong.

Priority 2: *strengthening disaster risk governance to manage disaster risk*

Priority 2 focuses on governance within and across relevant sectors at local, national, regional, and global levels for effective disaster risk reduction. This requires leadership, collaboration, and participation of stakeholders during all phases of a disaster. While the explicit reference to health limits to epidemic risk, a much wider health perspective is recommended. Health perspective should be integrated in national disaster risk reduction strategies and plans, relevant laws, regulations, and policies. Structures, roles, and responsibilities within the governments in relation to Health-EDRM should be defined, finances and manpower requirements be planned, and coordination mechanism for the operation of Health-EDRM be in place (WHO & PHE, 2017). Health-EDRM research should be planned with an aim to influence disaster policy and practice, and previous research should be reviewed to draw up practical policy recommendations (Lo et al., 2017).

Priority 3: *investing in disaster risk reduction for resilience*

Priority 3 concerns building up resilience through cost-effective structural and non-structural measures to reduce disaster risk, where health is featured most prominently. Resilience is defined as "the ability of a system, community or society exposed to hazards to resist, absorb, accommodate to and recover from the effects of a hazard in a timely and efficient manner, including through the preservation and restoration of its essential basic structures and functions" (UNISDR, 2009, p. 24). Specific references to health include safe hospitals, enhanced health system resilience, assured access to basic health services to maintain basic well-being and management of underlying chronic diseases. The Sendai Framework highlights that the significant role played by resilient health systems in reducing disaster risk cannot be overestimated, in particular the needs of chronic disease patients.

Safe health facilities help ensure that disruption to health services following a disaster is kept to the minimal. Issued by WHO in 2015, the Comprehensive Safe Hospital Framework and the Safe Hospital Index provide practical and detailed guidance for national governments to implement the relevant action recommended in the Sendai Framework (WHO, 2015a). However, health system resilience is more than safe health facilities. The six "building blocks" of health systems under the WHO framework include (i) service delivery, (ii) health workforce, (iii) health information systems, (iv) access to essential medicines, (v) financing, and (vi) leadership/governance, each with indicators and measurement strategies to track progress and evaluate performance (WHO, 2007, 2010). These WHO health system building blocks have been applied in devising a climate change-resilient health system operational framework (WHO, 2015b).

In addition, following the increasing global burden of chronic diseases and ageing population, chronic disease management has become an obvious health need post disaster (Aitsi-Selmi & Murray, 2015; Chan & Kim, 2011). Due to physical injuries, change in living conditions, or interruption of care post disaster, pre-existing chronic conditions could be exacerbated or new conditions may arise (United Nations Interagency Task Force on NCDs & WHO, 2016). The most crucial health need of people with chronic disease in a disaster is uninterrupted access to the medication and care, e.g. supply of insulin for diabetic patients and dialysis service for patients with severe kidney diseases.

Priority 4: enhancing disaster preparedness for effective response and to "build back better" in recovery, rehabilitation, and reconstruction

Priority 4 calls for preparedness in response, recovery, rehabilitation, and reconstruction through integrating disaster risk reduction into development programmes. The importance of resilient health facilities is reinforced under this priority area.

For a unique health perspective in community disaster resilience, the development of primary healthcare, which focuses on basic services to improve health status, may be a platform for further action. An effective primary healthcare system is critical to community resilience and is the foundation for emergency response, as it reduces vulnerabilities and improves preparedness. It also provides the capacity to attend to the needs of chronic disease patients, which is often not the focus in the acute phase of emergency response but contributing an increasingly large burden (WHO & PHE, 2017). A valuable but often forgotten lesson is that community resilience must involve empowerment, including participation of the vulnerable population. For example, older people could be active members in community disaster planning, as in the case of Bolivia, where there is a regular association of older people called the "White Brigades", which assist in registering older people, involving in emergency planning, participating in drills, and identifying the older people's needs during emergency. In fact, involving the vulnerable population in disaster planning and programming could be an effective way to avoid misconceptions and unfounded assumptions about their needs and capacities (United Nations Population Fund & HelpAge International, 2011).

New Urban Agenda Habitat III: urban housing and health challenges in the 21st century

Since 2007, more than 50% of the global population have been urban-based; the figure reached 54% in 2014 and 16 of the 28 global megacities were in Asia in the same year (United Nations, Department of Economic and Social Affairs, Population Division, 2014). Public health and needs of urban-based living depend on multifactorial determinants such as demographic characteristics (e.g. predominant young and healthy migrants, slum population, and ageing), underlying epidemiological disease burden, systems and services as well as macro-determinants of health (refer also to Chapter 2). Large cities, with their high-density living arrangement and dependency on lifeline infrastructure, are particularly vulnerable to a wide variety of hazards and are at the greatest risk of emergencies resulting from natural hazards. Large-scale natural hazards, regardless of being climate-related or not, if affecting urban-based environments, (e.g. Wenchuan Earthquake in China (2008), Tsunami in Japan (2011), Typhoon Haiyan (2013) in the Philippines, Nepal Earthquake (2015)) might bring catastrophic human impacts. In the urban context, although lifeline infrastructure has been emphasised as a key determinant of human well-being and security, the potential impact of lifeline infrastructure that may be affected by natural disasters (named as "NatTech disasters") becomes an increasing concern. In addition, in the developing urban context of Asia, over 40% of its urban dwellers are living in slums and squatter settlements. These suboptimal living quarters pose significant health risk to the residents due to the underdevelopment or absence of water, electricity, sewage, and sanitation systems. However, there is very limited scientific evidence that has been generated to examine or estimate the impact of how urban living might be affected by damaged infrastructure.

A person's health is affected by a range of water-related issues such as availability of safe drinking water, water for personal hygiene and food preparation, and the potential vector breeding-related risks of the stagnant puddle of water that is outside one's habitat. A safe, reliable, affordable, and easily accessible water supply is essential for good health but such water requirements might be affected by climate change. In cities, community well-being and public health protection rely heavily on the integrity and reliability of lifeline infrastructure that supports water supply and sewage systems.

Hong Kong is a city in southern China, which hosted 7 million urban habitants in 2018. It is characterised by being one of the most densely populated vertical cities globally with the highest number of high-rise buildings that exceed 150 metres. Public health and community well-being is extremely sensitive to water scarcity in this city (Chan & Ho, 2018). Although the city has its own rainfall catchment reservoir system, 80% of its lifeline water supply is imported from Dongjiang (the East River) of Guangdong province of mainland China via a dedicated aqueduct. Any potential industrial accidents that might lead to river pollution in its neighbourhood community, breakdown of lifeline water-related infrastructure (water, sewage pipes, and electricity that drives all the water-related pumps within its 316 ultra-high-rise buildings) would bring a major urban health crisis. In addition, as a dengue fever prone, seaside metropolis, stagnant water management and water quality of its beaches, marine, and rivers is crucial to human health, although Hong Kong has set up a safe, reliable, affordable, and easily accessible water supply overall. Complex infrastructure and water resources have been secured to support the health of the dense urban population adequately. However, the security of this water supply is vulnerable as it is highly dependent on the provisions of a working system. Any critical incidents can potentially have widespread effects, particularly if not managed correctly. Additional issues such as ecological stability, industrial pollution, and increasing drought due to climate change all pose risks to the water supply in the years to come.

Drainage, sewage, and water in the environment

Drainage refers to the removal of unwanted water from the human environment. Unwanted water originates from various sources: used wastewater, rainwater, floodwater from overflowing rivers, and other natural sources of surface water. In urban environments, proper drainage is necessary to maintain public health and reduce health risks, namely faecal-orally transmitted diseases and disease-bearing vectors. Faecal-oral diseases, as discussed in the earlier sections on common water-borne diseases (refer to Chapters 3 and 9), are generally of minimal outbreak risk in areas with well-established water and sewage infrastructure. However, a breakdown of the well-established system would quickly put the large urban population at risk. Besides, disease-bearing vectors, mainly referring to the presence of mosquitoes for Hong Kong, can easily find their way to breed and thrive in environments with stagnant water (see Case Box 13.6 and Knowledge Box 13.1). While working to secure a reliable water supply, Hong Kong was also simultaneously developing the infrastructure for drainage and sewage. Starting during its early colonial years in the 1840–1850s, the need for drainage infrastructure was linked with the unsanitary and overcrowded living conditions, particularly in the local working-class residential districts.

Hong Kong experiences high amounts of annual rainfall, averaging 2,400 mm annually. Of even greater importance are the uneven temporal distribution of this rainfall and the occurrence of extreme heavy precipitation events, which can overwhelm the drainage systems beyond their design capacities for an extent of time. Non-permeable surfaces such as roads and sidewalks, built-up districts near major waterways, older storm water drainage systems built with past protection standards, and the lack of green infrastructure to absorb precipitation cause flooding risks throughout the city (Drainage Services Department [DSD] of the Government of the Hong Kong Special Administrative Region, 2016). Debris, either litter or natural materials, may build up around drainage inlets, further inhibiting efficient drainage. Additionally, the city of Hong Kong is also built around steep slopes and mountains, resulting in accumulation of runoff in downstream areas. To tackle this problem, a flood prevention strategy has been implemented with long-term measures designed to expand the capacity of water drainage in three major aspects. Drainage tunnels, designed to withstand a flood with a return period of 200 years (or a 1-in-200-year flood), are constructed to intercept runoff at upstream locations and divert directly to nearby water bodies. Underground storm water storage tanks, built in low-lying areas, help reduce the peak flow rate during extreme precipitation events through the temporary retention of storm water. Finally, waterways have been reconstructed and revitalised to include widened channels and ecological elements to expand their flood control capacities. These drainage improvement works have enabled the city to be more capable of facing heavy rainfall events, reducing the number of flooding "blackspots" from 90 in 1995, down to 8 in 2016 (DSD of the Government of the Hong Kong Special Administrative Region, 2016).

Knowledge Box 13.1 Climate-related health risks: stagnant water and mosquitoes

Stagnant water can be accumulated when water is not properly drained away. Not only does this concern the drainage systems and outdoor environments, but particularly in and around people's homes. Retaining water can lead to unexpected breeding ground and the transmission of diseases such as dengue fever, malaria, Japanese encephalitis, and Zika virus. Particularly, dengue fever is often at risk of becoming endemic in Hong Kong and an enhanced surveillance as well as mosquito prevention and control system has been regularly managed by the government (Food and Health Bureau of the Government of the Hong Kong Special Administrative Region, 2017). Public announcements and health promotions urge residents in Hong Kong to help remove stagnant water sources around the home by:

- Tightly covering water containers
- Keeping drains clear and free from blockage
- Changing water in vases and clearing the water in the plates under flower pots weekly
- Proper disposal of empty containers
- Preventing accumulation of water in air-conditioner drip trays
- Placing mosquito larvae-eating fish in fish tanks
- Smoothing out uneven ground surfaces to prevent puddles

Source: Food and Environmental Hygiene Department of the Government of the Hong Kong Special Administrative Region (2012)

Flooding due to rainfall is only one of the potential disaster risks to the water infrastructure in Hong Kong. Other natural disaster risks include storm surges, tropical cyclones, landslides, and even potential tsunami or earthquake. Other man-made emergencies may cause accidents or damage to the infrastructure. These potential disaster risks do not only have direct impacts on health, such as loss of life, injury, illness, and disability (Chan & Murray, 2017), but also indirect impacts through breakdown of water infrastructure. Breakdowns may lead to contamination of drinking water supply or discontinued service of water. Bursting of water pipes would cause additional flooding in those locales. All of these would reduce the amount of safe reliable drinking water supplied to residents and such risks must be reduced to prevent a large impact on human health.

Water quality and sewage management

The water quality in the environment is often affected by the sewage as well as other sources of pollution. Rapid industrial development starting from the mid-20th century increased the domestic sewage and water pollution in Hong Kong. The increase rapidly deteriorated the marine and stream environments, as treatment of the wastewater and sewage were not common practice (DSD of the Government of the Hong Kong Special Administrative Region, 2008). Unregulated direct discharge added to the amount of water pollution as well. Whereas rainwater is comparatively cleaner, used wastewater that incorporates excreta disposal has a large load of infection-causing micro-organisms such as bacteria, virus, fungi, and protozoa (Blom, 2015). There is evidence that water drains can be a source of microbial infection for households and healthcare services (Blom, 2015). Poor sewage treatment can also result in deterioration of environmental water quality, as will be discussed later. In Hong Kong, a total of 300 sewage treatment facilities are in operation, treating over 1 billion cubic metres of sewage per year and averaging 2.8 million cubic metres daily (DSD of the Government of the Hong Kong Special Administrative Region, 2016). The system services 93% of the city's population and consists of a network 1,700 km long (DSD of the Government of the Hong Kong Special Administrative Region, 2016). The treatment process removes biochemical oxygen demand, suspended solids, nitrogen, dewatered sludge, screenings, and grits. Sludge is a semi-solid by-product of sewage treatment, which then undergoes further treatment of thickening, digestion, and dewatering (DSD of the Government of the Hong Kong Special Administrative Region, 2013). The treated sludge is then disposed of in landfills, as agricultural fertiliser or incinerated, to reduce the amount being dumped into the ocean. In efforts to diminish the amount of sludge dumped into Hong Kong's main harbour and to improve its water quality, a Harbour Area Treatment Scheme was constructed in Hong Kong over a period of 20 years and began full operations in 2015 (DSD of the Government of the Hong Kong Special Administrative Region, 2016). Sewage from all the districts around the harbour is conveyed to a centralised sewage treatment plant for treatment and disinfection before being discharged at the western end of the harbour.

Water stress and ecological limits sustainability

The increasing impacts of climate change, which lead to changes in rainfall distribution, frequency, and amount, will affect both the supply and demand of water (Shaw & Thaitakoo, 2010). The increased frequency and greater severity of drought periods, as well as greater rainfall intensity and flooding events will influence the quantity and quality of water available. In coastal areas, sea-level rise has the potential to cause salinisation of water sources. Additionally, the changes caused by climate change will influence the patterns of vector-borne diseases. As a densely populated urban area, Hong Kong will face difficulties in ensuring a sufficient water supply. Not only is Hong Kong naturally water-scarce, but the Dongjiang River, which Hong Kong relies on for 80% of its water, is the water source for seven other cities in the Pearl River Delta region, including Dongguan, Heyuan, Huizhou, Shaoguan, Meizhou, Guangzhou, and Shenzhen. Serving as a prominent example of inter-basin water distribution, altogether, the river sustains a total of 40 million people, with proportion of dependence varying between cities (Liu, 2013). The river has already experienced water stress, with water withdrawals since 2004 periodically exceeding the "ecological limit" established at 33% of the river's total water resources (He, Ma, Peng, & Li, 2009; Lee, & Moss, 2014). With continuing economic development in several of the less-developed cities, the demand for Dongjiang water is projected to increase and will lead to increasing competition among the region's cities.

Sustainable Development Goals

Adopted in September 2015 at the United Nations Sustainable Development Summit, the Sustainable Development Goals (SDGs) succeeded their predecessor the Millennium Development Goals (MDGs) that were a global effort between 2000 and 2015 to combat poverty, hunger, and ill health. The SDGs address three dimensions of sustainable development: economic growth, social inclusion, and environmental protection, with 17 goals and 169 targets to guide global and national actions from 2015 to 2030. See Knowledge Box 13.2 for the full list of SDGs.

As the SDGs are "integrated and indivisible", serving to balance one another (United Nations General Assembly, 2015). The SDGs and their targets aim to enable a sustainable and resilient development of all countries. The 2030 Agenda for Sustainable Development, also known as Sustainable Development Goals (SDGs), was adopted in 2015 to end poverty, protect the planet, and ensure prosperity for all as part of a new sustainable development agenda. Goal 13 commits all countries to take urgent action to combat climate change and its impacts and Goal 3 calls for the strengthening of national capacity for early warning, risk reduction, and management of national and global health risks, which are highly relevant to climate-related disasters. Given the far-reaching health impacts of climate change, its relevance cuts

---

Knowledge Box 13.2 The Sustainable Development Goals (SDGs)

Goal 1. End poverty in all its forms everywhere

Goal 2. End hunger, achieve food security and improved nutrition, and promote sustainable agriculture

Goal 3. Ensure healthy lives and promote well-being for all at all ages

Goal 4. Ensure inclusive and equitable quality education and promote lifelong learning opportunities for all

Goal 5. Achieve gender equality and empower all women and girls

Goal 6. Ensure availability and sustainable management of water and sanitation for all

Goal 7. Ensure access to affordable, reliable, sustainable, and modern energy for all

Goal 8. Promote sustained, inclusive, and sustainable economic growth, full and productive employment, and decent work for all

Goal 9. Build resilient infrastructure, promote inclusive and sustainable industrialisation, and foster innovation

Goal 10. Reduce inequality within and among countries

Goal 11. Make cities and human settlements inclusive, safe, resilient, and sustainable

Goal 12. Ensure sustainable consumption and production patterns

Goal 13. Take urgent action to combat climate change and its impacts

Goal 14. Conserve and sustainably use the oceans, seas, and marine resources for sustainable development

Goal 15. Protect, restore, and promote sustainable use of terrestrial ecosystems, sustainably manage forests, combat desertification, and halt and reverse land degradation and halt biodiversity loss

Goal 16. Promote peaceful and inclusive societies for sustainable development, provide access to justice for all, and build effective, accountable, and inclusive institutions at all levels

Goal 17. Strengthen the means of implementation and revitalise the global partnership for sustainable development

Source: United Nations General Assembly (2015)

---

across many other goals, e.g. Goal 2 on improving food security and nutrition (given that extreme temperatures and rainfall could result in crop failure and food shortage) (see Case Box 13.6), Goal 6 on water and sanitation (given that climate-related disaster like flooding could result in water contamination). The New Urban Agenda adopted in 2016 set out global standards for sustainable urban development through reforming the way that cities are built and managed. The New Urban Agenda recognised that unplanned urbanisation caused human settlement to be vulnerable to the impacts of climate change and climate-related disasters and called the adoption of climate change mitigation and adaptation efforts into urban development and planning processes.

Case Box 13.6 Impacts of climate change on food security and nutritional health

By Amos P. K. Tai

Future crop production is highly vulnerable to climate change, with implications for global food security and nutritional health. More frequent temperature extremes and more fluctuating occurrences of droughts and floods, as well as more severe ozone pollution that comes with higher temperatures, are all expected to increase the likelihood of crop failures in the future. Tai, Val Martin, and Heald (2014) presented an integrated analysis of the effects of 2000–2050 climate change and ozone pollution trends on the production of four major crops (wheat, rice, maize, and soybean) worldwide based on historical observations and model projections, specifically accounting for ozone–temperature co-variation. They found that warming alone could reduce global crop production by >10% by 2050, with a potential to substantially worsen global malnutrition in all scenarios considered. For instance, warming alone could increase undernourishment in developing countries from the current rate of 18% to 27% by 2050 in a business-as-usual scenario, ceteris paribus, representing an important nutrition-mediated link between climate change and human health. Ozone trends were found to either exacerbate or offset a substantial fraction of climate impacts depending on the scenario, suggesting the importance of air quality management in combating not only respiratory health but also climate-related food insecurity in the future. They also found that some crops (e.g. maize) are particularly sensitive to excess heat, and called for greater use of climate change adaptation, such as by breeding and selecting heat-tolerant cultivars, in current agricultural practices in response to the imminent climate threats.

The 2030 Agenda for Sustainable Development maintains that the primary responsibility for achieving the SDGs in national development lies within each country, while a global partnership helps ensure implementation (United Nations General Assembly, 2015). Aiming to empower the vulnerable groups in particular, the SDGs are well aligned with the prevention-focused Health-EDRM framework. On the one hand, disasters are inevitable inhibitors to sustainable development, causing damage and setbacks in communities and leading to mortality and losses to infrastructure, in economic productivity, human capital, and health. On the other hand, better development can reduce the impact of natural hazards and the need for emergency relief (Buchanan-Smith & Maxwell, 1994). In order for societies to attain sustainable development, it is thus necessary to increase health resilience and reduce vulnerability to health risks posed by hazards, a key to the preventative approach of Health-EDRM. The root of human vulnerability in disasters and emergencies rests with a complex group of "social, economic, health and cultural factors" (WHO & PHE, 2017). As the 17 SDGs aim to address these multifaceted factors, the vulnerability of at-risk populations in disasters could also be reduced by meeting these goals.

Research gaps

As illustrated by earlier chapters in this book, a number of scientific publications had already pointed out the evidence of how various climate-related environmental factors (e.g. temperature, rainfall) might affect health outcomes. There, however, remain a number of research and potential implementation challenges in health protection for policymakers.

Research methodology and relevance of findings to context

Many of the research study findings of Hong Kong, a subtropical city in Asia, presented in this book showed that various climate change-related adverse health impact thresholds, as well as environmental and behavioural variables might be different when compared with related scientific findings of other western contexts globally. The Hong Kong study series might help show more research studies are urgently needed to understand how climate change might affect communities beyond the traditional western city context. In Asia, where most of the global urbanisation is happening, findings might help facilitate better health protection policies that might address local needs in the densely populated Asian urban planning and high-rise building environment, as well as the behavioural and cultural context. New data collection methods (e.g. by digital devices), research methodologies, and relevant theoretical models should be developed to capture, examine, and explain the specific build environment (e.g. vertical city), communication and information-seeking patterns (e.g. in a digital-based environment), and emergency response and self-help patterns.

Translation of scientific evidence to actions

Figure 13.1 intends to show the various temperature thresholds as identified in the research studies mentioned in previous chapters (refer to Chapters 8–12). Although these findings might support health and well-being protection policies (such as public warning, hotline, and emergency services planning and protocols and patient management guidelines in extreme events), relevant planning and implementation might be subject to public and stakeholder awareness, institutional interest and policies as well as issues with suboptimal coordination of related services.

Monitoring of long-term health outcomes

The current studies remain largely related to retrospective data analysis. To clearly monitor and map out how future climate/environmental/behavioural factors might affect health outcomes and well-being, consistent and well-defined cohort data should be collected in an integrated manner. Although there is increasing recognition of the need for long-term data to examine climate change impact on health and the global digital and big data movement might

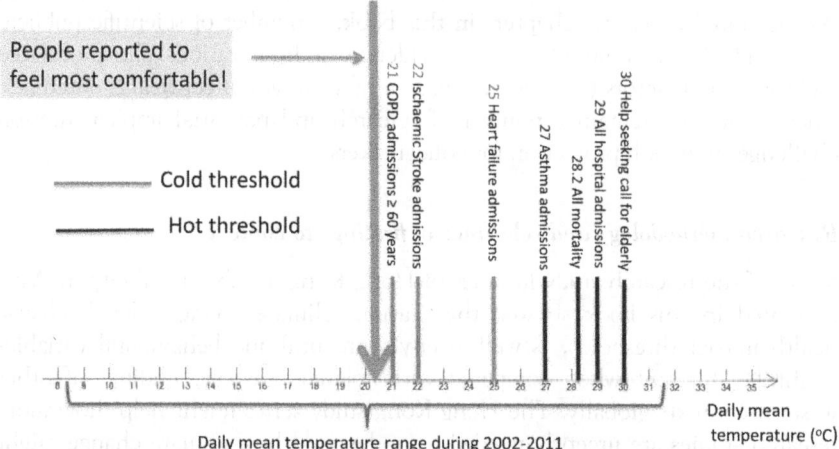

Figure 13.1 Threshold temperatures of increasing health risks in Hong Kong.

facilitate such development, issues such as patient privacy and rights to their own health outcomes, data confidentiality, population movement as a result of migration and extreme event impact are all examples of contexts that might present limitations to the overview tracking and monitoring of the future health impact of climate change.

Bridging of research agenda beyond climate change

Research and evidence generated for extreme events, disasters, sustainable development are useful to inform and facilitate handling climate change-related challenges that are posed for health. The paradigm Health-EDRM (refer to earlier sections in this chapter) might be an important research and policy theme to consider when building relevant research outputs and policy discussion. These research-policy collaborative efforts might be useful to maximise the effort to use science to mitigate or to support community adaptation to climate-related events.

Conclusion

This chapter shows health might be an essential component to consider when engaging in mitigation actions that target addressing the impact of climate change. Climate-related disaster management and Health-EDRM provided a comprehensive framework to improve the health outcomes. Climate change is no longer a subject solely about the environment, but a cross-cutting issue with significant impact on disaster management and wider sustainable development, which explains its prominence in international agreements covering a wide range of subjects: the Sendai Framework, SDGs, and the New Urban Agenda. It is worth noting that climate change, including its effect on climate-related disasters, is the focus not only under the climate change international agreements. It features prominently also in a few other instruments guiding global developments: the SDGs, the Sendai Framework, and the New Urban Agenda, indicating the cross-cutting effect of climate change on human development in different settings.

With the far-reaching impact of climate change over different aspects of human life and development, climate change adaptation now goes hand in hand with mitigation, which was traditionally the major focus of climate change policy. The number of climate-related disasters has been on the rise and climate change is considered a contributing factor to their increasing intensity and to increasing frequency in some cases. Flood, storm, and extreme temperatures are the climate-related disasters that lead to the highest death toll, while drought affects the most number of people. Different types of climate-related disasters are associated with different immediate health outcomes and with some longer-term health consequences common to all. Impact on chronic disease management and disruption to the health system have been the main concerns in recent years. Health-EDRM is applicable to the climate-disaster context and calls for a range of action to improve the health outcomes, in particular the building of a health system and community resilience and development of an effective early warning system, which are all advocated in the Sendai Framework. An understanding of the role of health in climate change and climate-related disasters naturally connects to the concept of health and environmental co-benefits (HECs), which provides additional justifications for climate change mitigation policies and has the potential to galvanise much stronger public support for climate actions across the globe.

References

Abroms, L. C., & Maibach, E. W. (2008). The effectiveness of mass communication to change public behavior. *The Annual Review of Public Health, 29*, 219–234.

Advisory Council on Food and Environmental Hygiene. (2013). *Report on consultancy study on organic food.* Retrieved from www.fhb.gov.hk/download/committees/board/doc/2013/paper20130220_02.pdf.

Aitsi-Selmi, A., & Murray, V. (2015). The Sendai Framework: Disaster risk reduction through a health lens. *Bulletin of the World Health Organization, 93*(6), 362. doi:10.2471/BLT.15.157362.

Banwell, N., Rutherford, S., Mackey, B., & Chu, C. (2018). Towards improved linkage of disaster risk reduction and climate change adaptation in health: A review. *International Journal of Environmental Research and Public Health, 15*(4), 793. doi:10.3390/ijerph15040793.

Blom, K. (2015). Drainage systems, an occluded source of sanitation related outbreaks. *Archives of Public Health, 73*(8), 1–8.

Buchanan-Smith, M., & Maxwell, S. (1994). Linking relief and development: An introduction and overview. *IDS Bulletin, 25*(4), 2–16.

Busch, V., VanStel, H. F., Schrijvers, A. J. P., & deLeeuw, J. R. J. (2013). Clustering of health-related behaviors, health outcomes and demographics in Dutch adolescents: A cross-sectional study. *BMC Public Health, 13*, 1118. doi:10.1186/1471-2458-13-1118.

CARe2018 Organising Committee (2018). *CARe2018: Hong Kong conference: Summary report and policy recommendations.* Hong Kong: Hong Kong University of Science and Technology.

Chan, E. Y. Y. (2017). *Public health humanitarian responses to natural disasters.* London: Routledge.

Chan, E. Y. Y., & Ho, J. Y. (2018). *Water security and disaster risk reduction* (CCOUC Working Paper). Hong Kong, CCOUC.

Chan, E. Y. Y., Ho, J. Y., Hung, H. H. Y., & Liu, S. (in press). Health impact of climate change in cities of middle income countries: The case of China. *British Medical Bulletin.*

Chan, E. Y. Y., & Kim, J. (2011). Chronic health needs immediately after natural disasters in middle-income countries: The case of the 2008 Sichuan, China earthquake. *European Journal of Emergency Medicine, 18*(2), 111–114.

Chan, E. Y. Y., & Murray, V. (2017). What are the health research needs for the Sendai Framework? *The Lancet, 390*(10106), e35–e36. doi:10.1016/S0140-6736(17)31670-7.

Chan, E. Y. Y., Wang, S. S., Ho, J. Y., Huang, Z., Liu, S., & Guo, C. (2017). Socio-demographic predictors of health and environmental co-benefit behaviours for climate change mitigation in urban China. *PLOS One, 12*(11), e0188661. doi:10.1371/journal.pone.0188661.

Chan, M. (2015). WHO Director-General addresses event on climate change and health [online]. Retrieved from www.who.int/dg/speeches/2015/climate-change-paris/en/.

Dietz, T., Gardner, G. T., Gilligan, J., Stern, P. C., & Vandenbergh, M. P. (2009). Household actions can provide a behavioral wedge to rapidly reduce US carbon emissions. *Proceedings of the National Academy of Sciences, 106*(44), 18452–18456.

Drainage Services Department of the Government of the Hong Kong Special Administrative Region. (2008). *Sewerage and flood protection: Drainage services 1841–2008.* Retrieved from www.dsd.gov.hk/EN/Files/publications_publicity/Publications/2008 book.pdf.

Drainage Services Department of the Government of the Hong Kong Special Administrative Region. (2013). Media briefing: DSD introduces Environmental Sludge Treatment Scheme developed on "Co-settling" [online]. Retrieved from www.dsd.gov.hk/EN/Publicity_and_Publications/Publicity/Events___Others/EventOther198.html.

Drainage Services Department of the Government of the Hong Kong Special Administrative Region. (2016). *Cleaner harbour, better life: 2015–16 sustainability report.* Retrieved from www.dsd.gov.hk/Documents/SustainabilityReports/1516/common/dsd_full_report_2015_16.pdf.

Environmental Protection Department of the Government of the Hong Kong Special Administrative Region. (2016). Environmental Levy Scheme on Plastic Shopping Bags [online]. Retrieved from www.epd.gov.hk/epd/english/environmentinhk/waste/pro_responsibility/env_levy.html.

Fisher, C., Bashyal, S., & Bachman, B. (2012). Demographic impacts on environmentally friendly purchase behaviors. *Journal of Targeting Measurement and Analysis for Marketing, 20*(3–4), 172–184. doi:10.1057/jt.2012.13.

Food and Environmental Hygiene Department of the Government of the Hong Kong Special Administrative Region. (2012). *Let's remove stagnant water: Eliminate mosquitoes for healthy living* [pamphlets]. Retrieved from www.fehd.gov.hk/english/pestcontrol/library/pdf_pest_control/mosquito_home.pdf.

Food and Health Bureau of the Government of the Hong Kong Special Administrative Region. (2017). *Enhanced mosquito prevention and control in face of threats from Zika Virus Infection* (LC Paper No. CB(2)531/16–17(03)). Retrieved from the website of the Hong Kong Legislative Council www.legco.gov.hk/yr16-17/english/panels/fseh/papers/fseh20170110cb2-531-3-e.pdf.

Global Heat Health Information Network. (2018). GHHIN Forum [online]. Retrieved from http://ghhin.org/programme-and-agenda.

Guha-Sapir, D., Hoyois, Ph., & Below, R. (2016). *Annual disaster statistical review 2015: The numbers and trends.* Retrieved from https://reliefweb.int/sites/reliefweb.int/files/resources/ADSR_2015.pdf.

He, T., Ma, X., Peng, X., & Li, T. (2009). Problems and contradiction in water resources environmental management of Dongjiang Basin [in Chinese]. *Water Resources Protection, 25*(6).

Herring, S. C., Christidis, N., Hoell, A., Kossin, J. P., Schreck III., C. J., & Stott, P. A. (Eds.). (2018). Explaining extreme events of 2016 from a climate perspective. *Bulletin of the American Meteorological Society, 99*(1), S1–S157. doi:10.1175/BAMS-Explaining ExtremeEvents2016.1.

Hutchinson, J., Prady, S. L., Smith, M. A., White, P. C. L, & Graham, H. M. (2015). A scoping review of observational studies examining relationships between environmental behaviors and health behaviors. *International Journal of Environmental Research and Public Health, 12*(5), 4833–4858.

Intergovernmental Panel on Climate Change [IPCC]. (2012). *Managing the risks of extreme events and disasters to advance climate change adaptation. A special report of Working Groups I and II of the Intergovernmental Panel on Climate Change.* Retrieved from www.ipcc.ch/site/assets/uploads/2018/03/SREX_Full_Report-1.pdf.

Intergovernmental Panel on Climate Change. (2014). Summary for policymakers. In *Climate change 2014: Impacts, adaptation, and vulnerability. Part A: Global and sectoral aspects. Contribution of Working Group II to the Fifth Assessment Report of the Intergovernmental Panel on Climate Change.* Retrieved from www.ipcc.ch/site/assets/uploads/2018/02/SYR_AR5_FINAL_full.pdf.

Intergovernmental Panel on Climate Change. (2015). Summary for policymakers. In *Climate change 2014: Mitigation of climate change: Working Group III contribution to the IPCC fifth assessment report.* Retrieved from www.cambridge.org/core/books/climate-change-2014-mitigation-of-climate-change/summary-for-policymakers/EE0E4ADA72 7454B77093DA3AE19533BB.

Kelman, I. (2015). Climate change and the Sendai Framework for Disaster Risk Reduction. *International Journal of Disaster Risk Science, 6*(2), 117–127.

Kelman, I. (2017). Linking disaster risk reduction, climate change, and the sustainable development goals. *Disaster Prevention and Management: An International Journal, 26*(3), 254–258.

Kurz, T., Gardner, B., Verplanken, B., & Abraham, C. (2015). Habitual behaviors or patterns of practice? Explaining and changing repetitive climate-relevant actions. *Wiley Interdisciplinary Reviews: Climate Change, 6*(1), 113–128.

Lee, F., & Moss, T. (2014). Spatial fit and water policies: Managing asymmetries in the Dongjiang River basin. *International Journal of River Basin Management, 12*(4), 329–339. doi:10.1080/15715124.2014.917420.

Liu, S. (2013). *Liquid assets IV: Hong Kong's water resources management under "One Country, Two Systems".* Retrieved from https://civic-exchange.org/report/liquid-assets-iv-hong-kongs-water-resources-management-under-one-country-two-systems/.

Lo, S. T. T., Chan, E. Y. Y., Chan, G. K. W., Murray, V., Abrahams, J., Ardalan, A., ... Yau, J. C. W. (2017). Health emergency and disaster risk management (Health-EDRM): Developing the research field within the Sendai Framework Paradigm. *International Journal of Disaster Risk Science*, 8(1), 145–149. doi:10.1007/s13753-017-0122-0.

National Academies of Sciences, Engineering, and Medicine. (2016). *Attribution of extreme weather events in the context of climate change*. Washington, DC: The National Academies Press.

National Bureau of Statistics of China. (2016). *China statistical yearbook 2016*. China: National Bureau of Statistics of China.

National Development and Reform Commission of China. (2007). *China's national climate change programme*. Retrieved from http://en.ndrc.gov.cn/newsrelease/200706/P020070604561191006823.pdf.

Phalkey, R. K., & Louis, V. R. (2016). Two hot to handle: How do we manage the simultaneous impacts of climate change and natural disasters on human health? *The European Physical Journal Special Topics*, 225(3), 443–457.

Remais, J. V., Hess, J. J., Ebi, K. L., Markandya, A., Balbus, J. M. Wilkinson, P., ... Chalabi, Z. (2014). Estimating the health effects of greenhouse gas mitigation strategies: Addressing parametric, model, and valuation challenges. *Environmental Health Perspectives*, 122(5), 447–455.

Rinchen, N. (2018). Students' knowledge and perception on climate change and disasters in two Universities in Asia: A comparison. Unpublished Master thesis, Chinese University of Hong Kong.

Rozin, P., Hormes, J. M., Faith, M. S., & Wansink, B. (2012). Is meat male? A quantitative multimethod framework to establish metaphoric relationships. *Journal of Consumer Research*, 39(3), 629–643.

Schösle, H., deBoer, J., Boersema, J. J., & Aiking, H. (2015). Meat and masculinity among young Chinese, Turkish and Dutch adults in the Netherlands. *Appetite*, 89, 152–159. doi:10.1016/j.appet.2015.02.013.

Shaw, R., & Thaitakoo, D. (2010). Water communities: Introduction and overview. In R. Shaw & D. Thaitakoo (Eds.), *Water communities* (Community, Environment and Disaster Risk Management, Vol. 2, pp. 1–13). Bingley, UK: Emerald.

Smith, A. C., Holland, M., Korkeala, O., Warmington, J., Forster, D., Apsimon, H., ... Smith, S. M. (2015). Health and environmental co-benefits and conflicts of actions to meet UK carbon targets. *Climate Policy*, 16(3), 37–41.

Smith, K. R., Woodward, A., Campbell-Lendrum, D., Chadee, D. D., Honda, Y., Liu, Q., ... Sauerborn, R. (2014). Human health: Impacts, adaptation, and co-benefits. In *Climate change 2014: Impacts, adaptation, and vulnerability. Part A: Global and sectoral aspects. Contribution of Working Group II to the fifth assessment report of the Intergovernmental Panel on Climate Change*. Retrieved from www.ipcc.ch/site/assets/uploads/2018/02/WGIIAR5-PartA_FINAL.pdf.

Spickett, J., Katscherian, D., & Brown, H. (2015). *Climate change, vulnerability and health: A guide to assessing and addressing the health impacts*. Retrieved from http://ehia.curtin.edu.au/local/docs/cc-guideline-10615.pdf.

Tai, A. P. K., Val Martin, M., & Heald, C. L. (2014). Threat to future global food security from climate change and ozone air pollution. *Nature Climate Change*, 4(9), 817–821. doi:10.1038/Nclimate2317.

Thomas, V., & López, R. E. (2015). *Global increase in climate-related disasters* (ADB Economics Working Paper Series No. 466). Manila, Philippines: Asian Development Bank.

United Nations, Department of Economic and Social Affairs, Population Division. (2014). *World urbanization prospects: The 2014 revision.* Retrieved from https://esa.un.org/unpd/wup/publications/files/wup2014-report.pdf.

United Nations General Assembly. (2015). *Transforming our world: The 2030 Agenda for Sustainable Development* (Resolution adopted by the General Assembly on 25 September 2015, A/RES/70/1). Retrieved from www.un.org/ga/search/view_doc.asp?symbol=A/RES/70/1&Lang=E.

United Nations Interagency Task Force on NCDs & World Health Organization. (2016). *Noncommunicable diseases in emergencies.* Retrieved from www.who.int/ncds/publications/ncds-in-emergencies/en/.

United Nations International Strategy for Disaster Reduction [UNISDR]. (2009). *2009 UNISDR terminology on disaster risk reduction.* Retrieved from http://ba.one.un.org/content/dam/unct/bih/PDFs/UNISDR%20Terminology%20%20English.pdf.

United Nations Office for Disaster Risk Reduction [UNISDR]. (2015). *Sendai Framework for Disaster Risk Reduction 2015–2030.* Retrieved from www.preventionweb.net/files/43291_sendaiframeworkfordrren.pdf.

United Nations Population Fund, & HelpAge International. (2011). *Manual for MIPAA plus 10 bottom-up, participatory approach: "The voices of older persons": A contribution to the state of the world's older persons 2012.* Retrieved from www.helpage.org/silo/files/manual-for-mipaa-plus-10-bottomup-participatory-approach.pdf.

Ürge-Vorsatz, D., Herrero, S. T., Dubash, N. K., & Lecocq, F. (2014). Measuring the co-benefits of climate change mitigation. *Annual Review of Environment and Resources, 39,* 549–582.

VanDooren, C., Marinussen, M., Blonk, H., Aiking, H., & Vellinga, P. (2014). Exploring dietary guidelines based on ecological and nutritional values: A comparison of six dietary patterns. *Food Policy, 44,* 36–46. doi:10.1016/j.foodpol.2013.11.002.

Wanner, M., Götschi, T., Martin-Diener, E., Kahlmeier, S., & Martin, B. W. (2012). Active transport, physical activity, and body weight in adults: A systematic review. *American Journal of Preventive Medicine, 42*(5), 493–502. doi:10.1016/j.ampepre.2012.01.030.

Water Supplies Department of the Government of the Hong Kong Special Administrative Region. (2015). *Let's save 10L water 2015* [leaflet]. Retrieved from www.lcdmc.edu.hk/wp-content/uploads/2013_2014/1314_save10litres.pdf.

Watts, N., Adger, N., Agnolucci, P., Blackstock, J., Byass, P., Cai, W., … Costello, A. (2015). Health and climate change: Policy responses to protect public health. *The Lancet, 386*(10006), 1861–1914. doi:10.1016/S0140-6736(15)60901-1.

Wiernik, B. M., Ones, D. S., & Dilchert, S. (2013). Age and environmental sustainability: A meta-analysis. *Journal of Managerial Psychology, 28*(7–8), 826–856.

Women's Commission of the Government of the Hong Kong Special Administrative Region. (2010). *"What do women and men in Hong Kong think about the status of women at home, work and in social environments?": Survey findings.* Retrieved from www.women.gov.hk/download/research/WoC-Survey-Finding-FAMILY_E.pdf.

World Bank, & Development Research Centre of the State Council of China. (2014). *Urban China: Toward efficient, inclusive, and sustainable urbanization.* Washington, DC: World Bank.

World Health Organization [WHO]. (2007). *Everybody's business: Strengthening health systems to improve health outcomes: WHO's framework for action.* Retrieved from www.who.int/healthsystems/strategy/everybodys_business.pdf.

World Health Organization [WHO]. (2010). *Monitoring the building blocks of health systems: A handbook of indicators and their measurement strategies.* Retrieved from www.who.int/healthinfo/systems/WHO_MBHSS_2010_full_web.pdf.

World Health Organization [WHO]. (2013). *Guidance to protect health from climate change through health adaptation planning.* Retrieved from http://apps.who.int/iris/bitstream/10665/137383/1/9789241508001_eng.pdf.

World Health Organization [WHO]. (2015a). *Comprehensive safe hospital framework.* Retrieved from www.who.int/hac/techguidance/comprehensive_safe_hospital_framework.pdf.

World Health Organization [WHO]. (2015b). *Operational framework for building climate resilient health systems.* Retrieved from http://apps.who.int/iris/bitstream/handle/10665/189951/9789241565073_eng.pdf;jsessionid=3EEB79ACE1ACE402CC14E48569D3E2F1?sequence=1.

World Health Organization [WHO]. (2017). *A strategic framework for emergency preparedness.* Retrieved from https://extranet.who.int/sph/sites/default/files/document-library/document/Preparedness-9789241511827-eng.pdf.

World Health Organization, & Public Health England. (2017). *Health emergency and disaster risk management: Overview.* Retrieved from www.who.int/hac/techguidance/preparedness/risk-management-overview-december2017.pdf.

World Health Organization, & World Bank. (2014). Access to modern energy services for health facilities in resource-constrained settings: A review of status, significance, challenges and measurement. Retrieved from http://apps.who.int/iris/bitstream/handle/10665/156847/9789241507646_eng.pdf?sequence=1.

World Organization of Family Doctors [WONCA]. (2017). *WONCA statement on planetary health and Sustainable Development Goals.* Retrieved from www.globalfamilydoctor.com/site/DefaultSite/filesystem/documents/policies_statements/Statement%20on%20planetary%20health.pdf.

Xia, T., Nitschke, M., Zhang, Y., Shah, P., Crabb, S., & Hansen, A. (2015). Traffic-related air pollution and health co-benefits of alternative transport in Adelaide, South Australia. *Environment International, 74,* 281–290.

Xinhua. (2017, 23 March). China reports highest sea level in 30 years [online]. Retrieved from the website of *China Daily:* www.chinadaily.com.cn/china/2017-03/23/content_28652843.htm.

Yi, W., & Chan, A. P. C. (2015). Effects of temperatures on mortality in Hong Kong: A time series analysis. *International Journal of Biometeorology, 59*(7), 927–936.

14 Conclusion

Climate change is one of the major global environmental changes (GECs) that will affect human beings and their urban living environment for the decades to come. Moreover, a majority of the natural disasters post-2000 are climate-related. The 2015 Lancet Commission on Health and Climate Change concluded that the effects of climate change "represent an unacceptably high and potentially catastrophic risk to human health" (Watts et al., 2017, p. 1861). The World Health Organization (WHO) calls climate change "the defining issue for health systems in the 21st century" (WHO, 2015, p. 1). Whilst the increased human activities are causing wide range of changes to the environment and climate systems, climate-related changes have also posed a great threat to human health and well-being.

The 21st century also marks the beginning of a global urban-based living pattern (United Nations, Department of Economic and Social Affairs, Population Division, 2014). The increased frequency of extreme weather events, the acceleration of urbanisation, and the dependency on lifeline infrastructure render the urban-based community and system vulnerable to the challenges of maintaining human well-being and minimising the potential health impact of the erratic climate change-related events. Rapid urbanisation is taking place in many developing countries and the scientific evidence discussed regarding the subtropical urban environment may serve to show the potential impact climate change may have for other places of similar latitude and level of socio-economic development. Health impacts of various climate events on individuals and health services utilisation in urban setting will continue to evolve. More scientific evidence is urgently needed to examine how health impact patterns might change and how the associated community health risk preparedness and response measures can be mounted in an evidence-supported way via both top-down and bottom-up approaches.

References

United Nations, Department of Economic and Social Affairs, Population Division. (2014). *World urbanization prospects: The 2014 revision*. Retrieved from https://esa.un.org/unpd/wup/publications/files/wup2014-report.pdf.

Watts, N., Amann, M., Ayeb-Karlsson, S., Belesova, K., Bouley, T., Boykoff, M., ... Costello, A. (2017). The *Lancet* countdown on health and climate change: From 25 years of inaction to a global transformation for public health. *The Lancet*, 391(10120), 581–630. doi:10.1016/S0140-6736(17)32464-9.

World Health Organization [WHO]. (2015). *Did you know? ... By taking action on climate change you can strengthen public health (Key facts): WHO message to health ministers.* Retrieved from www.who.int/globalchange/publications/didyouknow-health-ministers. pdf?ua=1.

Index

Page numbers in *italics* denote figures, those in **bold** denote tables